AIDS AND THE DISTRIBUTION OF CRISES

Edited by

DUKE UNIVERSITY PRESS
DURHAM AND LONDON 2020

AIDS AND THE DISTRIBUTION OF CRISES

Jih-Fei Cheng

Alexandra Juhasz

Nishant Shahani

Library of Congress Cataloging-in-Publication Data
Names: Cheng, Jih-Fei, [date] editor. | Juhasz, Alexandra, [date] editor. |
Shahani, Nishant, [date] editor.
Title: AIDS and the distribution of crises / edited by Jih-Fei Cheng,
Alexandra Juhasz, Nishant Shahani.
Description: Durham : Duke University Press, 2020. | Includes
bibliographical references and index.
Identifiers: LCCN 2019040582 (print) | LCCN 2019040583 (ebook) |
ISBN 9781478007777 (hardcover) | ISBN 9781478008255 (paperback) |
ISBN 9781478009269 (ebook)
Subjects: LCSH: AIDS (Disease)—Social aspects. | AIDS (Disease)—
Political aspects. | AIDS (Disease)—Historiography. | Health services
accessibility—Political aspects. | Neoliberalism—Health aspects. |
AIDS activists. | Health and race.
Classification: LCC RA643.83 .A358 2020 (print) | LCC RA643.83 (ebook) |
DDC 362.19697/92—dc23
LC record available at https://lccn.loc.gov/2019040582
LC ebook record available at https://lccn.loc.gov/2019040583

Chapter 3 is adapted from Jih-Fei Cheng, "AIDS, Black Feminisms, and the
Institutionalization of Queer Politics," GLQ 25, no. 1 (2019): 169–77. © 2019
Duke University Press.

Chapter 4 is adapted from Julia S. Jordan-Zachery, "Safe, Soulful Sex: HIV/AIDS
Talk," in Shadow Bodies: Black Women, Ideology, Representation, and Politics
(New Brunswick, NJ: Rutgers University Press, 2013), 76–100. © 2017 Reprinted
by permission of Rutgers University Press.

Chapter 5: Viviane Namaste, "AIDS Histories Otherwise: The Case of Haitians in
Montreal." © 2020, Viviane Namaste.

Chapter 11 is adapted from Juana María Rodríguez, "Activism and Identity in the
Ruins of Representation," in Queer Latinidad: Identity Practices, Discursive Spaces
(New York: New York University Press, 2003), 37–83. © 2003 Reprinted by permis-
sion of NYU Press.

Cover art: Zoe Leonard, Strange Fruit (detail), 1992–97. Orange, banana, grapefruit,
and lemon skins, thread, buttons, zippers, needles, wax, sinew, string, snaps, and
hooks. 295 parts: dimensions variable. © Zoe Leonard. Photo by Graydon Wood;
courtesy Philadelphia Museum of Art.

CONTENTS

FOREWORD

Cindy Patton

The world—and especially the places, issues, and people affected by US policy (which I suppose is nearly everyone, whether they know it or not)—moves too fast, and at the same time, if measured in terms of real improvement in people's lives, far too slow. Stable objects of analysis are hard to come by, in part because of the century-long project of critical theory, which steadfastly places the very idea of the object "under erasure."[1] But the careful work designed to document the fragile construction of "the real" has also been hijacked from the other side: the neoliberal claim that postmodernists do not believe in any truth has been symbolically discounted and transformed into a cynical assault on any notion of facticity. Whether the unreal is, for some people, real and vice versa is the condition that poststructuralists, reinvigorating the two-thousand-year-old debate between the sophists and emergent Platonism, tried to understand as effects of knowledge systems or truth systems: that is, truth is produced not discovered. The tweeter-in-chief and his companions exemplify almost the opposite, or rather, a new form of power that derives from selecting, in a completely obvious, self-interested way, which among a set of "facts" to assert, reassert, or, if I may coin a term, "de-assert." The flip-flop feeling of numbness and panic that results from agreeing with the logic of poststructural nominalism (that the names we apply are a result of the social and institution configurations available to create objects) and seeing "facts" de-asserted daily qualify as an existential crisis. Or it should: the most frightening aspect of the present may be the inability to feel anything at all.

Although perhaps neither more nor less than in other times and places, the present seems to qualify as a time of "crisis" but perhaps in a new way: the incommensurability of the forces of personified hate, and those who take the challenge of difference as a source of curiosity and promise, is so massive as to appear completely unbreachable. It is getting harder and harder to tolerate, ignore, hope to change, or engage those who live in what seems to be an alternate reality about human suffering and human *be*-ing. At the end of this brief foreword, I will come back to the problem of encountering the shock of the unforeseeable without sentimentalizing the vessels of that shock, nor averring from the personal responsibility to *act*, at a minimum, by calling out the ongoing-ness of racism, in particular.

First I want to ask: What work does it do to call *this* present—or any present, or past for that matter—a time of "crisis"? From the early 1980s through the present, people directly affected by "AIDS" often refer to the appearance and organization of the epidemic as a crisis of varying kinds—in every case medical, and most places moral and political, and in countries whose worker class was strongly affected, economic. The idea of crisis—the rational assertion of a time out of time—does both productive and reductive work, and the chapters in this volume are interested in considering the relationship between racism and the management of the "AIDS crisis," with a particular focus on what is left out in the abstraction of "crisis" from real places and people.

The authors in this volume rightly critique the use of the idea of "crisis," following the line of scholarship that extends through Giorgio Agamben's contemporization of Foucault's historical analysis of power and "truth effects" to consider the post-Nazi examples of "permanent state of exception."[2] They sidestep the question of whether "the crisis" is over, or whether "it" continues unacknowledged in places long affected and newly affected that lack the material, social, and political resources to replicate the movements and to distribute the medicines that have made "AIDS" an apparently natural feature of sexual life—something to be avoided but not something to be feared or to fear in others. The present volume re-raises the question of racism by thinking political economy, and by emphasizing the distribution of space and time rather than supposing that inequalities are a matter of financial power alone. Instead of becoming gridlocked in a debate about the bared-teeth capitalism of drug companies, the chapters and dispatches seek to reunderstand how racism works in tandem with global political structures to utilize medical concepts in order to obscure what is more properly, as the authors collectively point out, the uneven distribution of rights and relationships (including spiritual), and even the distribution of the idea of "crisis" itself.

The Traffic in Theories: The Trouble with History

Works that bring Agamben into play help us consider the role of "emergency" and "crisis" in creating links between otherwise distinct medicopolitical and social/cultural economies. However, like Foucault, his work conscripts *longue durée* histories to analysis of a "very near history," occluding possible "other histories" that are simultaneous with the history that takes the foreground. The central problem of all the works following Foucault (and now Agamben) has been to fail to take history *itself* as an object of analysis, a proposition that Pierre Bourdieu makes in his later works on the state and on science. In the case of the AIDS epidemic, the uses of Foucault generate a doubled inattention to historicity, which continually embeds epidemiology's historiography as the driving motor of any histories of AIDS, and constructing a teleology where postmodern theories had tried hardest to eradicate them: the idea of "first occurrence of the epidemic" is apparently intransigent, even if the place and time of that "first" is subject to revision.

As has been widely noted, because the AIDS epidemic was scientifically and sociologically visible in US gay male communities *first*, the experience there—here—has overdetermined the conceptualization of the epidemic in "other places." It is not simply that histories of AIDS have ignored women, or Black people, or children, as if inserting these groups into the founding narrative solves the problem. It is not even so much that groups or locals have tried to bend their local to the US story. The larger problem is the interplay between the idea of the "first occurrence" and those other places, many of which immediately take up their local understanding of the epidemic in the terms of the presumed experience of gay communities in the United States—either to say "the same thing is happening here" or to contest the relevance of the US gay experience of the epidemic. There is no privileged place from which to understand "AIDS," but there is most definitely a privileged place from which to refuse knowledge about AIDS.

From the get-go, the very perceptual apparatus in locales is forced to orient to the "first occurrence" and the specific historicity that *becoming incorporated into the story* effects. This historicity of the local formed much of the state and suprastate response to the epidemic "from the beginning." For example, there was political utility for Europeans in adopting some of the US gay community's discursive construction of the epidemic. Similarly, it was not such a bad idea for groups who could reinvent themselves as constituencies to take up the Orientalist mirror implied in the "first occurrence" in order to articulate the idea of "Other" epidemics, notably, a "heterosexual" epidemic in the already Orientalized spaces.

The "first occurrence" idea—grounded in epidemiological privileging of time over space—thus produced a comparative conceptualization that was overly focused on temporality. Situated as a problem of temporal transfer, the sheer size of the United States and Africa made it seem like the two were spaces at a similar scale, but this was the *result* of scientific activity, not a "natural" feature of the geography of disease. In fact, there was no particular reason not to make comparisons on a city-to-city basis rather than a continent-to-continent basis. Indeed, it is only a fixation of the physics of scale that prevents coherent comparisons across scale and geopolitical definition to consider, say, a small city in India with a country in Europe, a contra-scale comparison that would historically situate migration outside the story of "sending" and "receiving" nations.

In order to deal with these problems, I have intermittently and now in a quite sustained way used Pierre Bourdieu, who late in his career paid more explicit attention to historical analysis within his sociological work. Bourdieu was willing to set provisional time brackets on temporal fragments, in order to consider *the struggle over securing a specific history* as a stake in the political field.[3] This might take us out of the position of posing short-timeframe counterhistories as correctives to longer timeframe histories or "histories proper," producing cycles of revisionist histories that support the most dangerous forms of political relativism. If and when we discover battles over histories, we should pin these down for a moment to consider how these battles and successes repositioned the agonists within their fields of struggle. For example, whose interests were served in the initial convergence of epidemiology's historical narrative and the narrative of the genesis of AIDS activisms as a particular form of response seen only in gay communities? Who fought to place that narrative at the center, and what other narratives were eliminated and when?

The Text

The works collected in AIDS *and the Distribution of Crises* take up different terms and methodologies en route to presenting historical, ethnographic, and critical accounts of specific locales where "AIDS crises" may be said to be occurring. At a moment in history when the glare of racism and sexism are omnipresent and even celebrated as moral postures newly liberated from a harsh regime of political correctness, it requires a little bit of attention span to read works that return us to the often hard-to-identify structural features (the consolidation of capital in forms that are monetary, social, cultural, and bureaucratic) that enable the ugliness to proceed.

The chapters in this volume (particularly the ones by Bishnupriya Ghosh, Marlon M. Bailey, and Andrew J. Jolivette) try to ferret out the inextricable relationship between globalized health phenomenon—both the "disease itself" and the political economy formed around and through "it"—and the local instantiations of "a disease" in specific contexts that is also, but not only, formed by political relationships. It is in these spaces that we most clearly see the structures of mutual recognition and aid (to use Bourdieu's definition of social capital, at once minimalist and capacious) that have always been capable of thwarting capital's aims, even if this is through the apparently self-destructive acts that loop individuals and their networks into renewed structures of colonization: for example, when groups of men engage in countersafe practices as a means of finding intimacy and connection against the grain of advice that may once have had their interests at heart but has become its own mechanism of control. (Preexposure prophylaxis [PrEP] is a tragic example of something said to be offered to help individuals by those who are positioned to "act on behalf" of a whole that pretends to include Black brothers but who are seen as recalcitrant members of that whole who put others at risk. For more on PrEP, see chapter 1.) In these "situations," we also see the practices that are reworked from cultural forms in order to talk over, under, and around the much louder voices of established organizations. These works find the middle ground between rendering locales as dots on an epidemiologic map of practices that might aid or disrupt a temporal chain of infections and the sentimentalizing of spaces of agency as sufficient to the problem of constructing personhood in the context of overwhelming colonial forces. (I am reminded of the way that claims of "indigenous resilience" served as an excuse to fail to respond to First Nations' needs in the epidemic.)

A Taste for Method

The political stance of refusing established historical and epidemiological narratives about where the "time" of epidemic starts and how the "space" of epidemic unfolds requires strict discipline if new histories ("revisionist") hope to avoid collaborating in yet other histories that are proposed as less invested and more objective. Here, we have a double problem—vilifying earlier gay communities' lifeways and responses to state violence, a problem that stems in part from the perpetual adoption of the narrative put forward in the overexposed (because its popularity as a journalistic account redoubled by being made into an HBO special) *And the Band Played On*. How can we sustain critical theory's conviction that critical analysis must be perpetual but without pursuing critique for the sake of critique (or career)? How can we revitalize the normative impulse of critical theory (even in its post-Marxist, antihumanist versions) in the age of an assault on facticity (as a product of shared values that broaden who participates in their production) and the rise of a new form of highly dispersed fascism? Jean-François Lyotard, especially in his critique of Holocaust deniers and collaborator apologists, offers a very austere method for remaining perpetually attuned to "the wrong."[4]

Similarly, Emily Bass's emphasis on scattering in this volume usefully offers a method for approaching AIDS scholarship that is "perpetual." She counteracts the notion of static "populations" by considering bodies-in-motion through ideas similar to the "transversal politics" of earlier phases of the AIDS epidemic. In this context, we might also usefully recall Monique Wittig's theorization of "the lesbian" not as a type of sexuality but as a parallel marker for bodies that "run away." She constructs an analogy between serfs who moved beyond the city-state definition, slaves who ran away from plantations to netherworlds, and "lesbians" as figures who have run away from heteropatriarchy. Forms of intentional and forced deterritorialization produced both the US gay communities of the 1970s (formed from demobilizations after World War II that attracted new queers) and the Black communities in decayed former industrial centers (which had attracted southern African Americans to northern cities during the World War II domestic industry mobilization). These histories and those of the ragged construction of many other cities help us understand the spatialization of race that underwrites the epidemiological centers of the AIDS epidemic and its activisms.

The works in this volume consider specific non-Euro-American places (what the medical publishing establishment refers to as ROW—"rest of the world") as well as considering places in (but not "of") variously conceived "centers," a move that foregrounds the role of race and empire in locating Black and Brown bodies as "in and of" a different space and time. This necessarily disassembles the master narrative from within the master's house, even if or perhaps especially since the master is at present wildly out of control and the minions who enact the master's work are at odds with themselves and within themselves. The "structures of depth" that require working within what I might call multidimensional localities without borders helps untangle in a new way the link between the gay movement and the public health system in the United States that emerged through the 1960s and 1970s and the poorly understood foundation of the American response to HIV at both the local institutional levels (gay, feminist, and sympathetic staff within the public health system) and at the political levels. In the absence of an internet as a mode of networking, very few young activists in the many cities that had "gay movements" had much of a sense of the hidden activism—the "scattered" and "scattering" activisms that were occurring in their same time, if not always in their same spaces. We must consider that those activists were working along-side antiracist activists, whom they considered exceptional because they, too, could not privilege their own experience over the larger epidemiological narrative that labeled "the first cases" by sexuality and race. Certainly where I was active (in Boston) in the early 1980s, activists were completely aware that Black gay men were among those who were dying, but we had only a fractured lens through which to understand the situation around us.

The chapters here rework the emphasis on colonialism's primary logic of enlisting the colonized into their own oppression. The authors resist senti-mentalizing locally meaningful practices that were repurposed in the nexus of aspiration and colonial management. In these clear descriptions of "locales," we see the distribution of "space" but also of time—lifetimes, the time of epidemic, the time of individual illness (often called a "course," as if an individual's illness is a small tributary that eventually dumps into a larger body), time "in time," and time "out of time." Bishnupriya Ghosh, in particu-lar, shows how "waves" of an epidemic are read against geopolitics to under-score political economy but also to produce and redistribute time, what she calls "nonlinear discontinuous histories of HIV/AIDS epidemics attuned to global viral emergences."

Traffic in Theory: Thinking Now

Producing more nuanced accounts of places and times is, of course, impor-tant in its own right—never more so than now, in the present of an apparent refusal of anything like a history lesson. But this places the problem of pro-ducing description (historical, anthropological, and critical), the problem of the present of history writers and readers, into the domain of ethics. Readers must take up the ethical task of making use of the works they read; they must consider the distribution of moral responsibility by raising a few questions about the practice of reading or, more broadly, the practice of seeking more or refusing any knowledge about racism.

Many readers of this volume will already have spent many years working through (and on) the complex issues raised by the epidemic. Such readers may in some cases find that the chapters present information that "we al-ready knew." In these cases, we should ask ourselves: What work am I doing to categorize the new cases as "just like" other cases I know about? That is, what is the process through which we set aside local specificity in service of global claims? How do new localizations allow us to invite the concept of distribution to identify new solutions to undoing the inflection of racism in AIDS policy? Readers new to scholarship on AIDS might notice that they have heretofore resisted reading critical analyses of AIDS. Here, we might ask: When do we stop reading AIDS *as AIDS itself*, as people themselves, and read the epidemic situation as a symbol for something else?[5]

As readers consider the new histories and critical assessments that are the substance of this volume, I hope they will also inculcate their disposition to notice whether, and when, they occupy what Eve Kosofsky Sedgwick in 1988 succinctly described as the "privilege of unknowing," a term that asks us to ponder the difference between "not (yet) knowing" and refusing to know.[6]

The writings of Jean-François Lyotard, especially his work in relationship to the assault by the French right wing on Holocaust memory and memorialization, give us some guidelines as readers of works like those in this volume. Notions of crisis and exception can be augmented to sharpen their moral relevance by reconsidering Lyotard's reworking of the notion of "anamnesis," in which the play of space and time afford the subject but especially that subject capable of doing harm (let's call it a "postliberal" subject). Here, the "event" eludes time because the organism has no means to "place" it in a context. Moments—or "some time"—later, the event emergences contexualized but also misrecognized. What remains in the event (time emplaced) is a trace of the bare reception of the shock, a slight glimmering shred of decency (in this age when apparently no decency is powerful enough to overcome the indecent) that can be pressed toward a future recognition of "about to do harm" before the harm is done. Combined with the idea of reading, writing, thinking "under erasure," we become more attuned to the possibility that the thing, this special place-time that we encounter with surprise, requires that we attend to the present, not as something knowable as such but as a potentiality, thus dampening the effect of crisis's misuse by holding space for the recognition of doing harm: "Reflection requires that you watch out for occurrences, that you don't already know what's happening. It leaves open the question: *Is it happening?*"[7]

In the fissure between history and critical historiographies, on the one hand, and art- and worldmaking, on the other, lies something like ethics. Darius Bost's chapter revisits the problem of racism and empire that has vexed oppositional politics, by underscoring the significance of racism and its elision of the figure of Assotto Saint, New York activist and artist whose very definition (gay, Haitian, lover of white men at a time of reemphasis on blackness) is impossible within the city plan and concepts of epidemiology of New York at the height of the AIDS epidemic. Bost teases out the multiple threads of pain and suffering that Saint experienced because of his disease but also because of the inadequacy of the extant narratives to enable his voices. Resisting a sentimental reading of Saint's artistic production and biography, we can see the value of being attuned to the inarticulable, and we can more quickly recognize that it is the poverty of our "hearing" rather than a problem on the side of those who wish to utter their individual and collective pain. Before the violence of categorizing must come the question: Is it happening?

Notes

1 We inherit the concept of "writing under erasure" via Gayatri Chakravorty Spivak's postcolonialist translations and implementations of Jacques Derrida's reuse of a concept found in Martin Heidegger's work as *sous rature*. For Heidegger, the words describe an analytical strategy in which one marks a word that is inadequate to a concept but for which there is no better word. For Derrida, all language (but especially those to do with representing representation) is inadequate to concepts. For Spivak, this is attenuated under conditions of coloniality: the "master's words" refer to the master's conceptualization of the world, which the colonized have no resort but to utilize, inflecting the master's world through use of the master(s') language. See Heidegger, *Fundamental Concepts of Metaphysics*; Derrida, *Of Grammatology*.

Writing under erasure is not the same as "lacking visibility": the early work of the epidemic came on the heels of work by gay and homophile activists to create gay visibility, thought to be the crucial first step for a "minority" that was harder to see than those that were racially demarcated. The subsequent consolidation of identity—"gay identity"—was either a movement success or a case of self-description using the master's worldview. For the form of postcolonial theory that influenced the "first generation" of writing about the AIDS epidemic's figurative racialization and literal distribution, this "writing under erasure" meant using medicine's language to accomplish the double gesture of critique of medicopolitics and extension of medicine's promise to suffering. Perhaps beginning with the apparent success of first-generation antiretrovirals, the idea that AIDS was an "idea" (and not a thing) became nearly impossible to sustain, even in the critical discourses about "AIDS." Some of the many results of taking "AIDS" out from under erasure appear as the objects of critique in the new chapters in this volume, which once again raise the question of who defines the meaning of "AIDS."

2 See Agamben, *State of Exception*.

3 See Bourdieu, *Practical Reason*; Bourdieu, *Sketch for a Self-Analysis*; Bourdieu, "Social Space and Symbolic Power"; Bourdieu, "Rethinking the State."

4 See Lyotard, *Differend*; Lyotard, *Heidegger and "the Jews."*

5 I would like to remind readers of this important and early critique of some of the artistic and critical work on AIDS in the late 1980s: Nicholas Nixon's photographs of the dying, Susan Sontag's *AIDS and Its Metaphors*, and Louise Hay's *You Can*

Heal Your Life and Helen Schucman's closely associated *A Course in Miracles*, which were popular in the 1980s and early 1990s before the advent of vaguely successful pharmaceuticals replaced the hope of "healing the self" with the hope of surviving by means of drugs. These works (and others like them) were all criticized for deflecting the "reality" of people trying to get through the medical system and society stigma in favor of seeing in AIDS a silver lining, an opportunity to rework the self or come to an understanding of some larger forces.

6 Sedgwick, "Privilege of Unknowing."

7 Lyotard, *Differend*, xv.

Bibliography

Agamben, Giorgio. *State of Exception*. Chicago: University of Chicago Press, 2005.

Bourdieu, Pierre. *Practical Reason: On the Theory of Action*. Stanford, CA: Stanford University Press, 1998.

Bourdieu, Pierre. "Rethinking the State: Genesis and Structure of the Bureaucratic Field." *Sociological Theory* 12, no. 1 (1994): 1–18.

Bourdieu, Pierre. *Sketch for a Self Analysis*. Chicago: University of Chicago Press, 2002.

Bourdieu, Pierre. "Social Space and Symbolic Power." *Sociological Theory* 7, no. 1 (1989): 14–25.

Derrida, Jacques. *Of Grammatology*. Translated by Gayatri Chakravorty Spivak. Baltimore: Johns Hopkins University Press, 1976.

Hay, Louise. *You Can Heal Your Life*. Carlsbad, CA: Hay House, 1984.

Heidegger, Martin. *The Fundamental Concepts of Metaphysics: World, Finitude, Solitude*. Translated by William McNeill and Nicholas Walker. Bloomington: Indiana University Press, 2001.

Lyotard, Jean-François. *The Differend: Phrases in Dispute*. Minneapolis: University of Minnesota Press, 1988.

Lyotard, Jean-François. *Heidegger and "the Jews."* Minneapolis: University of Minnesota Press, 1990.

Nixon, Nicholas, and Peter Galassi. *Nicholas Nixon: Pictures of People*. New York: Museum of Modern Art, 1989.

Schucman, Helen. *A Course in Miracles*. Omaha: Course in Miracles Society, 2009.

Sedgwick, Eve Kosofsky. "Privilege of Unknowing." *Genders* 1 (1988): 102–44.

Sontag, Susan. *AIDS and Its Metaphors*. New York: Farrar, Strauss, and Giroux, 1989.

Spivak, Gayatri Chakravorty. "Translator's Preface." In Jacques Derrida, *Of Grammatology*, translated by Gayatri Chakravorty Spivak, ix–lxxxix. Baltimore: Johns Hopkins University Press, 1976.

Wittig, Monique. *The Straight Mind and Other Essays*. Boston: Beacon, 1992.

PREFACE

Jih-Fei Cheng, Alexandra Juhasz,
and Nishant Shahani

To understand the networks of AIDS and its distribution of crises, it seems useful to recount the social, organizing, and creative affinities that inspired this anthology. In 2014 the three editors of the collection presented papers at the Society for Cinema and Media Studies (SCMS) conference in Seattle on different panels. Alexandra (Alex) and Nishant attended Jih-Fei's panel discussion, where he presented his work on the documentary *How to Survive a Plague* (2012). On a panel titled "Queer Contexts," organized and facilitated by film and media studies scholar Lucas Hilderbrand, Jih-Fei's presentation grappled with the contemporary cultural revisitations of the early years of the US AIDS crisis and the erasure of women and people of color in the telling of white male heroism leading up to the advent of antiretrovirals—an intervention that drew upon Alex's scholarship on AIDS media activism and historiography. The paper resonated with Nishant's own work on the whitewashing of AIDS history in relation to the same documentary. Alex and Jih-Fei first became acquainted at that conference, with Alex mentoring Jih-Fei thereafter as he completed his doctoral dissertation and works toward completing his forthcoming monograph. Following the conference, Lucas Hilderbrand initiated a more formal email introduction between the three of us, given our common political and scholarly investments.

Since two of us were in the process of working on essays that grappled with a critique of whiteness and the redemption of biomedical discourse in AIDS representations in the context of the same film, we began to share our work and offer each other feedback. Both our essays were subsequently published in 2016—Jih-Fei's piece in WSQ: *Women's Studies Quarterly* ("How to Survive: AIDS and Its Afterlives in Popular Media," vol. 44, nos. 1 and 2) and Nishant's article in QED: *A Journal in GLBTQ Worldmaking* ("How to Survive the Whitewashing of AIDS: Global Pasts, Transnational Futures," vol. 3, no. 1). While both essays used *How to Survive a Plague* as the focal point to make a larger argument about the representational terms of AIDS historiography and its impacts on the ongoing nature of crises, our broader goals extended beyond recentering the very objects of our critique. Given our shared investments in drawing connections between AIDS and exercises of racism, sexism, homo- and transphobia, global capitalism, and colonialism, Nishant proposed to Jih-Fei the idea of curating a larger collection of essays. We both agreed that asking Alex to coedit the volume with us would shape the project in crucial ways, given her pioneering work on (and production of) AIDS representations, particularly around the investments of feminism, lesbians, and women of color in AIDS activist videos. At this time and since, she has been collaborating with the AIDS cultural activist Theodore (Ted) Kerr (and before that with Marty Fink, Bishnupriya Ghosh, and David Oscar Harvey) on a series of written conversations about cultural phenomena, what Kerr named "AIDS Crisis Revisitation"—the sudden, rather unexpected deluge of representations of HIV/AIDS in popular media, after the period of discursive quiet that he has called the "second silence"—the same one that Nishant, Jih-Fei, and so many of our colleagues are also considering in their work.[1]

Building on a growing analysis naming whitewashing and other shortchanges that seem to be defining many of these revisits, Alex could testify that other stories, people, images, and actions—profoundly linked to the needs and struggles of gay men and also moving in other directions—had occurred in the interlocked and sometimes contestatory interchanges within activist communities, and between that multifaceted alliance and larger institutions, at least during the first outset of American AIDS (video) activism in the late 1980s. Such interventions, from those who had been there and done that, intermixed with research by those who came later or from elsewhere— testifying to or researching other emergences, timelines, and responses—are central to the dynamic flows and interchanges that our collection seeks to engage and draw out.

At this early stage, the three of us discussed our collective commitments to grapple with both repetitions within as well as newer forms of insecurity that were informing and shifting the enduring nature of the pandemic. We thought that a new collection on AIDS could offer a social and political barometer of the present state of the pandemic at precisely the historical moment when dominant scripts insisted on its pastness. We were particularly interested in how frequent and nearly dominant stories of the "end of AIDS," of AIDS obsolescence, were part of a larger narration bent upon illuminating the supposed "recovery" of the United States from its crisis as a means to resurrect the exceptionalism of empire and retool the engine of global capitalism. Many of our conversations thus returned to considering how the labor of AIDS activism in contemporary narratives was being assimilated into national fictions of democracy, neoliberal cure, and linear teleologies of progress. As Marita Sturken has pointed out, at stake in AIDS studies, politics, and art, including their embedded place within national and imperial constructions, are the ideological terms by which the epidemic's history is constantly being remembered, deployed, and marketed—not simply as a matter of dispelling a singular and authentic AIDS story but because the memories and political economy of AIDS continue to shape the present and future of the pandemic, as well as the lives of those who remain disproportionately exposed to its impacts.[2] Drawing on our collective and varied interests in women of color feminisms, queer of color critique, AIDS media production, globalization, activism, and decolonization, our discussions around the book's conceptual scope revolved around how we could focus these connected but diverse investments into a single volume. In many respects, the potentially sprawling scope of the project reflected the very nature of the subject matter under consideration—not just through epidemiological categories (i.e., the unstable viral life of contagion and transmission) but also in structural terms—that is, how HIV travels socially by merging the quotidian with the global in a web of unpredictable and precarious arrangements.

Furthermore, the three of us were personally and spatially scattered in some of the many senses that define the topic and approaches at hand. Namely, we live and thus work on our collaboration across three US time zones (although often one or more of us might also be abroad); we inhabit three states of rank within US higher education; we are trained and situated within different disciplines and intellectual generations albeit all within the humanities; we span multiple possible alignments of gender, sexuality, race, ethnicity, and HIV status; and we enjoy varied and changing states of personal and professional intimacy. These arrangements between the productive tensions experienced through our labor, personal histories and embodiments, and lived places and ideological affiliations paralleled and informed our approach to contemporary AIDS scholarship as we grew the intellectual framework and anticipated the network of authors and their attendant issues that would become this anthology. Of course, they too would be distributed in these many and even more senses (by careful design), although perhaps not as intimately. We asked: How are the durations and intensities of crises experienced in specific contexts, by real people, in their lives, communities, and cultural and political practices? We hope that sharing one personal/

professional anecdote will prove demonstrative of how our own local and lived durations, intensities, and uneven distributions both sustained and stymied our (and any) distributed reckonings with AIDS.

In the late stages of our work on this collection, we organized just one of countless Skype calls, this time to create a to-do list that would respond to our invigorating readers' reports. Nishant was in Mumbai, Alex at home in Brooklyn, and Jih-Fei in Los Angeles without internet access while toggling with phone apps to take notes and thus unable to fully access our Google Drive. We have all been in this scattered "there": interacting via skewed technologies, temporalities, and platforms that should be too familiar to most scholars and many collaborators in the early twenty-first century. We decided that it might be useful for Alex to write a paragraph, much like this one, because she remarked that when we had started working together, we barely knew each other outside our shared scholarly commitments, and that taking the risk of collaborating with near strangers had proven to pay off, even as you never quite know. We agreed: we work together very well, in a productive, professional, and friendly fashion, contributing our discrete skills as writers and editors, our varied networks of colleagues, connections, and foundational texts, all the while staying mindful and respectful of our differences in perspectives and position.

Then, Alex took a tentative step in a new direction. She named her sense of place as a white, middle-aged, cisgender, HIV-negative queer woman who had been working on AIDS, in particular women of color and AIDS, for more than thirty years. Her move was not much of a risk in itself as Alex is often more effusive, self-reflexive, or outgoing (in professional contexts) than are Jih-Fei or Nishant, and she is the senior scholar in this group. This risk was theirs. And as is true across this effort, this risk was further differentiated by our distinct experiences. Alex's words served as an implicit invitation, but given the tender state of our collaboration and individual selves, it was not a demand. Even so, Jih-Fei engaged. He narrated his own coming to HIV/AIDS—as an (as of this writing) HIV-negative and East Asian American queer cisgender–presenting man; his first sexual experience after high school with an older HIV-positive white gay man who had an Asian fetish; followed with his involvement in HIV/AIDS social services and research, cultural productions, and activism during the late 1990s to mid-2000s; and his later decision to continue to focus on AIDS in his doctoral research. There was a pause, a rather lengthy one, and, as might be expected, Nishant began to speak. But then, something unexpected happened. He did not disclose. Instead, Nishant glazed forward, saying something benign or polite; his words served as a graceful transition elsewhere. It seemed that the sensitivities lived between us were too real, too alive, too important to engage through the scatterings of technology and place and personhood that underwrote this conversation. Alex felt like she had made an inappropriate gesture; Jih-Fei, with his inimitable grace and reserve, moved the conversation forward.

We got back to work. There were places of AIDS we would not share, at least not this time; there was a time for HIV that was not this one. The next day, Nishant sent an email written with his characteristic gentle, professional attentions. He explained that the felt pause had been real. However, it was precipitated not by a withholding but by the unexpected entrance of his father into the room, just as the conversation had become more personal, and just out of our camera sight. He apologized for not being able to contribute some details about his own positionality during this moment of shared vulnerability and possible openings. The lessons of this one small and subtle interaction—how lived, personal, interpersonal discordances and connections will produce what we can know and learn about HIV; bound by technology; happening in space; as tender as an unspoken word; as deep as cultural norms; as powerful as rank and fathers and friends; how possible or missed interactions and connections sit in alignment and tension with more scholarly ways of speaking, writing, and making sense of HIV/AIDS; how AIDS is an everyday phenomenon ever ready to inspire new crises or cures (big and small)—reflect the shared and building understanding of the AIDS crises that we hope this anthology might help to reveal by distributing approaches, as well as authors, topics, places, and connections.

Given our many investments in theorizing the ongoing nature of AIDS crises, we thus decided there would be several scattered logics for our volume— temporal and spatial, ethnographic and political-economic, local and global, many voiced and differently oriented—that would frame attention to the distribution of the pandemic by thinking about AIDS not simply as "the most perfect metaphor for globalization" but as globalization's most apposite and indexical expression.[3] In this regard, our volume would be distinct from AIDS scholarship that conceptualized its "local" and "global" distributions as discrete entities. For example, in theorizing memory politics subtending the "unremembering" of AIDS, Christopher Castiglia suggests that the global turn in AIDS scholarship comes at the cost of attention to the material specificities of crises that are more "homegrown" in nature. He contends:

When AIDS in the United States disappeared from queer theory, it vanished from American Studies as well because of a move toward the transnational, the hemispheric, and the global. Although focusing attention on transnational paradigms correctly stretches our understanding of the border crossings of capital, populations, and ideology (allowing us, for instance, to understand the global spread of HIV/AIDS), it has also made local freedom struggles within the United States seem provincial and narrow, tainted with the bad smell of national exceptionalism.[4]

The idea of local erasure ostensibly performed by a transnational turn in AIDS studies, however, fails to account for the inextricable relation between the two, especially when considering the global political economies of neoliberalism and their impacts on activist practices and local communities. American studies critics such as David Eng and Jodi Melamed have pointed to the importance of considering how neoliberal multiculturalism in the United States assumes transnational proportions by obscuring race—locally and globally—in the service of "an ever-increasing global system of capitalist exploitation and domination" that is predicated on the "hyperextraction of surplus value from racialized bodies."[5] In considering the mutual imbrications of local and global, we thus collectively ask: How is the advent of AIDS structured by and structuring of the neoliberal logic of crisis as it remains autochthonous but also as it migrates across various transnational, cultural, and geopolitical sites and legal institutions? How have AIDS' aesthetic expressions and political practices been linked, delinked, and taken up across national, transnational, and diasporic contexts to shift the terms for blame, "risk," and responsibility? What social, material, political, and cultural circumstances have enabled AIDS crises to become global and yet, in a sense, unremarkable? And, in which moments are the historical, cultural, and political contexts of AIDS erased, repackaged, incorporated into, and wielded by US empire?

In keeping with the capacious scope of these questions, we decided that the forms of writing in the book needed to reflect the wide array of voices in AIDS scholarship and activism not only in terms of who would be theorizing but also the subject positions who, or subject matters that, were being theorized. We began the process of identifying contributors by each creating lists of scholars, activists, and artists who have and continue to importantly signal the broadly defined field of "AIDS studies" (while simultaneously recognizing that the constitutive boundaries of such a field have and will always, of necessity, be contingent and amorphous). We culled names from our personal, activist, and artistic webs as well as by scouring conference abstracts and published scholarship from at least the late 1990s, when AIDS studies seemed to dwindle, to the present. Not surprisingly, we began with a combined list of more than seventy names. One of the reasons for organizing three "Dispatches" in addition to the nine full-length chapters, original and reprinted, was to expand the number of contributors to the volume, thus including as many of the insights available from our impressive list. Needless to say, a list of this magnitude itself represents something about the current shape, places, and persistence of AIDS. Additionally, and more significantly than a simple accommodation of numbers, we felt like the dispatches would allow conversations regarding the past, present, and future of AIDS to take place at a different register—one that would be more dialogic and less formulaic in scope. We each "ran" one of the dispatches: naming the questions, communicating with our contributors, editing their responses, and writing an introduction. Thus, these three efforts represent not simply diverse approaches to the temporalities of AIDS but also our unique (if connected) orientations and commitments.

It is also important to note, and begin to attend to here, that no matter the force behind our close care, commitment, and attention, Black women kept sliding off, disappearing from, or moving ever so slightly out of our sight lines. We name who we could not always see in the most capacious and fleeting ways: women representing the complex diasporic histories of Africa, including African women, African American women, Black women from other locales and nations, as well as gender nonconforming Black people who identify with femininity. These subjects were not being adequately centered or seen by our processes—as authors, agents, interlocutors, or collaborators—despite our best intentions and many efforts. While it might appear that this has been somewhat "corrected" through our selection of chapters and authors, an invitation for all the participants in the anthology to attend as thoroughly to Black women as is appropriate for their topic and method, and our discussions of our attempts at full attention here and elsewhere, we did not want this structuring absence to be paved over and obscured. It was only late (although every conversation we had about the anthology attended to this "issue") that we understood our ongoing predicament as indicative of yet another tender disruption, mistemporality, or disalignment of power, privilege, and position from which we must learn about AIDS: socially, professionally, theoretically, structurally, in ways that matter most for the health of all people and communities affected by HIV. Recentering Black women is not simply a tactic, gesture, or commitment because it starts with a center that cannot hold: an absent presence that throws the work and forms of scholarship and other forms of writing into crisis, lack of focus, or inability to attend to carefully. But why is this?

In her reprinted piece for this anthology, Julia S. Jordan-Zachery demonstrates how some Black women's writing about HIV/AIDS—from politicians, popular magazines, and blogs—itself creates gaps and disappearances. She asks, "Is it a crisis if it is not seen?" We are certain that this is perhaps one of the most severe crises underlying the (im)possibilities of good health for all individuals and communities impacted by HIV. Thus, recentering our attention to Black women and HIV returned us, again and again, to the central preoccupations that motivated this book—that is, an attention to the impacts of AIDS beyond the demographic centrality of cisgender white gay men who have become, and still are, the primary default setting for academic theorizations, public health and medical initiatives, and popular culture revisitations. But we learned that recentering is only the first step of a much more nuanced, refined, and systematic process. So, we selected and engaged with contributors whose work reflects what Cathy J. Cohen calls "cross-cutting" activist practice[6]—that is, an understanding of AIDS that challenges the confines of single issue politics in order to consider exploitative measures, including the upward distribution of resources and downward distribution of suffering, land dispossession, occupation, gentrification, surveillance, policing, border patrols, criminalization, an extensive carceral apparatus, the mass buildup of arms, antiterrorism and the suspension of rights, slavery, various forms of under- and no-wage labor, the lack of housing and food security, privatized health care and inadequate medical care, and more. And our selections also took into account the generational shifts in AIDS scholarship, activism, and cultural production—not to privilege the "new" over "old," or vice versa, but to address different temporal registers, historical repetitions, and age- and place-specific interpretations. Our goal with these selections from different generational perspectives was to investigate how the presences (and futures) of AIDS encountered its pasts through the persistent distributive networks of crises and connections. We wanted to inquire about what remained (of use) from earlier theorizations and modes of political action, and also what warranted continued critique and perhaps different forms of collective imagining and organizing.

And still we had more work to do. Readers will find traces of our efforts and successes at working with our authors and focusing ourselves on the meanings of Black women's visibility and erasure, as well as their presence and power, across the anthology. But we wanted this to remain visible as an effort, rupture, process, ongoing problem, and gratifying solution. Once selected and loosely aligned through the offering of the terms discussed above or by way of the questions we posed for our three dispatches, our authors got to work. At the end of the process, we asked the authors of our seven original chapters to engage with Black women and other women of color, each other's now completed chapters, and the vibrant, diverse fields of contemporary AIDS cultural studies in which this anthology sits. Although our authors' disciplinary fields and training differ, as do their generations and the situations of their attention, one shared starting point and focus for the contributors emerged and grew. Our many contributors break down into local, marginal, and discrete studies something that otherwise had and has been more commonly understood to be overwhelming (crisis-like) in its scale and costs and ominous in its force of devastation. Each of the anthology's efforts draws its larger conclusions from close attention to a specific, grounded study of one outbreak of crisis for one local community. The methods and conclusions drawn in each contribution are distinct but complementary: theoretical about the state of HIV/AIDS and crises; practical in the sense of addressing collective cure, well-being, or better health; political in their rousing calls for effective formats for and outcomes from shared struggle; artistic in their voice and ongoing interventional efforts; spiritual in their compassion; or a unique amalgam of these approaches to best outline the crises under consideration. Notably, by honoring specificity, another definitive move is shared and performed: the distance traveled from the local exceeds individualism, exceptionalism, and myopia in order to foster much-needed collectivity, continuity, and connection.

Notes

1 Juhasz and Kerr wrote six conversations about AIDS crisis revisitation and the second silence between 2015 and 2017. Those form the basis of their forthcoming book on these topics, *We Are Having This Conversation Again: The Times of AIDS Cultural Production*. See also Fink et al., "Ghost Stories."
2 Sturken, *Tangled Memories*, 145–47.
3 Cazdyn, *Already Dead*, 117.
4 Castiglia, "Past Burning," 102.
5 Eng, *Feeling of Kinship*, 6; Melamed, "Spirit of Neoliberalism."
6 Cohen, *Boundaries of Blackness*, 15.

Bibliography

Castiglia, Christopher. "Past Burning: The (Post-) Traumatic Memories of (Post-) Queer Theory." In *States of Emergency: The Object of American Studies*, edited by Russ Castronovo and Sandra Gillman, 69–87. Chapel Hill: University of North Carolina Press, 2009.

Cazdyn, Eric. *The Already Dead: The New Time of Politics, Culture, and Illness.* Durham, NC: Duke University Press, 2012.

Cohen, Cathy J. *The Boundaries of Blackness: AIDS and the Breakdown of Black Politics.* Chicago: University of Chicago Press, 1999.

Eng, David. *The Feeling of Kinship: Queer Liberalism and the Racialization of Intimacy.* Durham, NC: Duke University Press, 2010.

Fink, Marty, Alexandra Juhasz, David Oscar Harvey, and Bishnupriya Ghosh. "Ghost Stories: An Introduction." *Jump Cut* 55 (Fall 2013). https://www.ejumpcut.org/archive/jc55.2013/AidsHivIntroduction/index.html.

Melamed, Jodi. "The Spirit of Neoliberalism: From Racial Liberalism to Neoliberal Multiculturalism." *Social Text* 89 (2006): 1–25.

Sturken, Marita. *Tangled Memories: The Vietnam War, the AIDS Epidemic, and the Politics of Remembering.* Berkeley: University of California Press, 1997.

ACKNOWLEDGMENTS

In times of crises, we turn toward collaboration. Our deepest thanks to the Duke University Press team—especially Elizabeth Ault for being such an encouraging and supportive editor, and Kate Herman for all the help with complicated logistics. Many thanks to Ellen Goldlust for her assistance with the book's production. We are also very grateful to the anonymous peer reviewers, who offered such careful criticism and constructive feedback. Their engagements and suggestions for revision have truly strengthened the vision of this collection. Much gratitude to Heather Ramos for assistance with citations and bibliography and to Anita Welbon for her careful work on our helpful index. Thank you also to Zoe Leonard, who gave us permission to use Graydon Wood's photo of her installation at the Philadelphia Museum of Art, *Strange Fruit*, for our cover.

INTRODUCTION

Jih-Fei Cheng, Alexandra Juhasz,
and Nishant Shahani

Crisis

The Acquired Immune Deficiency Syndrome (AIDS) is not merely a crisis in epidemiological terms; rather, it is the uneven and varying spatialization and temporalization of crises. As a term, *crisis distribution* brings into view the eerie distresses of this scattered dispersal. Crisis distribution also builds on recent theorizations of spatiotemporal logics that underwrite the classification of crisis.

> *crisis* (n.) early 15c., from Latinized form of Greek *krisis* "turning point in a disease" (used as such by Hippocrates and Galen), literally "judgment, result of a trial, selection," from *Krinein* "to separate, decide, judge," from PIE root *krei- "to sieve," thus "discriminate, distinguish." Transferred non-medical sense is 1620s in English. A German term for "mid-life crisis" is *Torschlusspanik*, literally "shut-door-panic," fear of being on the wrong side of a closing gate.[1]

By definition, crisis is exception. A crisis necessarily involves a diagnosis: in the sharp decline of individual and/or group health, presumably in a singular time, and perhaps a place or places. It is an occasion for judgment, an opportunity to render power. Yet a crisis is not meant to last. Judgment is meant to lead to justice, to reparation. We are meant to heal. Significantly, the etymology of *crisis* conjugates temporal and epidemiological meanings as the "turning point in a disease." In *Anti-Crisis*, Janet Roitman similarly preserves the medical and temporal connotations of the term by foregrounding the ubiquity of "*feverish* crisis pronouncements."[2] While her analysis is most germane to crisis in the context of financial and housing markets, the phrase once again invokes its temporal urgency through language associated with virality, infection, or sickness.

Roitman's critique is part of a larger scholarly attempt in the last decade to critically examine the rhetoric of illness and the temporality of crisis production. The "contemporary canon of crisis," as she terms it, engenders only those forms of critique that expose the scandal of crisis through logics of exceptional time.[3] "Feverish crisis pronouncements" thus fail to address the reorganization of the broader structures that subtend the makings of crisis. Like Roitman, Eric Cazdyn's work on illness and time cautions against the spectacular rendering of crisis as a temporal phenomenon existing out of lockstep with the ordinary. He contends, "Crisis is not what happens when capitalism goes wrong, but when it goes right." The precarity of exploited labor, for instance, is not symptomatic of capitalism's unfulfilled potential or unintended consequence. Rather, precarity and the production of an underclass are integral to the seamless cycles of crisis "when contracts are obeyed and factories are clean and safe."[4] Sharing the critical skepticism around the shock and awe of endless crisis pronouncements, Lauren Berlant offers the concepts of *slow death* and *crisis ordinariness* to address the counterintuitive registers through which crisis forms the historical present via the quotidian or even banal. Against what she calls "the inflated rhetoric and genre of trauma," a focus on the ordinary attends to "the problem of the forms heightened threat can take as it is managed in the context of living." Berlant proposes a "ballast of ordinariness" in order to "*distribute* our analyses of 'structure' as a suffusion of practices throughout the social" if we are to avoid the exceptionalization of crisis that both Roitman and Cazdyn warn against.[5]

By invoking the terms *crises* and *distribution* in the title of this volume, we draw from and reflect on AIDS: How is it one (or many) of the outcomes and expressions of crises that are made ordinary and exceptional at the same time? How are these durations and intensities of crises experienced in specific contexts? For AIDS, the critical suspicion around the inflation of crisis rhetoric might appear to brush up against historical and political refusals to recognize the catastrophic consequences of the virus. In spite of initial declarations that the AIDS crisis is over, given the invention of antiretroviral drug combination therapies, crisis rhetoric regarding the pandemic continues to be mobilized in the context of the Global South and communities of color in the Global North. Thus, as ongoing events, AIDS and global crises are intertwined, recursive, and unrelenting. Insisting on feverish pronouncements of crises in these contexts could possibly operate as antidotes to the myopias that mark both institutional neglect and false narratives of progress. For, with AIDS, we find ourselves in the midst of long-term and still ongoing global crises. As protracted global crises, we might even consider AIDS fundamental to procuring and sustaining what Giorgio Agamben names the *state of exception*.[6] The global emergency of AIDS occasions Global North nations to exercise power, exploit international asymmetries, and retrench individual rights at will.

Yet, as if staid in due course, AIDS remains the longest enduring modern pandemic without a cure and without widespread access to preventative care or treatment for the majority of those infected with HIV. In the context of racialized communities and societies, the heavy burden of AIDS constitutes what Achille Mbembe terms *necropolitics* to describe the management of subjugated populations whereby "new and unique conditions of life confe[r] upon them the status of living dead."[7] Drawing upon Mbembe and Agamben, Subhabrata Bobby Banerjee conjures the concept *necrocapitalism* to name the forms of dispossession and "'the subjugation of life to the power of death' . . . in the organization and management of global violence through the increasing use of privatized military forces and conflicts over resources between transnational corporations and indigenous communities."[8] Eric A. Stanley theorizes the notion separately to mean the dead labor extracted to produce massive wealth for global pharmaceutical companies that participate in the structured abandonment of racialized subjects.[9] For those living with HIV and with access to medication, the virus can be suppressed to the point of being undetectable. However, that person's health status is permanently labeled HIV positive and remains in the balance, underscoring poet Justin Chin's description of today's biochemical health management as a *microscopic war* internalized by the patient and sustained by the pharmacological regulation of time and space.[10] And all—healthy, dying, worried, fighting—face this contemporary exception: a cultural deep freeze of denial in the form of "AIDS is over" so long as one remains tethered to this chemical battle.[11] Those who are structurally abandoned are laid to waste on this battleground. Thus, AIDS-related deaths are exceptionalized and normalized vis-à-vis dual processes of racialization and the spatiotemporalization of one's proximity to communities in crises.

The continued asymmetrical warfare of AIDS means that the period for judgment remains protracted, rendering the judgment levied against those rendered at risk for, or living with, an HIV or AIDS diagnosis self-justifying. In turn, justice is delayed, overdue, maybe even foreclosed for some. What if we, instead, think about crises—of AIDS—as globally networked and without beginning or end?

A consideration of crises ordinariness in the context of AIDS invites another pressing question: Does the ordinariness of crises correspond with the very historical moment when its effects become scattered among populations whose proximity to death is naturalized as inevitable or axiomatic, or whose access to representation or representability allows their crises to go unrecognized and/or misrepresented? Many of our volume contributors contest the supposition that the AIDS crisis began in the United States in 1981 among a cluster of white gay men and ended around 1996 when effective antiretrovirals hit the market and extended lives. Yet, as we have been arguing, AIDS crises and their profitability rely upon women of color, queer and trans people of color, and peoples of the Global South—particularly those from the sub-Saharan Africa region—to continue to be infected, experience delayed access to care and treatment, develop serious illnesses, and/or pass at rates that demonstrate that the pandemic is unending.[12] In this sense, racialized, gendered, queer, and trans subjects, and Global South peoples generally, remain exceptional; they remain *in* crises.

So, it matters where we locate the crises, how we temporalize their multiple durations, and when and how we identify, name, and categorize their impacts. Originally AIDS was not AIDS—it was Gay-Related Immune Deficiency (GRID), until scientists looked beyond the cluster of white gay men in the United States and considered Haitian-born immigrants in Florida who had shown symptoms of the disease as early as 1980.[13] The viral etiology for AIDS—HIV—was not clinically isolated until 1983.[14] In short, what we have come to know pithily as HIV/AIDS was never a linear or singular history with one simple subject. The crises are bound up with histories of race, racialization, globalized yet uneven development, and widespread economic inequity. The popularized medical terms for illness and the troubling epidemiological categories for race, nation, gender, sexuality, and so on reveal the limited and contradictory ways that meaning has been quickly and hastily fashioned with enduring consequences for comprehending and addressing the pandemic. Meanwhile, the public health classifications for risk behaviors (e.g., men who have sex with men [MSM]) and transmission categories (e.g., mother to child) simultaneously presuppose race and gender while disavowing the causes for its continued impact. Black people (especially Black men) are most often presumed sexually dishonest and predatory. Meanwhile, Black people are thought of as available to white men with historically systemized sexual violence exacted upon Black women and transfeminine peoples.

This hypersexualization, hypervisibility, and criminalization of blackness vis-à-vis HIV/AIDS epidemiology and the US state make invisible the specific effects of the pandemic among Black communities, other communities of color, and the Global South in general while absolving white-dominated heteropatriarchal institutions and white supremacy itself. Yet the reduction of the pandemic to risk behaviors and transmission categories only obscures how race, gender, sexuality, economics, global policing, militarism, and incarceration are inextricably tied to the virus and its lived outcomes—particularly as they are exercised against those who are racialized as Black. Thus, the epidemiology and popular conceptions of AIDS rely on race while denying the proliferation of racism.

More to the point, why must we constantly appeal to HIV/AIDS infection, morbidity, and mortality statistics in order to highlight the crises among people of color and the Global South? Indeed, the overlap between epidemiology and geopolitics to highlight sub-Saharan Africa as the region most devastated by HIV/AIDS underscores how colonial categories for race, gender, and sexuality persist in our contemporary maps for nation, peoples, and global health. The term *sub-Saharan* is often drawn to succinctly name an origin for the historical "scattering of peoples . . . as a result of the slave trade and European colonialism."[15] Although this history is crucial to geopolitical and epidemiological analyses, its knee-jerk deployment often reproduces uncomplicated, essentialized, and depoliticized notions of Black, Africa, African, and African diaspora.[16] Sub-Saharan invokes the linked histories of colonialism, slavery, and global capitalism but promises no relief from these. Neither has AIDS found much relief as it has been experienced through overlaps between settler colonialism, Native dispossession, slavery, and the globalization of capitalism.

What if we understand Africa as not only a place that is racialized and hypervisibilized as Black on colonial maps but also a series of representational absences and epidemiological crises? Women of color, especially Black and Indigenous women, are often rendered statistically less significant than their male counterparts with respect to either a local or global epidemiology of AIDS. The sum cases of women of color infected with HIV or living with AIDS do not exceed men of color. When epidemiologists instead turn to rates of infection to measure the impact, it is often the case that women of color are compared to each other. This makes rigid the categorical distinctions between Black, Indigenous, woman, man, and so on. Meanwhile, women of color continue to be a statistical afterthought and increasingly disappear in the rear view.

Public health surveillance of AIDS insists that the further delineation of such categorical distinctions holds the promise for a more accurate depiction of global AIDS. However, what is simultaneously obfuscated is the way that, in the words of Brent Hayes Edwards, "*diaspora* points to difference not only internally (the ways transnational black groupings are fractured by nation, class, gender, sexuality, and language) but also externally . . . in terms of a complex of forced migrations and racialization . . . a history of 'overlapping diasporas.'"[17] Likewise, AIDS, as global crises, is an interlinking of Black, Indigenous, and other nonwhite groupings that are simultaneously fractured by nation, class, gender, sexuality, language, and more. Rather than abandon these epidemiological distinctions, or insist on ever-more-finite categorizable differences, what if we notice the absences themselves as articulations of ongoing crises?

It takes all of this anthology's nine original scholarly chapters (including the foreword and afterword), two reprinted book chapters with new introductions and/or postscripts, and three carefully amalgamated dispatches of asynchronous conversations between scholars, artists, and activists to glimpse, study, and map some of the many linked and distributed crises rendered ordinary. In total and in distinction, the collected writings in *AIDS and the Distribution of Crises* work to bring into focus and conversation what contributor Bishnupriya Ghosh names "nonlinear discontinuous histories of HIV/AIDS epidemics attuned to global viral emergences."

AIDS Distribution and the Scattering Effects of Globalization

Given this volume's attention to how HIV/AIDS is unevenly distributed across space and time, it seems critical to consider if, or how, connection is possible across the specific, racialized genealogies of scattering that define Berlant's and our own use of crisis ordinariness. Relying upon Berlant's use of ordinariness *does not* imply diminished impact or tempered scale but instead attends to how structural problems are unevenly distributed. Berlant's call for attending to distribution—that is, of analyzing structures of power as a kind of suffusion practice—is particularly relevant to this book's attention to the scattering effects of contemporary HIV/AIDS.

Each of this volume's three dispatches—atemporal conversations between AIDS activists, artists, and scholars built to complement the more traditional scholarly chapters of this anthology—is led and edited, respectively, by the three volume editors. Jih-Fei Cheng organizes a conversation on the past, Alexandra Juhasz tackles the future, and Nishant Shahani initiates his groups' thinking on globalization. In "Dispatches from the Futures of AIDS," AIDS activist Emily Bass offers a useful way to grasp all our efforts to theorize crisis distribution as a kind of scattering effect. Responding to Alex Juhasz's question about the future of AIDS activism under Donald Trump, Bass poses a seemingly tangential hermeneutical question: How can the English translation of the Holocaust-themed *A Memoir of the Warsaw Uprising* capture the nuances and varied use of the verb *run* that recurs throughout the text to describe the movement of terrified rebels fleeing Nazi occupation? Bass asks, "In 2017, how many ways are there to run?" The varied linguistic uses of *run* confound the possibility of an easy English translation; the different political responses to attacks on the poor and the Global South, especially surrounding health care, under Donald Trump make it impossible to articulate any singular solution of activist practice. "I'm scattered here," writes Bass, "and that's the point. . . . Everybody run." This scattered running is not political nihilism (she never suggests running *away*). Instead, her invocation of *scattering* serves as methodological imperative for our book's many attempts to cognitively map the effects of and responses to the AIDS crises that mark its distributive logics across space (local and global, North and South) and time (present, past, future, now, then, and beyond). While attending to these different temporal registers and spatial scales, scattering as a distributive method also challenges the neat paradigm shifts and simple separations that disaggregate these categories.

In a different context, the image of scattering recalls an epistemic moment of AIDS activism referenced in another activist intervention—David Wojnarowicz's memoir, *Close to the Knives* (1991), where he called for friends and lovers of the dead to drive through the gates of the White House "and dump their lifeless form on the front steps."[18] Then there were the Ashes Actions in 1992 and 1996. The 1996 Ashes Action of ACT UP was inspired by the political funerals of activists killed in anti-apartheid South African movements—complicating the linear trickle-down temporality through which North/South Hemispheric relations are conventionally (and colonially) theorized. But beyond this most literal invocation of scattering, the word also captures uneven distributive logics of globalization particular to the presences and pasts of AIDS. Scattering as methodological anchor allows for an attention to the fractal logics that inform the globalization of AIDS. While globalization has often been understood via temporal registers of hyperconnectivity and immediacy, these seamless narratives of enhanced speed obscure structures of delay, stagnancy, and deferral that are tethered to matters of life and death. For example, acute shortages of medicines at antiretroviral therapy (ART) centers in India have caused extended breaks in drug access, challenging the official narratives of progress around prevention and health care presented by the National AIDS Control Organization (NACO). Yet another instance of temporal lag can be witnessed in the prolonged duration of legal cases where pharmaceutical companies launch patent custody battles over generically produced drugs. The volume's theorization of what Dredge Byung'chu Kang-Nguyễn calls *multiple epidemics* and Bishnupriya Ghosh defines as *high-crisis pockets* points to the proliferation of crises at varying scales and sites of intensity. The distributive logics of crisis ordinariness thus enable an attention to what Ghosh calls the "discontinuous space-times of HIV/AIDS epidemics—in the plural."

The fractures in temporality that mark these discontinuities are intimately tied to what Eric A. Stanley refers to in this volume as the geopolitical investment in globalized racial capitalism. Take, for instance, the literal invocation of time by Andrew Natsios (head of the United States Agency for International Development [USAID]) to justify the use of global funds on prevention rather than life-saving drugs: "[Africans] don't know what Western time is. You have to take these drugs a certain number of hours each day, or they don't work. Many people in Africa have never seen a clock or a watch their entire lives. . . . They know morning, they know noon, they know evening, they know the darkness at night."[19] In a different context, the temporality of global racial capital can be read as represented in the ACT UP documentary *How to Survive a Plague* (dir. David France, 2012) in the form of a running ticker that recurs throughout the film, intended to illustrate the rise in fatalities with the lapse of time. With every year that passes, the rapidly increasing numbers, as highlighted by the ticker, function as a temporal index of urgency and crisis. While these numbers draw on global statistics, *How to Survive a Plague*'s focus remains almost exclusively tethered to the needs and associated heroism of mostly white gay men in the United States. The film's triumphant conclusion—in which most of its white male protagonists survive due to the availability of the very combination therapy drugs that they fought to make available—marks the historical moment in the mid to late 1990s when multinational drug companies began to secure intellectual property patents on life-saving drugs to preempt cheaper generic availability in countries like South Africa and India. While not as explicitly egregious as the racist logic of primitivism that informs Natsios's comments, time in *How to Survive a Plague* can only be measured in accordance to its subjects in the Global North—even as a global unconscious constitutes the film's absent center through the ticker's feverish crisis pronouncements.

In attending to the distribution of AIDS as it is scattered through global space-time discontinuities, our volume is invested in refusing a kind of unreflexive and ethnographic voyeurism in which the non-West is simply a site of essential difference or crisis. Thus, even while chapter authors and contributors to the dispatches address the specificities of crisis distribution in the context of the People's Republic of China (Catherine Yuk-ping Lo), India (Ghosh), Haiti and the Haitian diaspora (Viviane Namaste, Darius Bost), exhaustive geographical coverage is not our goal. Instead, we are interested in mapping the relations between global and local that avoid making the Global North the default referential point in understanding the political economy of AIDS. It will not do then to approach an analysis of AIDS globalization through what Arjun Appadurai calls *center-periphery models* that foreclose the place of nonstate local actors in shaping the global imaginaries of AIDS crises.[20] In her analysis of the unbundling of national sovereignty that marks globalization, Saskia Sassen points to the importance of recognizing the place of local actors—immigrants, health advocacy groups, environmental activists, indigenous peoples, refugees—in recalibrating local-global connections.[21] Thus, in our volume, AIDS becomes the site through which "congeries of money, commerce, conquest, and migration" can be mapped and theorized.[22] For some of our authors, AIDS is situated in specific, local communities (including immigrants who were once from) outside the Global North (Ghosh, Bost, Namaste), while others locate these congeries smack-dab in the many peripheries of this sometimes center (Andrew J. Jolivette, Jih-Fei Cheng, Cait McKinney, Marlon M. Bailey, Julia S. Jordan-Zachery, Juana María Rodríguez). Jordan-Zachery suggests: "We need to come back to the question of who gets to be in the center. Specifically, we need to explore how Black women work to bring other Black women from the margin to the center." Yes, people can help themselves move and be moved. It thus seems necessary to detail how the center-periphery model cannot completely hold any of these chapters, as the pull of global capital and pharmaceuticals, the migration of peoples, and the movements enabled by ideas, art, and politics serve to connect any discrete local under consideration with other orbits of crisis and activism.

The displacement of or outward linkages to US-centric perspectives in mapping these global/local relations is accompanied by what "Dispatches on the Globalizations of AIDS" contributor Stanley calls an attention to "grappl[ing] with these thick histories so that connections of depth might be made through locations and not simply over them." To get at these thick histories, the Global South cannot be simply theorized through what Ghosh calls a *cartographic projection*; such a monolith must be replaced instead by recognition of an *ameboid geography* that marks the material particularities of regions across the globe. Thus our collection's approach to understanding the globalization of AIDS resists unilateral symmetries in which the hegemonies of global capitalism simply impose themselves on a passively abject local. While the distribution of crises is marked by the fracturing or unbundling of national sovereignty, such a mode of deterritorialization does not simply displace the role of the nation-state. In fact, the nation has assumed a more pronounced regulative function precisely under the aegis of its putative disappearance, often manifesting itself through parochial nativisms that most severely impact Black and Brown women and sexual minorities. Global capitalism might enable what Aihwa Ong calls *flexible citizenship* for some entities within the Global South, but it also produces crisis pockets of boundedness, inflexibility, and immobility for others.[23] Our volume thus attempts to address the contradictions and calibrated specificities through which AIDS consolidates and produces unequal connections of depth across the globe.

Without an attention to these structures of depth, we merely repeat history as we know it, as Ghosh reminds us in her chapter in this volume. Globalized crises generally, and viral pandemics and AIDS crises in particular, can then simply be retooled for more cycles of capitalism. Ghosh astutely observes that health, as we currently define and measure it, "is not a universal human right but an economically adjudicated enfranchisement at both national and global scales. Hence states and global institutions back big pharma and insurance companies in their parsing and valuation of life in terms of risk aggregates; and state and interstate legal systems continue to protect their interests." If we invest singular hope in a medical cure or in individuals' access and adherence to the once-a-day preventative pill preexposure prophylaxis (PrEP) instead of diagnosing a failing globalized system and, in turn, renewing strategies for collective survival, then we ignore the lived realities under stark systems of globalized inequality that have made AIDS a nexus of ongoing crises. Stanley beseeches us to consider the role of the West in spurring racial capitalism such that "what we have come to know of 'HIV/AIDS' are the haunts of conquest and chattel slavery," especially when considering the punishment exacted upon Haiti for staging the "first successful slave revolt in the Western Hemisphere." Similarly, within the same conversation, provocations by Sarah Schulman on Russia and Catherine Yuk-ping Lo on China remind us that HIV/AIDS forms what Lo calls a *security nexus* that stems from Cold War politics, if not earlier, and governmental policies embedded in nationalism, military defense, willful ignorance, and enduring AIDS stigma.

Theorizing the Distribution of Crises from the Gaps of Histories

An attention to these transnational dispersals and hemispheric implications, however, cannot replace the focus on regional particularities within the West—an equally generalized cartography. In "America's Hidden H.I.V.

Epidemic," Linda Villarosa's *New York Times* feature on gay and bisexual Black men in the US South, she points to accelerated rates of HIV-related deaths in Louisiana and Mississippi in the last decade. While the United States President's Emergency Plan for AIDS Relief (PEPFAR) legislation provided $15 billion global funds for treatment and prevention in African nations, Villarosa writes, "Black America, however, never got a Pepfar." The citizens she encounters exist out of national time, within states of exception that are paradoxically mundane. They appear to have "stepped out of the early years of the epidemic," inhabiting "a present that looks like the past."

How it feels to step into a Black future falling into the past, for visitors to and residents of the American South, is what is depicted in *DiAna's Hair Ego Remix* (2017), a short video that Juhasz worked on with fellow queer/feminist videomakers Cheryl Dunye and Ellen Spiro (and editor and coproducer Jennifer Steinman). Visual AIDS commissioned the video as part of their annual Day With(out) Art 2017 series, Alternate Endings, Radical Beginnings, that prioritized Black narratives within the ongoing AIDS epidemic by commissioning seven videos by and about Black Americans. When Cheryl was invited to contribute, she connected to her friend Ellen, and then the two of them reached out to Alex. They conceived of a video where Cheryl and Ellen would go to South Carolina to find out the following: "What has changed here, in the context of HIV/AIDS, from thirty years ago until today?" The answer was as clear and ominous as the subject was invisiblized: "There was a white epidemic, and there is an African American, person of color epidemic," answers Dr. Bambi Gaddist on camera. "There was an interest when it was a white epidemic. But somehow over these past thirty years, as it's changed its face, there's a lack of discussion and interest."

Bambi and fellow activist DiAna DiAna began organizing together in the 1980s in their local community of African American feminists in South Carolina, later building connections across the South and the United States, because at that time support from governmental agencies was not available. DiAna and Bambi first revved up their AIDS educational efforts in DiAna's beauty salon, DiAna's Hair Ego. Ellen's video (1989), of this same name, tracked a group of AIDS activists from NYC who visited the salon to learn about the radical, Black female-focused, local activism happening there. A friendship and commitment to sharing this work outside South Carolina ensued.

As is true for many AIDS activists, everyone's work continued and adapted over the three decades of the struggle. Some of these women moved on to other local or social issues, while Bambi stayed the AIDS course. She is currently the executive director of the South Carolina HIV/AIDS Council, one of the only AIDS nonprofits still extant in the region and currently under real peril because of the ongoing defunding efforts of that state's republican leadership. With the only mobile outreach unit in the state, her nonprofit has provided free, confidential HIV testing to more than 8,600 people. That, and much more, is under attack.

Ellen had made two videos about the hair salon and the safer sex parties that DiAna and Bambi were throwing in the 1980s. The images, activities, and energy of these women, engaging on the local level with bravado, humor, and power, felt and still feels game-changing. The choice, in 2017, to revisit Ellen's friends and comrades is consistent with the logic of AIDS Crisis Revisitation, a term we credit to Theodore (Ted) Kerr: a hope to herald, remember, and learn from the powerful efforts of the past (including, in this case, her own video footage and experience). This time, however, Ellen partnered with Cheryl (figure I.1). Given what we have learned about the perils of appropriation and the powers of collaboration to build the insights, experience, and energy we need to best learn from Black women's power, Cheryl's contributions as a Black lesbian artist, on screen and off, invested the remix project and visit with a dynamism and authenticity crucial for this moment. The videomakers were most interested in asking DiAna and Bambi, as well as their local Black friends and activists who dropped by the salon while Cheryl and Ellen were in town—Bailey, Greg, Ernest, Stacey: activists, people living with HIV, AIDS-prevention educators—about their experiences as Black women and queer people in today's South: What are the experiences of HIV for Black women in your community today? Does this align with Black Lives Matter? How do the changing norms of gender identity and sexuality affect Black/queer women's experience and understanding of HIV and AIDS activism at the salon, in your town, AIDS service organizations, and organizing?

In a compelling cry to be asked, heard, and understood, Bambi Gaddist explains in her interview from 2017 that there are two AIDS crises in America—or more precisely one, the other having receded from view: one for white people and one for Blacks. The timeline and analysis she relays, from her own work over three decades, breaks along color lines: "In the '80s we were talking about gay people, but we were talking about white gay people. Everything that we did in the '80s, when she and I went out, had to do with looking into the future and knowing that if we did not do something it was going to be Black people." And they did something monumental and profound, and the AIDS crisis in the South "is still Black people." According to DiAna, Bambi, and their crew, the toxic brew of anti-Black defunding efforts on the state and

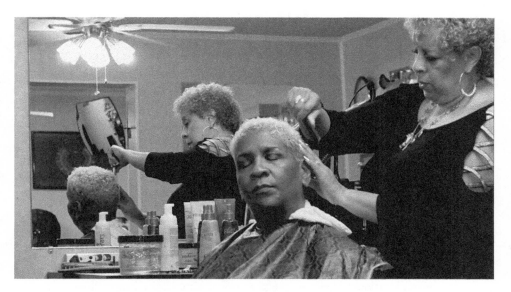

FIGURE I.1 Salon owner DiAna DiAna and Dr. Bambi Gaddist discuss their HIV-prevention work thirty years prior. Film still from *DiAna's Hair Ego Remix* (dir. Cheryl Dunye and Ellen Spiro, 2017). Courtesy of Alexandra Juhasz.

national level, mixed with antiqueer and also sexist patterns of socialization among religious Black folks in the South, has decimated the very AIDS services, community, and visibility that these devoted activists and their cadre of friends have worked and work for: "I'm really frustrated. You spend thirty-five years of your life doing a body of work, only to sit here in 2017," says Gaddist at the video's conclusion, "and I'm sitting with my colleagues in all these national meetings and we're all saying the same thing: 'This sounds like déjà vu. This sounds like 1985.'" The clear vision of Black women about their AIDS temporalities—this sounds like 1985—attests to the ways that crisis ordinariness both constructs and is constructed from multiple temporalities, situations, identities, affinities, and possible connections: those who are left out of progressive time (due to blackness, or region, or education, or gender, or funding priorities) and those who have been "fortunate" to survive, however tenuously within it, in the shadows of a plague.

In attempting to make sense of these contrasting but coexisting temporalities, several contributors mobilize different interpretations of political economy and neoliberalism to attend to topics as varied as settler colonialism, internet regulation, forced migration, the war on drugs, and the pathologization of Black bodies. Throughout the volume (and the dispatches in particular), contributors point to putative forms of progress that are, in fact, inextricably linked to neoliberalism's investments in the privatization of public goods, the gutting of social safety nets, an enhanced investment in surveillance and security regimes, the professionalization of activism, and the gentrification of populations.

These legacies of the Ronald Reagan, George H. W. Bush, Bill Clinton, and George W. Bush eras assumed new and more insidiously multicultural forms under the Barack Obama years, so that neoliberal forms of *capitalist apartheids* appeared to be more benevolent, benign, and even progressive.[24] For example, in "Dispatches on the Globalizations of AIDS," Ian Bradley-Perrin points to the self-serving reciprocity between pharmaceutical companies and mainstream AIDS service organizations as well as Pride Parades, in which the latter were sponsored by drug profits, which in turn offered up target populations for market expansion and clinical trials. The amelioration of crisis thus becomes the narrative and epidemiological framework through which multinational pharmaceutical companies manage chronic illness. At the same time, large corporatized US AIDS service organizations (ASOs), such as the AIDS Healthcare Foundation, act as rainbow or activist alibis for drug profiteering, patent law evergreening (i.e., the minor molecular modification of drug composition that legally justifies patent monopoly), and/or exerting an ever-growing sphere of influence on local and global politics. While critiques of gay assimilation are conventionally associated with marriage equality and military inclusion in the new millennium, it is crucial to historicize contemporary mainstreaming and commodification of lesbian, gay, bisexual, and transgender culture and politics in relation to the creation of niche markets for people with HIV/AIDS, cultivated and maintained as consumers. Such marketing includes not just drugs and medicine but also the construction of lifestyle politics and brand loyalty, as Sarah Schulman has pointed out in her book *Stagestruck*.[25]

To intervene into such market-driven global(ized) views, this volume heeds the local and specific struggles that are often rendered invisible by master narratives. The aim is not to simply represent marginalized perspectives or bring these struggles to light. Rather, the volume proceeds under the belief that the political will and strategies of those most vulnerable to violence, illness, and death yield insights into the enduring, immeasurable, and impactful ways of being and organizing for collective survival. As Roger Hallas points out in "Dispatches from the Pasts/Memories of AIDS," the particularities of "local micronarratives provide powerful, comparative testimony to the global inequities of access to health care." Thus, we recognize the importance of antiracist intersectional feminisms to many of the authors' thinking as a powerful means to address the localizations and globalizations of crises. In the words of Black feminist and queer intellectuals and activists recorded in the 1977 Combahee River Collective Statement, "We realize that the liberation of all oppressed peoples necessitates the destruction of the political-economic systems of capitalism and imperialism as well as patriarchy."[26] They continue: "We realize that the only people who care enough about us to work consistently for our liberation are us. . . . We might use our position at the bottom, however, to make a clear leap into revolutionary action. If Black women were free, it would mean that everyone else would have to be free since our freedom would necessitate the destruction of all the systems of oppression."[27]

It is important to note that AIDS would not be a crisis if we did not dismiss, as exceptions, the experiences of Black women, Black queer women, Black trans subjects, and those racialized and gendered as Black women and/or trans people in the Global South. As Black feminists have long argued, when we center Black women we are faced with the challenge of innovating upon our epistemological, methodological, and political interventions to generate new ways of knowing, acting, and organizing. As antiracist feminists continue to clarify that intersectionality is a critique of oppression and power and not just about identity and difference, Jih-Fei Cheng's chapter reflecting upon the crises in knowledge production reminds us to keep in view how historical and ongoing AIDS activism reflects the calls by today's #BlackLivesMatter movement founders Alicia Garza, Opal Tometi, and Patrisse Cullors; the #MeToo movement founder Tarana Burke; and the #NoDAPL movement founded by the Women of the Oceti Sakowin, or the Seven Council Fires, among many other contemporary movements, to remember and reclaim women of color feminist scholar-activisms as historically and continuously central to addressing global crises, including AIDS.[28]

Viviane Namaste underscores how historical antiblackness and the falsified origins for HIV/AIDS have been fundamental to the decades-long proliferation of the pandemic. Furthermore, the repetition of white men's centrality to AIDS history elides the variety and effectiveness of Black political struggles and resistances. Namaste asks us to reconsider the definitions and salience for the terms AIDS, (white) *gay men*, and AIDS *activism* in the context of Haitian political organizing across national boundaries. Collectively, our authors demonstrate how AIDS origin stories can and must be challenged, and call for further interventions that center people of color, especially Black diasporic peoples. To do so, Marlon Bailey's contribution invites us to think beyond AIDS Inc.'s stultifying and vilifying categories for risk by considering how Black gay/queer men eroticize sexual intimacies and community in the midst of, in spite of, and through multiple crises.

Who is the exception and who is the rule? Whose words and experiences define safety and/or risk? As editors, we remained attentive to our own role in distributing attention or in reproducing known and yet persistent gaps in AIDS knowledge within the volume. When we attend closely, as we do here across a series of chapters, to Black gay/men's sexual intimacies, do other practices and pleasures evaporate from view? We keep Cathy J. Cohen's *Boundaries of Blackness: AIDS and the Breakdown of Politics* as a foundational and continually edifying frame, centering, as she does, blackness, AIDS, and Black queer women's AIDS activism. While referencing the Combahee River Collective Statement, Cohen has argued in her influential 1997 essay "Punks, Bulldaggers, and Welfare Queens: The Radical Potential of Queer Politics?" that in order for queer scholarship and activism to challenge white supremacy and heteropatriarchy, it must historicize the production of blackness, Black sexuality, Black families, Black women, and Black motherhood as deviant and queer. By tying together intersectionality and queer theory and politics, Cohen documented the history of AIDS activism and its multi-issued approach to the pandemic, ranging from its involvement in needle exchange programs to antiprison movements to women's health-care rights.

We attend to the boundaries of blackness and wonder how this distributes to other linked crises of identity, activism, care, and community in the enduring shadow of AIDS for those most affected. Thus, we also chose to republish from *Queer Latinidad: Identity Practices, Discursive Spaces,* Juana María Rodríguez's chapter "Activism and Identity in the Ruins of Representation," accompanied here with a postscript that revisits her earlier assertions on how identity politics is creatively "reimagined and negotiated" by foregrounding "marginalized cultural production."[29] In the present, Rodríguez deliberates on the end of organizations, such as the ones on which she once wrote, and the "failed" efforts that, like relations(hips), come to an end. Instead, she finds traces of the hauntings of ghosts attending to the rituals of mourning as today's cultural workers call back the earlier Latinx queer and trans artists-activists, who have since been displaced by the Bay Area tech boom, to counter the tidying of history and memory by the onslaught of gentrification.

While Cheng argues that the co-optation of women of color feminisms into the academy also yields pedagogical and praxis-oriented interventional tools, Julia S. Jordan-Zachery proclaims that "in the face of #BlackLivesMatter, we see the assertion of #Sayhername, which is a call to insert Black girls and women into the narratives of Black death that result from state-sanctioned violence." Both Jordan-Zachery and Cheng remark upon the insidious manner in which—even as Black women actively engage in scholarship, electoral politics, and direct action—they are, in the words of Jordan-Zachery, "somehow . . . simultaneously disappearing." Thus, Jordan-Zachery continues, "while it is important to study the mechanics of this disappearance, we need to come back to the question of who gets to be in the center." As argued by Evelynn Hammonds, the "'culture of dissemblance'" and a "politics of silence by black women on the issue of their sexuality" are a form of resistance to historical sexual and medical violence practiced on Black women during and after the formal period of chattel slavery, and continued through the stereotypes and states of policing and surveillance that oversexualize, pathologize, and criminalize Black women.[30] Hammonds writes: "The identification of a black hole requires the use of sensitive detectors of energy and distortion. In the case of black female sexualities, this implies that we need to develop reading strategies that allow us to make visible the distorting and productive effects these sexualities produce in relation to more visible sexualities."[31] Thus, in recognizing and forwarding Black and other women of color feminisms that have been foundational to queer and AIDS theory and politics, this volume foregrounds the disturbances that seem to operate in the periphery or in tangential ways to the centering of North American white men.

Ethics of Care, Healing, and Radical Love

The intention of this volume to mark and then theorize from historical, regional, political, and representational gaps is not intended to generate more master narratives about HIV/AIDS. To repeat: AIDS is not *a* crisis. It is the global distribution of networked *crises*. In attending to these modes of globally distributed moments of extraordinary and yet persistent rupture, our volume does not, however, lose sight of what is being done and what must become different across the vast array of space, time, and experience represented here. In one of the most provocative statements expressed in this anthology, Dredge Byung'chu Kang-Nguyễn sets forth a reversal of terms that has helped him, and others, understand the changed stakes of some of our most contemporary iterations of the AIDS crisis: "HIV is not just about what you do but who you are." This statement is stunning in its almost sacrilege, at least for activists from the first (and later) generations, against a well-known, commonly held, activist-created belief system.

One of the primary orientations of the earliest segments of the AIDS crisis was a go-to analysis, and its associated set of procedures, policies, and politics, that insisted on the disarticulation of disease or infection from identity. At the time, and moving forward across the crises, this became a fundamental orientation and response to the bigoted and scientifically unsound underpinnings and ongoing manifestations of the epidemic where stigma was the underserved outcome for entire classes of humans, producing immense violence and oceans of bad information in one stupid, lasting swipe (initially about and against homosexuals, heroin users, hemophiliacs, and Haitians but eventually and quickly crystallizing and sticking to gay men). The earlier activist credo—AIDS is not about who you are but what you do—armed people to better understand that safer sex practices, attempts at healthy living, and clean-needle use (to name a few of what you do) mattered above identity categories. When Kang-Nguyễn turns this doctrine on its head, he sets the stage for much of what defines the analysis and action described throughout this anthology. Jessica Whitbread reminds us that personal health—who you are—is the first step to individual and then communal well-being: "When we talk about wellness, where do self-care and self-preservation fit in?"

Working from the belief that AIDS is who you are allows for much that follows: chapters built from close attention to disenfranchised communities who have been and continue to be unduly impacted by HIV/AIDS because it is inextricably linked to poverty, and poverty's attendant denials of access to education, health care, and well-being. Hence Bailey's explanation of his ethnographic method: "I query what sexual health actually means to Black gay men on their own terms and what it looks like in their quotidian lives from their own perspectives." Of course, for Black gay men, and the many other disenfranchised and heavily impacted communities attended to in this anthology, this who you are, while highly and decidedly personal and commonplace, is the result of systematic, ongoing colonial and racist oppressions.

What to do as HIV/AIDS seems intractable for so many of humans damaged as much if not more from the systematic violence and dismantling of collective care by racism, colonialism, poverty, and ill health? A good many of our authors suggest that healing, ritual, teaching, radical love, and sexuality become necessary responses to this, a racist crisis manifested as damaged humans. If AIDS is who you are, and you are unwell because of poverty and/or racism and/or colonialism, there is work to be done. Many of our authors attest that finding positive personal health outcomes in these seemingly unmanageable environments might initiate from working toward a core sense of self-love and self-knowledge, and its attendant connection to others, which remains hard to find and harder still to maintain.

Our authors attest that this work must move deeper than the local and wider than the personal. The chapters thus theorize and practice forms of knowing—artistic, sexual, spiritual, interpersonal—that not only remain homegrown and private but are modeled in proximity and intimacy with others. These practices of well-being commencing from who you are—a proud, self-aware, defiant person with AIDS (PWA) who is Haitian in Montreal, indigenous in San Francisco, or Chicano from Los Angeles—are built and maintained by a hard-learned sense of where you come from, historically, culturally, and spatially, and then the harder work of expressing beyond yourself and to/with your community. Darius Bost, for example, explains: "The languages readily available to [Assotto] Saint are insufficient because they deny him access to selfhood." Saint and his creative praxis demand that we take stock of "memories of resistance and alternative modes of being that already exist," which reveal the potential ends to capitalism and crises. Through his testimony on HIV seroconversion and ceremony, Andrew Jolivette prompts us to regard how the sacred leadership of Two-Spirit Native peoples is necessary for addressing histories of Indigenous dispossession as well as the individual and communal healing of those most affected by the pandemic.

Given that a central method of racist colonialism is to rip away and destroy local tradition, culture, knowledge, and self-love from the colonized, a core tactic of contemporary AIDS analysis and activism is to better understand, reinstate, and honor local knowledge and experience. Thus Jolivette suggests: "Ceremony is an art. It requires balance, good intentions, and people who participate must be willing to move away from colonial perspectives that reduce the experiences of those at risk for HIV to Western constructs of heteropatriarchy." Many of our authors locate sex itself as one such radical ceremony. Overcoming obstacles to sexual pleasure and joy are a necessary step in gaining good health. Bailey writes about the ways that "unsafe" sexual practices are in pursuit of something core to well-being: "a deep intimacy, a closeness and a 'being desired and wanted' in a world in which Black gay men are rarely desired and wanted." These connections and intimacies are open, promiscuous, fun, joyous, and necessary. Feminism, including the work of poet, intellectual, and activist Audre Lorde, reminds us that these personal, sexual, private, local forms of being, erotics, and knowing are also always political and structural, and are produced and experienced in ways and places well beyond, if including, the agency of the individual.[32]

Our authors, on their own, but more so as a working collection, draw discrete maps that model how to link time, place, and people who need each other locally, sexually, spiritually, politically, and artistically as they also need each other across borders of nation, space, and time. As just one example, in the second set of dispatches in the anthology, focusing on the uses and meanings of the past, Pablo Alvarez contributes some of his doctoral research into, and daily knowledge of, the experience of Latinx gay men, AIDS, and Los Angeles. Rereading "There Are Places You Don't Walk at Night, Alone," a poem by Gil Cuadros published in the book *City of God* in 1994, Alvarez writes how Cuadros, one of the authors Alvarez's work considers, "documents the reality of AIDS signification, homophobic violence, love, and Chicano desire on the streets of Los Angeles. Written in three parts, each part locates main intersections of Los Angeles that are located near my home. These are the streets that I have traveled throughout my life." In the original version of her chapter, Rodríguez seems to respond: "Maps are useful guides but they are site-specific ideological constructions and are quickly dated by the earthquakes of history."[33] Our collection connects across earthquakes. In "Dispatches from the Pasts/Memories of AIDS," Cecilia Aldarondo explains her AIDS pedagogy to young students who seem almost fully unaware of the history or ongoing reality of the epidemic: "[Their] questions are openings—cracks in time that allow for transformation."

The many places of rubble, the tiny and large fissures in time identified here, have important and notable connectivities. Each interaction between an author (as activist, researcher, scholar, and/or artist) and a community manifests a particular, refined answer to Viviane Namaste's founding question: "How do we tell the history of AIDS, locally and globally?" As diverse as are the answers to this question and the approaches of our authors to get there, we can highlight one characteristic move and another distinguishing place: our authors invest in the local, the daily, and the quotidian experiences of HIV/AIDS by attending to histories, people, and places in the world and across time that have hitherto been understood as "marginal" for reasons that feel almost too painful, common, or self-evident to restate here. And yet state, explain, embellish, disqualify, respond to we must and we will. As stated by Ghosh: "Mothers, working people, tax-paying citizens, and property owners have the right to medical recourse, and can demand it—not so easy for those who live on the edge, [and] migrate constantly for employment." Citing Cohen, Bost reminds us that "Black leaders could have used their bully pulpits to make AIDS a priority for their constituency, but instead they pursued a more aggressive campaign of denial and distance that marked

Black people with AIDS as outside the community." In "Dispatches on the Globalizations of AIDS," Theodore (Ted) Kerr explains what emerges from the cracks, the ruptures, and the margins of crises thus: "How might we think, which is say how might we respond to HIV/AIDS differently, if these were among the places we began questions of globalized AIDS?" When we start with migrants, or Black gay men, or Latinx peoples in Los Angeles or in San Francisco, what do we learn, what do we see, what can we know, and best yet, what can we do about the crises of AIDS? As Cait McKinney writes about the formative years of the public use of the internet in AIDS organizing, "Critical Path's model placed vulnerable users at infrastructure development's center." Bost continues, "Writing from the shadows also provides possibilities for reimagining the racial, class, gender, and sexual ideologies that undergird the neoliberal urban landscape."

Summaries of the Chapters and Dispatches

By "writing from the shadows" and looking to new centers or "pockets of crisis" that have been too-little attended to thus far, the collected work of this anthology does much more than simply accumulate a set of new, varied, and less-attended-to perspectives or subjects. Instead, our aligned but distinct orientations allow us to see AIDS with a chilling shared clarity: as an ongoing, global crisis—experienced locally and with specificity—of enduring, structuring colonialism and racism, and all the violence to person, place, health, and self-knowledge that such systems wreak. As Namaste explains, "If we take for granted the conventional framework for writing history, we risk neglecting entire populations of people and their experience with this disease." And of course, it is not coincidental that "the historical telling of an epidemic in which white male bodies are at the center is, to say the least, not the best model for understanding the complex relations between Black bodies, migration, and infectious disease."

Bishnupriya Ghosh, a scholar of English and media studies, begins our anthology with "The Costs of Living: Reflections on Global Health Crises," by performing the kind of decentering that Namaste calls for. Her chapter holds the uses and values of large-scale, global economic and political cost-benefit analysis systems against a series of specific, local health emergencies and their resident responses in the northeastern Indian state of Manipur. Ghosh examines how local NGOs and activist networks have responded to the region's long state of exception to work on their own local calculus of health, one that counts the loss and value of even one life as incalculable.

To follow, feminist, queer, and science studies scholar Jih-Fei Cheng considers why and how women of color feminisms is foundational to AIDS scholar activism and yet why women of color—particularly Black and Indigenous women—rarely remain the subjects of AIDS historiography and studies. In "AIDS, Women of Color Feminisms, Queer and Trans of Color Critiques, and the Crises of Knowledge Production," Cheng maintains that we cannot address the AIDS pandemic by focusing on it as such. Rather, we must center attention on how AIDS can be better and more comprehensively known. For instance, women of color feminisms, taught within academic institutions and drawn upon by a number of social movements, can enable us to follow already existing roadmaps laid out by intersectional feminists to navigate a host of structural violences that shape their lives, including AIDS.

In "Safe, Soulful Sex: HIV/AIDS Talk," political scientist and professor of public and community service Julia S. Jordan-Zachery shares a new introduction to her reprinted chapter, which traces how Black women commonly address AIDS through electoral political stumping and corporate welfare rather than through the structural discrimination they experience as Black women, lesbians, and transfeminine peoples. Jordan-Zachery's inquiry into media and media images highlights the dual hypervisibility/invisibility experienced by many Black women, especially those who are constituted as *shadow bodies* (i.e., HIV positive, lesbian, trans, poor) of public discourse and the politics of respectability.

In "AIDS Histories Otherwise: The Case of Haitians in Montreal," Vivian Namaste, a scholar of HIV/AIDS and sexual health, learns from "research located in sites of migrant communities themselves" by looking at epidemiological statistics, clinical observations, and community organizing around the impact of AIDS in Montreal's Haitian communities during the first years of the epidemic.

Several close looks at the work of radical activists follow. In his chapter, "'A Voice Demonic and Proud': Shifting the Geographies of Blame in Assotto Saint's 'Sacred Life: Art and AIDS,'" Darius Bost, a scholar of sexuality studies, works through readings of Saint's 1980s and 1990s writings. Bost finds Saint's radical project—gaining selfhood and self-respect while grounded within local community—as a necessary response to the stigma, ill-health, and risk bred by systematic racism, homophobia, and marginality. Cait McKinney, an information and media studies scholar, also engages in close readings in the chapter "Crisis Infrastructures: AIDS Activism Meets Internet Regulation." Looking at one early AIDS activist internet website, and the court testimony about its structuring logic given by Kiyoshi Kuromiya, director of Philadelphia's Critical Path AIDS Project, in a field-defining case against it, McKinney connects activists' demands for critical paths to AIDS knowledge and another struggle, one for open routes to information online. Of course, paths can open or close knowledge. Several of the chapters in this volume perform a genealogical retracing written through a spatial logic. They consider how any unfolding of the history of AIDS forced to commence in Africa or Haiti will create frameworks that fuel and perpetuate ongoing crises within Black communities.

How then do people of color take care given this violence? Marlon M. Bailey, a scholar of African American and gender and sexuality studies, in his contribution "Black Gay Men's Sexual Health and the Means of Pleasure in the Age of AIDS," studies local cures in relation to the racialized distribution of risk and sexual (ill-)health. By focusing on the suffering disproportionately felt by African American gay men, Bailey's work homes in on desires for intimacy and love and suggests that an erotic subjectivity and autonomy based in pleasure can serve as a foundation for a Black gay male epistemology of self-care. In "HIV, Indigeneity, and Settler Colonialism: Understanding PTIS, Crisis Resolution, and the Art of Ceremony," Andrew J. Jolivette, a scholar of American Indian studies, continues this focus upon causes and ever more imaginative remedies for the uneven distribution of ill-health, trauma, and HIV risk with a particular focus on Indigenous communities. He maps the clear through lines between the *longue durée* of colonialism and the local, present, and personal manifestations of risk behaviors, including his own. Juana María Rodríguez, a professor of gender and women's studies, engages in similar, if entirely differently situated, work, by looking to the promotional and educational efforts and materials of one local AIDS activist nonprofit, "Proyecto ContraSIDA Por Vida," serving Latinx and Chicanx communities in San Francisco's Mission District since the earliest years of the crisis. In this reprinted chapter, "Activism and Identity in the Ruins of Representation," from *Queer Latinidad* (2003) and also in her timely update, Rodríguez challenges the relations between theories of postmodern identity and politics and practices of community-based projects of well-being.

Interspersed between these chapters, our dispatches similarly engage with the anthology's core interests through three interactions focused, at least ostensibly, around the themes of HIV/AIDS and globalization, the past, and the future. Our dispatches on the globalizations of AIDS, from the pasts/memories of AIDS, and from the futures of AIDS are critical to our larger project because they provide alternative pathways for talking, engaging, and knowing HIV/AIDS (to learn from Kuromiya in McKinney's chapter), attending to diverse knowledge frameworks (à la Namaste), and making use of tabulations and calculations at other scales and registers (Ghosh's hope) than have been true for more typical scholarly essays on what Ian Bradley-Perrin names the *neoliberal pharmaceutical state industrial complex*. The three editors each led, edited, and introduced one of the dispatches, although we selected and invited our participants with a shared understanding of the reach of the volume as a whole. Given our core orientation to the crises of AIDS as always local, situated, and changing, we felt it was imperative to open out into the density of HIV/AIDS by including a range of voices, approaches, and styles. The dispatches also offer a time capsule of sorts since they were conducted either right before or in the aftermath of the Trump election in 2016. However, their order of appearance in the collection does not necessarily replicate the sequence in which they were conducted, so that the anxieties, frustrations, and fears of this moment are scattered in different moods, scales, and registers throughout the three dispatches. Perhaps there is something apposite about these peaks and dips in that they replicate the logics of crises, which by definition are uneven in temporal scope—heightened and intensified in some moments and attenuated and atrophied in others.

Given the definitive diversity of these voices, many of whom we have already quoted in this introduction, it seems less useful to try to summarize here the rich and definitive variety of what can be discussed in a conversational format and instead simply signal that our contributors (some of whom are scholars and professors, many of whom are not) have been authorized to speak about broad topics as they wish while using the range of vernaculars that best suit their (and our) HIV/AIDS practice. Their diverse voices add to our anthology the urgency and energy of fellow activists who engage in the theorizing and the doing of AIDS culture. For instance, in "Dispatches from Pasts/Memories of AIDS," Jim Hubbard rallies: "Finally, if you are dissatisfied with the media being made now about the AIDS crisis, there is a solution—make your own. That's what AIDS activists did in the 1980s and '90s and with the ubiquity of cell phones and computerized editing systems, it's even more possible today." Just so, scholar, activist, and poet Margaret Rhee creates her vision of limitless care by quoting others' words from the "Dispatches from the Futures of AIDS."

> For a world of limitless care for Indigenous people,
> We fight for care, resist the cutbacks, and the incarceration.
> (Elton Naswood)

"I believe acts of kindness are stronger than acts of fear."
(Jessica Whitbread)

Your words are kindness. So I release, fear. Fear runs as
We organize, convene, disseminate,
". . . and follow the lead of new waves of leadership . . ."
(Pato Hebert)

Given our core understanding that the crises of AIDS are always local, situated, and changing, we felt it was imperative for our collection to open out into the density of this diversity, multiplicity, and specificity by including a range of voices, approaches, and styles, while also thereby modeling in the anthology's structure the possibility and need for dialogue and community across the specific and local knowledge frameworks and experiences of AIDS.

Conclusion

"Dispatches from the Futures of AIDS" focuses on voices, projects, and contributions, like Rhee's above, that learn from, share, and imagine the best for and of us. We hope that this can also be read across the volume as a whole even as it is being written and edited during remarkably bleak and terrifying times for all humans, and particularly for those impacted by HIV/AIDS. Thus, rather than ask, Where did AIDS begin? or When will it end? the dispatches—like the entire volume—ask, How has it come to scatter and proliferate? and What will we do? Drawing a parallel between the development of Christianity and the development of the AIDS pandemic, Kerr inquires in the first dispatch: "How did a religion started as a cult of outsiders in the Middle East come to be so closely associated with dominance and white supremacy within the southern United States?" and "How has a virus that began in a southeast corner of Cameroon possibly as early as the late nineteenth century come to be so closely associated with white gay men living on the coasts of the United States in the late twentieth century?" By stringing together past, present, and future in the dispatches and chapters, the volume does not merely supply etiological, temporal, spatial, or etymological corrections to HIV/AIDS. Instead, the book's intent is to leave its readers with what Stanley calls a dreaming project—one that continues to challenge the limits of our artistic and political imaginations around HIV/AIDS. Even while resisting the temporalities of global capitalism that demand instantaneous solutions or magic bullet cures, these dreaming projects are not simply deferred to speculative moments of postponed futures. They exist in the here and now beyond the normative logics of state-driven "solutions," drugs into bodies "victories," whitewashed gay hagiographies, and AIDS service industries. They exist in Zoe Leonard's call for "a president who lost their last lover to AIDS" as well as the image on our cover of her installation "Strange Fruit" which so beautifully manifests the scatterings, distributions, and crises that we consider; in Marlon Riggs's reminders about the revolutionary possibilities of "black men loving black men"; in Kiyoshi Kuromiya's promiscuous media pedagogies; in Assotto Saint's "otherwise possibilities"; in the rejections of "homosex-normativity"; in the demands to be realistic by asking for the impossible; in the healing practices of Two-Spirit communities; in Quito Ziegler's injunctions to "live the future now," to "imagine liberation," to imagine futures without HIV, and without prisons.[34]

This volume thus seeks epistemological and political connections, and new horizons for understanding and addressing the globally networked crises of AIDS without false promises derived from false premises.

Notes

1 *Online Etymology Dictionary*, s.v. "crisis," accessed July 18, 2017, http://www.etymonline.com/index.php?term=crisis.
2 Roitman, *Anti-Crisis*, 6, emphasis added.
3 Roitman, *Anti-Crisis*, 43.
4 Cazdyn, *Already Dead*, 2.
5 Berlant, *Cruel Optimism*, 101, emphasis added.
6 Agamben, *State of Exception*.
7 Mbembe, "Necropolitics," 40.
8 Banerjee, "Necrocapitalism," 1542.
9 Stanley, "Blood Lines."
10 Chin, "Undetectable," 11.
11 Chin, "Undetectable," 12.
12 Centers for Disease Control and Prevention, "HIV in the United States"; "Global HIV and AIDS Statistics."
13 Centers for Disease Control and Prevention, "Opportunistic Infections."
14 Barré-Sinoussi et al., "Isolation of a T-lymphotropic Retrovirus"; Gallo et al., "Isolation of Human T-cell Leukemia Virus."
15 Edwards, "Diaspora," 77.
16 Edwards, "Diaspora," 77.
17 Edwards, *The Practice of Diaspora*, 12.
18 Wojnarowicz, *Close to the Knives*, 122.
19 Herbert, "In America."
20 Appadurai, "Disjuncture and Difference," 50.
21 Sassen, "Local Actors in Global Politics," 649.

22 Appadurai, "Disjuncture and Difference," 47.
23 Ong, *Flexible Citizenship*.
24 Berlant, *Cruel Optimism*, 55.
25 Schulman, *Stagestruck*, 138.
26 Combahee River Collective, "The Combahee River Collective Statement," 29.
27 Combahee River Collective, "The Combahee River Collective Statement," 29–30.
28 On Women of the Oceti Sakowin, see TallBear, "Badass (Indigenous) Women Caretake Relations."
29 Rodríguez, "Activism and Identity," 47–48 (original publication).
30 Hammonds, "Geometry of Black Female Sexuality," 128.
31 Hammonds, "Geometry of Black Female Sexuality," 144–45.
32 Lorde, *Uses of the Erotic*.
33 Rodríguez, "Activism and Identity," 38.
34 Leonard, "I Want a President"; Riggs, *Tongues Untied*.

Bibliography

Agamben, Giorgio. *State of Exception*. Chicago: University of Chicago Press, 2005.
Appadurai, Arjun. "Disjuncture and Difference in the Global Cultural Economy." In *The Anthropology of Globalization: A Reader*, edited by Jonathan Xavier Inda and Renato Rosaldo, 47–65. Malden, MA: Blackwell, 2002.
Banerjee, Subhabrata Bobby. "Necrocapitalism." *Organization Studies* 29, no. 12 (2008): 1541–63.
Barré-Sinoussi, F., et al. "Isolation of a T-lymphotropic Retrovirus from a Patient at Risk for Acquired Immune Deficiency Syndrome (AIDS)." *Science* 220, no. 4599 (1983): 868–71.
Berlant, Lauren. *Cruel Optimism*. Durham, NC: Duke University Press, 2011.
Cazdyn, Eric. *The Already Dead: The New Time of Politics, Culture, and Illness*. Durham, NC: Duke University Press, 2012.
Centers for Disease Control and Prevention. "HIV in the United States: At a Glance." Accessed July 25, 2017. https://www.cdc.gov/hiv/statistics/overview/ataglance.html.
Centers for Disease Control and Prevention. "Opportunistic Infections and Kaposi's Sarcoma among Haitians in the United States." *Morbidity and Mortality Weekly Report* 31, no. 26 (1982): 353–54, 360–61. https://www.cdc.gov/mmwr/preview/mmwrhtml/00001123.htm.
Chin, Justin. "Undetectable." In *Harmless Medicine*, 11–12. San Francisco: Manic D, 2001.
Cohen, Cathy J. "Punks, Bulldaggers, and Welfare Queens: The Radical Potential of Queer Politics?" *GLQ: A Journal of Lesbian and Gay Studies*, vol. 3, no. 4 (1997): 437–465.
Cohen, Cathy J. *The Boundaries of Blackness: AIDS and the Breakdown of Black Politics*. Chicago: University of Chicago Press, 1999.

Combahee River Collective. "The Combahee River Collective Statement." In *Theorizing Feminism: Parallel Trends in the Humanities and Social Sciences*, edited by Anne C. Herrmann and Abigail J. Stewart, 29–37. Boulder, CO: Westview, 1994.

Edwards, Brent Hayes. "Diaspora." In *Keywords for American Cultural Studies*, edited by Bruce Burgett and Glenn Hendler, 76–77. 2nd ed. New York: New York University Press, 2014.

Edwards, Brent Hayes. *The Practice of Diaspora: Literature, Translation, and the Rise of Black Internationalism*. Cambridge, MA: Harvard University Press, 2003.

Gallo, R. C., et al. "Isolation of Human T-cell Leukemia Virus in Acquired Immune Deficiency Syndrome (AIDS)." *Science* 220, no. 4599 (1983): 865–67.

"Global HIV and AIDS Statistics." Accessed July 25, 2017. https://www.avert.org/global-hiv-and-aids-statistics.

Hammonds, Evelynn. "Black (W)holes and the Geometry of Black Female Sexuality." *Differences: A Journal of Feminist Cultural Studies* 6, nos. 2–3 (1994): 127–45.

Herbert, Bob. "In America; Refusing to Save Africans." *New York Times*, June 11, 2001.

Leonard, Zoe. "I Want a President." 1992. Accessed June 25, 2016. https://iwantapresident.wordpress.com/i-want-a-president-zoe-leonard-1992.

Lorde, Audre. *The Uses of the Erotic: The Erotic as Power*. Tucson: Kore, 2000.

Mbembe, Achille. "Necropolitics." *Public Culture* 15, no. 1 (2003): 11–40.

Ong, Aihwa. *Flexible Citizenship: The Cultural Logics of Transnationality*. Durham, NC: Duke University Press, 1999.

Riggs, Marlon, dir. *Tongues Untied*. Culver City, California: Strand Releasing Home Video, 2008. DVD.

Rodríguez, Juana María. "Activism and Identity in the Ruins of Representation." In *Queer Latinidad: Identity Practices, Discursive Spaces*, 37–83. New York: New York University Press, 2003.

Roitman, Janet. *Anti-Crisis*. Durham, NC: Duke University Press, 2013.

Sassen, Saskia. "Local Actors in Global Politics." *Current Sociology* 52, no. 4 (2004): 649–70.

Schulman, Sarah. *Stagestruck: Theater, AIDS, and the Marketing of Gay America*. Durham, NC: Duke University Press, 1998.

Stanley, Eric A. "Blood Lines: AIDS, Affective Accumulation, and Viral Labor." Paper presented at the Gender Studies Symposium, Lewis and Clark College, Portland, OR, March 13, 2015.

TallBear, Kim. "Badass (Indigenous) Women Caretake Relations: #NoDAPL, #IdleNoMore, #BlackLivesMatter." Hot Spots, *Fieldsights*, December 22, 2016. https://culanth.org/fieldsights/badass-indigenous-women-caretake-relations-no-dapl-idle-no-more-black-lives-matter.

Villarosa, Linda. "America's Hidden H.I.V. Epidemic." *New York Times*, June 6, 2017.

Wojnarowicz, David. *Close to the Knives: A Memoir of Disintegration*. New York: Vintage, 1991.

ONE DISPATCHES ON
THE GLOBALIZATIONS OF AIDS

A Dialogue between Theodore (Ted) Kerr,
Catherine Yuk-ping Lo, Ian Bradley-Perrin,
Sarah Schulman, and Eric A. Stanley,
with an Introduction by Nishant Shahani

As the first of three "dispatches" that are interspersed throughout this volume, the juxtaposition of voices gathered below serves to highlight the multiplicity of approaches among thinkers who are academics, artists, journalists, and activists (in many instances not mutually exclusive categories). Besides initial prompts, the lack of editorial curation hopes to preserve these differences in register rather than paper over them in the service of smooth consistency in style or tone. The term *dispatches* (or *palimpsests of insights*, as one of the volume reviewers usefully called them) captures these truncated glimpses or musings that are not always in direct or explicit dialogue with one another but still generate the kinds of scattered collectivities that lie at the core of the volume's conceptual emphasis on the multiple scales and calibrations of distribution.

The five contributors to this particular dispatch—Theodore (Ted) Kerr, Catherine Yuk-ping Lo, Ian Bradley-Perrin, Sarah Schulman, and Eric A. Stanley—were put together from a broader list of thinkers that we carefully curated, consisting of those whose ideas centralized AIDS scholarship and activism while also circling around writings on AIDS in more oblique and, at times, even seemingly unrelated directions. The rationale was to allow for the cross-cutting of ideas beyond the traditional frames of what could be understood as scholarship on HIV and AIDS, so that the writings in this volume (and the dispatches in particular) could create connecting threads between sites conventionally thought of as discrete and discontinuous. From the congeries of names we created, the five selected for this "dispatch" offered precisely this combination of expertise on AIDS scholarship along with interests that could particularly offer a set of provocations in thinking through global frameworks. These include investments in ethics and theology (Kerr), security studies and Asian-Pacific foreign policy (Lo), the neoliberal politics of pharmaceutical marketing (Bradley-Perrin), critiques of homonationalism and gentrification (Schulman), and prison abolition and trans resistance (Stanley).

In terms of the form these dispatches would take, we arranged asynchronous rather than real-time exchange of writings, framed by two prompts for each dispatch. Such organizing had as much to do with logistical necessities, such as differing time zones and conflicting schedules, as with the critical orientations of the book. It is undeniable that such a non-coeval format has its limits—a potential loss of spontaneity that subtends the unpredictability of "live" exchange or the communal intimacies that can be forged with face-to-face or at least coinciding encounters. And yet there is something apposite about navigating the difficulties of achieving real-time connectivity in these dispatches on AIDS and globalizations. Globalization, after all, has been described as a phenomenon of hyperconnectivity that axiomatically transgresses space and time. But the celebration of its putative spatial and temporal condensations ignores the often alienating ways in which globalization also fragments and isolates, so that certain populations are left out of "real time" even as others benefit from economies of instantaneousness more immediately. Perhaps our inability to meet in real time constitutes a kind of instructive pedagogical failure. We might begin to understand globalization's compressed spatiotemporalities as those that truncate and "scatter" even as they purport to always connect and unite.

While the other two dispatches in this volume on the pasts and futures of AIDS are explicitly framed around logics of time, the "dispatches on the globalizations of AIDS" appear, at least superficially, as the anomaly. But in many ways, its intent is not dissimilar to the temporal structuring of the other two, by considering how globalizations implicate both "pasts" and "futures" (just as the dispatches on pasts gesture to futures and the dispatches from the futures often shuttle back to pasts). Framing these dispatches in temporal terms allows an understanding of both globalizations and AIDS as "nothing new," that is, as operating through long and prior geopolitical histories of imperialism and colonization but also as a flexible transnational practice that is constantly shifting and morphing through novel and reorganized mutations. In different ways, the contributors simultaneously recognize these recursive repetitions and updated permutations through theorizations of the politics of time: for example, Kerr's attention to the "urgencies of time" so that we can unpack global histories of AIDS prior to the 1980s, Schulman's retrospective framing of AIDS before and after the fall of the Soviet Union, and Stanley's contention that our present definitions of AIDS and HIV are predicated on traces of the past that are imbued with the "haunts of conquest and chattel slavery."

Relatedly, the prompts to contributors were proposed with the intent to brush up against narratives of globalization's purported elastic transgressions (where the role of the nation-state seemingly disappears from view) so that we might begin to articulate how systems of management are calcified and intensified at precisely the moments in which they are thought to weaken or diminish in their sovereign scope. It is not without significance then that a recurring preoccupation through several responses below is a consideration of how the flow and exchange of liquids—blood, plasma, drugs, vaginal fluids, breast milk, semen—become sites of governmentality saturated by anxieties around contagion (most explicitly foregrounded in Lo's analysis of the nexus between the state and blood banks that precipitated an HIV outbreak in the Henan province of the People's Republic of China). Blood, as Stanley has similarly pointed out in another context, is charged with meaning "beyond its cellular capacity," telling us "stories" that "are as much about blood banks, platelets, and centrifuges, as they are about race, kinship, sexuality, contagion and the force of exile."[1]

The management of "dangerous" liquids thus informs the logics of globalization under which the fluid movement of capital functions in tandem with, and as an alibi for, the magnification of boundaries and fixities. The contributions in this dispatch thus explore how capital's liquid-like flows are predicated on the geopolitical governing of fluids in order to allow for surplus accumulation—"liquidity" in another sense—of easily accessible capital that ostensibly guarantees market stability, and which must therefore be inoculated from the unpredictable contaminations of bad blood. Since blood is crucial to biopolitical logics of slavery, dispossession, and antiblackness, it is not a coincidence that several contributors allude to the central place of racial capitalism in how AIDS crises get distributed. The term *racial capitalism* itself has its genealogies in Black Marxist traditions of Cedric Robinson, who pointed to the ways in which the "development, organization, and expansion of capitalist society pursued essentially racial directions."[2] In considering these "racial directions" in the context of AIDS, the contributors explore its dialectical operations. Mobilizing Ruth Wilson Gilmore's theorizing of racial capitalism, Jodi Melamed analyzes how Gilmore's definition of racism points to seemingly oppositional logics of connection and disconnection. For Melamed, the implications of Gilmore's understanding of racism as the "group-differentiated vulnerabilities to premature death, *in distinct yet densely interconnected geographies*," are not fully grappled with, if the italicized quali-fication is bracketed as a parenthetical afterthought.[3] Racial capitalism thus operates through both "dense networks" and "amputated social relations" that disconnect racial subjects from their humanity precisely "so that they may be 'interconnected' to feed capital."[4]

The antinomies of racial capitalism explain the contradictions at the heart of globalization—its supposed capacity to shrink and connect while actually exacerbating fragmentation and isolation. Ironically, the critique of global-ization as a mode of "time-space compression" is often refracted through the lens of neoliberal multiculturalism, reducing it to the benign platitude of simply "the world becoming smaller." But as contributors in these dispatches usefully remind us, these "compressions" assume more literal and violent dimensions when considered in the context of racial capitalism's draconian projects of state-building—for example, imprisoned AIDS activists (Lo) as well as the carceral logics of prison expansion that have criminalized the HIV-positive Black body (Schulman). The bracketing of racial capitalism from the "stories" of globalization thus creates fictions of relationality and corporate largesse—for example, the pharmaceutical sponsorship of Pride parades or the "charitable" distribution of medicines by multinational companies that secure patents over generic HIV medications (as analyzed by Bradley-Perrin).

Melamed concludes her analysis of racial capitalism by suggesting that its dialectical contradictions "reveal its weakness as much as its strength."[5] For Melamed, a return to Robinson and Black Marxist thought allows for an understanding of relationality between past, present, and future that is not in the service of monetization and Black dehumanization. The "response of African people to being ripped out of webs of Indigenous social relations" continues to be one of "collective resistance . . . [in] the form of (re)consti-tuting collectivities," writes Melamed.[6] The dispatches below, despite their asynchronous formats, are attempts to imagine collectivities beyond the truncations of globalizations' fragments. When Schulman contends that "we have not yet found" answers amid "fragments of stories," or Kerr writes of "alienating waiting rooms" that embody how "there is no privacy in living with HIV" even while "HIV has largely been privatized," they document the technologies of globalizations and racial capitalism that disconnect and sever us from the reconstitution of collectivities. But in these scattered fragments are also "dreaming project[s]" (Stanley) of other times and places, of alterative genealogies of the past, and of reparative projects that gesture toward seemingly impossible futures.

—*Nishant Shahani*

Prompt 1

Nishant Shahani: From the very outset, discourses around HIV and AIDS have been implicated in global processes that impacted its cultural and epidemiological meanings. If AIDS, as Eric Cazdyn has pointed out, is not simply "the most perfect metaphor for globalization" but *is* globalization itself, what challenges do artists, activists, and scholars face in mapping the links between local and global AIDS in the twenty-first century?[7] How have these challenges morphed and shifted over time, but in what senses have they also persisted and remained the same?

Sarah Schulman: My first thought about international AIDS took place in September 1985, when I wrote the following piece for the *New York Native*:

AIDS Reported in the Soviet Union
Sarah Schulman

According to a story filed from the Soviet Union by United Press International, Soviet doctors have admitted that an undisclosed number of AIDS cases have been diagnosed there. The doctors are reportedly searching for a cure.

Although the Soviet Union does not admit to the presence of homosexuals or drug addicts among its population, official press reports have blamed the spread of the disease on these groups. They have also warned against sexual contact with foreign visitors including a forty-member homosexual contingent from the Netherlands to the International Youth Festival in Moscow this summer.

One doctor, Leonid Filarov, chief of the Odzhinkidze Sanatorium in the Black Sea resort of Sochi, said that some doctors believe that AIDS results from "mixed marriages." According to Dr. Filarov, "Mixed marriages can create genetic mutations, and it is possible AIDS could be a result of these marriages."

An annoyed woman at the office of the *Daily World*, the New York newspaper of the Communist Party, USA, told the *Native* that she had "no information" and referred us to the official Soviet news agency, Tass. A representative there said that three or four articles on AIDS had been published in the Soviet Union, but that he had "no information." He did remember, however, that "a leading Soviet spokesman" believed that AIDS was the result of mixed marriages, but he could not recall which race the doctor had referred to.

Well, there is no more Soviet Union. The racist assumptions at the foundation of AIDS thinking are still active and dynamic, although they have shifted from race-mixing to the concept of the predatory Black male being targeted by HIV criminalization in the United States and Canada. The long-standing mythologies that Africa gave the world AIDS, instead of the other way around, have recently been addressed by studies showing that mass inoculation efforts carried out by the West in the Global South using multiple inoculations on one needle helped create the epidemic. But what really stands out for me is my own tentative voice in this piece. I am disturbed, annoyed, and offended that the Soviet Union is so prejudiced, but I also, clearly, have no idea that there will soon be a global epidemic of cataclysmic proportions. In a sense, this—my first glimpse of international AIDS—was experienced as an oddity. It also becomes apparent, upon rereading, that at this point in AIDS journalism, four years into the crisis, we were entirely grasping at straws. Any news could be important or irrelevant. There was chaos, not only in the newsroom where journalists themselves were dying but in our minds. We were sifting through glimpses, fragments of stories, eclectic sources, and endless overwhelming new information, trying to discern what really mattered, and what would take us to an answer to the problem of how to get AIDS out of our lives. This answer is something we have not yet found.

Catherine Yuk-ping Lo: Chinese president Hu stated in a 2003 public speech that "HIV/AIDS prevention, care and treatment is a major issue pertinent to the quality and prosperity of the Chinese nation." Similarly, Premier Wen asserted that "dealing with HIV/AIDS as an urgent and major issue is related to the fundamental interests of the whole Chinese nation."[8] The HIV/AIDS-security nexus was restated in the official 2004 "State Council Notice on Strengthening HIV/AIDS Prevention and Control." This document explicitly demonstrated the determination of the Chinese authorities in framing HIV/AIDS as a security problem of the country, stating that "HIV/AIDS prevention and control is linked to economic development, social stability, and national security and prosperity."

The HIV/AIDS-security rhetoric adopted by China in addressing HIV/AIDS can be contextualized in relation to the scandal of the "AIDS Village" (*aizibing cun*) in Henan, which garnered global attention by the international community in the early twenty-first century when Elisabeth Rosenthal published a series of reports in the *New York Times* revealing the government-supported blood-selling incident in the 1990s that caused a massive outbreak of HIV/AIDS in Henan. Since then, the Chinese government has been criticized and condemned on its capacity to attend to HIV/AIDS in China, raising questions about the legitimacy of the Chinese Communist Party (CCP). When I asked a human rights lawyer in Beijing whether HIV/AIDS remains politically sensitive several years after Henan, his answer was full of sarcasm: "HIV/AIDS is no longer a sensitive issue in China, because most of the infected individuals in Henan were perished with HIV/AIDS."[9]

The failure of the Chinese authorities in grappling with HIV/AIDS in the public health setting has exacerbated the prevalence of global HIV/AIDS-security discourse in China. Two respondents working in HIV/AIDS-related nongovernmental organizations (NGOs) based in Beijing and Shanghai, respectively, told me in 2011 that they are pessimistic that HIV/AIDS problems could be fully addressed in public health settings where the disease has stigmatized connotations. In China, the first cases of HIV/AIDS occurred among foreigners and homosexuals in the 1980s. Therefore, the Chinese authorities in the early years promoted the idea that HIV/AIDS only affected marginal populations and non-Chinese people. Zeng Yi, the chief of the Chinese AIDS Research Program, asserted that HIV/AIDS was a foreign threat. In this regard, the authorities perceived HIV/AIDS as a foreign disease and did not consider it a health threat to the nation. The misperception hence hindered the allocation of necessary resources to address the problem, causing the continuous spread of the epidemic in China.

The general population and even the well-educated Chinese middle class have an inaccurate understanding of how HIV/AIDS is transmitted even today. A university professor in Beijing told me, "One of my colleagues told students that HIV/AIDS is an airborne disease." A program manager of an HIV/AIDS-related NGO in Beijing explained, "HIV/AIDS-related stigma and discrimination is still severe in medical and employment settings. . . . Medical practitioners refuse to conduct surgeries for HIV/AIDS-infected individuals. In addition, infected individuals cannot work as teachers, civil servants; some companies or enterprises do not hire HIV-positive individuals." An HIV/AIDS specialist working in an international NGO in Beijing commented on the problem of HIV stigma in China: "Discrimination against HIV/AIDS-infected individuals is obvious in some workplaces, such as hotels and schools. . . . A lot of work has been conducted to help HIV/AIDS-infected children to be admitted by universities. However, they will not be employed as teachers, medical doctors, or government officials after graduation because of their positive status." Infected individuals anticipate discrimination in health service provision; doctors in general hospitals refuse to operate on HIV/AIDS-infected patients. The university professor in Beijing again revealed, "HIV/AIDS-infected individuals can receive operations in only two hospitals in China; both of these are located in Beijing. A local doctor in Chongqing told an HIV-positive patient that he should take a train to Beijing in order to receive operations."

In line with the global HIV/AIDS-security practice (i.e., increasing the engagement of civil society in global HIV/AIDS responses), Chinese leaders have repeatedly acknowledged the importance of the role of HIV/AIDS-related NGOS in national policy implementation since 2004. Having said that, the HIV/AIDS-related "third sector" development is nevertheless restrictive in scope. Explaining the relationship between the authorities and NGOS, a university professor in Beijing suggested: "In normal circumstances, local CDC staff hand over treatment delivery work to community-based organizations. Nonetheless, CDC officials intend to keep these CBOS small, giving them just enough money to run the programs, so that they wouldn't grow too strong to pose potential threats to the government. . . . These CBOS are usually very small, operated by one or two people, on a part-time basis." An HIV/AIDS specialist working in an international NGO in Beijing further stated, "During a 2011 HIV/AIDS NGO meeting, the Chinese government clearly claimed that the authorities would like to work with NGOS/CBOS conducting service delivery, but not with those working on HIV/AIDS-related human rights or gender issues." Considering the nature of NGOS and CBOS working on HIV/AIDS, service providers are preferred by the state, whereas groups serving as advocates of human rights and agencies providing legal services for HIV/AIDS-infected people would be subjected to prosecution and coercion. To illustrate this point, Chinese leaders publicly praised a Guangxi-based NGO named AIDS Care China, recognizing the work the organization had done in HIV/AIDS prevention. Meanwhile, an HIV/AIDS-related legal aid NGO, Beijing Yirenping Centre, was raided, and two of its activists were detained in June 2015. In this regard, the continuous inclusion/exclusion process would weaken HIV/AIDS advocacy groups that were conceived as threats to the legitimacy of the authoritarian regime while preserving NGOS and CBOS that are willing to be under control by the state apparatus and prepared to accept the regime's policy measures.

Eric A. Stanley: If we are to take as a point of departure that AIDS is globalization, then the two questions that, for me, follow are: How is HIV/AIDS written through globalized racial capitalism; and related, what is the relationship between colonization and HIV/AIDS? These questions are far too large for me to begin to answer here, but in the US context I'm thinking back to the CDC's 4HS (hemophiliacs, heroin users, homosexuals, and Haitians) that signified the real and imagined "high-risk" groups of people living and dying in the early 1980s. This marker of Haiti as vector cannot be divorced from the ways the white state (especially the United States and France, who both have a colonial and para-colonial relationship with Haiti and were doing much of the early publishing on the pandemic) has produced Haiti, by way of spectacle and exclusion, as always in need of punishment for its original and founding sin of decolonization. In other words, that Haiti was born from the first successful slave revolt in the Western Hemisphere, a success that then placed, and now continues to place, into jeopardy US exceptionalism, cannot be overlooked. This is a point made by many Haitian activist/scholars, but I am returning to it here because it seems important to understand how the epidemiological foundations of what we have come to know as "HIV/AIDS" are the haunts of conquest and chattel slavery.

This white fantasy of the unruly Black body, which is to say the fantasy of the US unconscious echoed through the Haitian narrative, is again reverberated through the attention paid to HIV infection rates in Black communities in the United States. There seems to be never-ending streams of money to study, chart, graph and report on HIV and Black communities, and yet the structured abandonment, which is among the mechanisms of racial capitalism, ensures the tools necessary to support Black HIV-positive people and slow new infection rates are always missing. Perhaps this point is too obvious, but nonetheless, when we think "globalization" we must attend to the histories and futures of forced movement (enslavement, migration, genocidal depopulation and repopulation). Or, one way we might think about the globalization of AIDS is by looking at uranium mining on the Navajo reservation, or gentrification in Fruitvale, California. How might we think, which is say how might we respond to HIV/AIDS differently, if these were among the places we began questions of globalized AIDS?

This is not to suggest a kind of US centrism, but what I'm interested in is thinking deep situatedness alongside geopolitics. For those of us primarily based in what is sometimes called "the West," the move toward thinking the globe too often leads us to seeing the processes of extraction and constriction in geographies far away. Among our challenges, as those who differently inherit the spoils of empire, is to work collectively to grapple with these thick histories so that connections of depth might be made through locations and not simply over them.

Ian Bradley-Perrin: When thinking about the local and global of HIV/AIDS, I cannot help but consider how the pharmaceutical industry seamlessly inhabits these juxtaposed frames for the epidemic. At the local scale, pharmaceuticals are ever present. They are the daily personal reminder of difference for the positive person with access to medication, and they are the local struggle of access and adherence that culturally and socially define difference among positive people. At the global scale, they define globalized capital. The trials that validate a pharmaceutical's efficacy are funded from high-income, high-cultural-capital centers and they are administered and undertaken in impoverished areas. The global and the local of pharmaceuticals are always embedding themselves in one another as well. The money made from the drugs that successfully pass these trials is invested in community projects, like Pride Parades and AIDS Service Organizations. These spaces then serve as recruiting grounds for further trials and target markets for the products they produce. Pharmaceuticals hold local power through their biological necessity and fear of their absence and mobilize global power through the capital they acquire through local centers as numerous as the populations they serve, growing every day through perpetual market expansion.

PrEP (preexposure prophylaxis) is a striking example of this phenomenon. In *Drugs for Life*, Joseph Dumit proposes that we have entered a new biomedical paradigm. The previous paradigm understood the body as essentially healthy, with intermittent medical intervention to return to that natural state. Dumit claims we have entered a new medical conception of the body as essentially ill, requiring medical intervention to stave off our natural state as diseased. If asked, most would say that disease is symptomatic (real and experienced). However, the new paradigm approaches disease as the risk of becoming symptomatic (and if we paused, most could clearly see this playing out in our lives). The efficacy of interventions in the new paradigm is determined by randomized control trials, and these trials, which require huge subject participation and capital investment, are undertaken either by the pharmaceutical industry or with funding from them. This produces a system of disease identification and remedy that is not accountable to the public but only to shareholders.

The risk paradigm expands markets and creates new ones. Since disease is no longer defined solely as symptomatic, the pharmaceutical industry is positioned to create new consumers for products whose necessity is defined by the very trials they undertake to determine the efficacy of their products. Everyone is a consumer in a world where everyone is at risk.

In January 2016, AIDS Healthcare Foundation (AHF) brought a formal Food and Drug Administration (FDA) complaint against Gilead for promoting the situational use of Truvada when the drug is only approved for daily use. The complaint centers on an ad called "I Like to Party." Of the complaint, Michael Weinstein said: "Gilead, which we believe has been deliberately mounting an under-the-FDA-radar, guerilla-style marketing and media campaign for PrEP for the past three years by funding scores of community and AIDS groups across the nation to promote PrEP, has run afoul of the FDA by funding this ad promoting off-label use of PrEP."[10]

Responding to this, *The Advocate*'s Tyler Curry wrote in January:

> Gilead had no part in the creation or development of the advertisement or any other PrEP advertisement by an independent organization. To date, Gilead has yet to release a single ad for PrEP. Instead, the drug company has left it up to HIV service organizations to educate those at-risk for HIV about the benefits that the prevention strategy has to offer. The movement to spread awareness has been an uphill battle, primarily because Weinstein, via AHF, has spent thousands buying ad space in local publications, shaming those who would use the prevention drug, purporting false claims of dangerous side effects, and calling Truvada, in its revolutionary HIV prevention use, a mere "party drug."[11]

I am no great lover of AHF or Michael Weinstein. They are repeatedly and correctly accused of using fear and stigma to promote their brand and using the weight of the law to diminish or destroy smaller dissenting voices in their market. But I find the exchange here regarding the cultural construction of PrEP enlightening.

First, PrEP does need to be taken daily. The IPreX study results, published in the *New England Journal of Medicine* on December 30, 2010, found that there was a 44 percent reduction in HIV infections among those randomized to Truvada rather than the placebo. The 90 percent-plus figure we bandy about is the product of a case control study within the IPreX, which demonstrated that those who did seroconvert despite being randomized to Truvada were not adhering to their medication. Thus the FDA complaint addresses this gap between the corrected results of the RTC (randomized control trial) study and the results of the case control study.

Second, AHF is described by Curry as an obstacle to "the movement." Gilead and its product Truvada are characterized as a movement, likening them to previous health movements such as the women's health movement and AIDS activism. Weinstein is characterized as obstructive. This is not unusual. The medical establishment has long been the target of health movements. But AHF is a HIV/AIDS community clinic, something that AIDS activism desired. Given that Weinstein's trajectory is one not of activism but rather of professionalization, he took an approach to HIV/AIDS not unlike that taken by many advocates and activists as AIDS service became professionalized and bureaucratized. Curry alleges that AHF's $1.1 billion budget is thrown behind its obstruction of the movement, but this characterization of Gilead as the movement and AHF as the obstruction is a false dichotomy.

Gilead is not a person (except in the corporate sense); nor is it a movement. Founded in 1987, Gilead immediately recruited Donald Rumsfeld to the board of directors, as well as Harold Varmus, who later became the head of the National Institutes of Health (NIH). These powerful connections have been essential to the rise of Gilead's profits. As reported by Dr. Joseph Mercola, when George W. Bush demanded in 2004 that the US Congress pass $7.1 billion in emergency funding to prepare for the possible bird flu pandemic, $1 billion of this funding was to be allocated solely to the purchase of Tamiflu, a patent owned by Gilead. Rumsfeld, who prior to his role as secretary of defense had risen to chairman of the board, retained his stocks despite his appointment and profited $12 million from Tamiflu.

Gilead again came under intense criticism from ACT UP Paris in 2004 when activists stormed the stage of the International AIDS Conference holding signs claiming that Gilead "uses sex workers for free." The protesters argued that nine hundred HIV-negative "beer girls," working the bars of Phnom Penh, were recruited for a placebo study (which is illegal for HIV in the United States since the standard of treatment is much higher).

The early PrEP trials received much less attention. However, Kirsten Petersen argued, in a paper given at the Second International Conference for the Social Sciences and Humanities in HIV, that the trials on HIV-negative women in Nigeria were facilitated by the military intervention of the United States, which displaced Nigerian communities off oil-rich land, destabilizing these communities. These same communities were then identified as being at high risk for HIV due to their violently reconfigured social structures produced by displacement and were proposed as the ideal site for PrEP trials. Peterson argues that US Africa Command (AFRICOM) and the United States President's Emergency Plan for AIDS Relief (PEPFAR), both controlled and established by

Bush and Rumsfeld, tied together US foreign health policy with military policy to the benefit of, among others, Gilead Sciences. With these connections and power, it is unsurprising that Gilead is currently valued at $32.4 billion with $27 billion of revenue a year, dwarfing AHF's $1.1 billion.[12]

Weinstein's claim that Gilead is engaged in "under-the-FDA-radar, guerilla-style marketing" is not addressed by Curry; instead, Curry states that Gilead is not to blame in the situational promotion of PrEP because Gilead has not produced any advertisements for the drug but provides unrestricted funds as part of a comprehensive prevention strategy. They are saying the same thing. PrEP is not advertised by Gilead but the marketing of PrEP has relied on hundreds of NGOs using Gilead's unrestricted funds to promote the drug within a community framework. A perfect example is the Stigma Project, which is a marketing- and advertising-oriented website, producing flashy visuals to counter the stigma of HIV. The website has an entire section devoted to PrEP as well as having it integrated into the project's other campaigns. Gilead cannot be at fault for the misleading situational dosage recommendations because it has designed a marketing strategy that intentionally divests it of that responsibility. Through the funding of these various organizations, PrEP is marketed to our community by our community. And by a clever sleight of hand, Gilead becomes the éminence grise while we "speak for ourselves," using "unrestricted" funds. And as a side note: the provision of the costly drug for free in exchange for trial enrollment is a marketing tactic, as it both verifies its efficacy to a consumer public and expands the market for the product, producing consumers who will have to purchase the medication when the trial ends.

These campaigns adopt the risk-based understanding of disease, and identification with this risk becomes the consumer drive to acquire the product. The mainstream media coverage is revealing of how the dominant culture interprets the PrEP phenomenon. A great example of this is the *New York Magazine* article "Sex without Fear," in which the implicit point is that "before we were afraid of sex with HIV+ people and now we are not." PrEP does nothing to reduce the legal burdens on poz people and does not mitigate the nondisclosure laws, thus the reduction of fear is a one-sided process. Because HIV stigma drives this product, at its very core, it *is* the product. The fear that we could become that which we define ourselves against is the fundamental motivation to take preventative medications. Under the claims that sex negativity and HIV stigma prevent HIV-negative people from accessing PrEP is the mobilization of stigma to create new markets and consumers for commodities that respond to this fear. The promise of a newly guaranteed future is marketed and consumed by our community, for our community. But it is not owned by our community.

In the words of Sarah Schulman, "It normalizes the fact of people's lives without actually addressing any of their special needs."[13]

Theodore (Ted) Kerr: As the historicization of HIV started to increase in the second decade of the twenty-first century, I found myself looking for a structure of thinking, feeling, and believing to better understand the virus, its impacts, and its history. This, in part, led me to attend seminary, where I studied Christian ethics. I wanted tools to see HIV not only as a twentieth-century event but as a longer moment. Informing my education was liberation theology, a belief system rooted in the idea that God is always with the oppressed, and that the material and contextual matter.

As a white, cis, HIV-negative gay guy from Canada living in the United States, working at the intersection of culture, AIDS, and activism for the last fifteen years, I began thinking more about the virus as its own thing, considering the global moves HIV has made through space and time. It's this I want to bring to our dispatches, specifically the when, where, and ideas of how HIV went from a localized virus to a worldwide pandemic, and what questions thinking about the long moment of AIDS bring up in thinking about how to respond and map the ongoing epidemic.

THE WHEN: The oldest HIV-positive sample we currently know of comes from a sample of blood plasma from a Bantu man who lived in Leopoldville in 1959. When this sample was sequenced by scientists in 1998, they discovered HIV had been circulating longer than previously thought, maybe as early as the 1930s. Ten years later, sitting on a laboratory shelf, the second-oldest HIV sample was found: a paraffin-saved biopsy of a lymph node from a woman living in 1960 who, like the man from 1959, had also been living in Leopoldville. This led to a whole new timeline.

Like you can learn the age of a tree by observing the cross-section of a trunk and counting the rings, you can learn the age of a virus by charting its mutations. After HIV has entered the body, latched onto a cell, replication of the virus begins through recombination. This is where mutation occurs, and HIV's high genetic variability becomes important. The reproduction of HIV never results in a perfect replica, so the longer the virus has been around, the more recombinations there will have been. In sequencing the 1960 sample and then comparing it with the 1959 sequenced sample, scientists were able to determine that people have been living with HIV even earlier still: since around the late 1890s—give or take a decade.

THE WHERE: To determine where HIV began, more comparing would be needed, this time looking at sequences of Simian Immunodeficiency Virus

(SIV), HIV's nearest zoological neighbor—the idea being the location where they find chimps living with a strand of SIV that most closely matches HIV will be the home of HIV or at least be a point in the right direction.

By now it is accepted that HIV is a result of spillover, a term to describe what happens when a virus spills over from what we may call an animal to what we may call a human. Through a series of studies with samples from captive chimps, a research team was able to establish that the closest SIV/HIV match came from a subspecies of chimpanzee that live only in western Central Africa—already a narrowing down of possible locations. To get more specific, researchers went into the field using noninvasive techniques to gather more samples of SIV from the chimps. What they found was, just like HIV is not evenly distributed across the world, neither is SIV. And in fact, the area where there were the highest rates of SIV was also where SIV and HIV most closely matched: the Southeast corner of Cameroon, now accepted within scientific communities as the cradle of HIV.

THE HOW: The most common theory is that the fateful spillover occurred during routine chimp hunting, a messy affair in which the blood of the prey and of the hunter comingle though struggle. At first, HIV stayed local and seemingly unnoticed within a contained community in rural Cameroon, with a replication rate most likely of 1.0—meaning one person passed it on only to one person. After the first few decades of the virus's slow circulation in Cameroon, HIV traveled south, via folks moving to urban centers such as Leopoldville, where by the end of the 1950s the virus had already been circulating long enough and at a heightened replication rate that remarkable recombinations had been made.

By then the capital city, founded less than fifty years earlier, was a thriving African metropolis amid much upheaval. In 1960 what had been the Belgian Congo achieved independence from Belgium, being renamed the Republic of Congo under the leadership of Patrice Lumumba. Within five years, Lumumba was dead, Joseph-Désiré Mobutu was in power, and Leopoldville was renamed Kinshasa, part of Mobutu's Africanization efforts. Amid the upheaval, European nationals were sent packing. But since the colonial leaders had withheld education from the natives of the country, world powers working with leaders from the Republic came in and peopled the country with doctors, teachers, and other professionals from Haiti.

Within a similar life span of HIV, Kinshasa went from a small colonial trading post to an African capital with direct links to the rest of the world, a place overcrowded, thick with political tension and too many men, and ever changing due to shifting social—and therefore sexual—norms. Within all this, HIV was being shared, causing death, and at a quickening pace moving far beyond where it came from.

AIDS in the United States: We don't know yet how HIV came to the United States. We do know that HIV was circulating in the United States as early as the late 1960s. The life and death of Robert Rayford, a Black teenager who died of AIDS-related causes in 1969 in St. Louis—confirmed in 1988 in the *Journal of American Medicine*—shows us this. This is further supported by an article published in the October 2016 issue of *Nature* that states HIV can be seen within sexual networks in New York as early as 1970.[14] And like its first few decades in Cameroon, HIV's first few years in the United States were probably marked with a relatively low reproduction rate, slowly increasing over time as it began to ingratiate itself in situations where bodily fluids are more readily shared: sexual encounters, intravenous drug use, and medical procedures.

The epidemic as we know it now was not discovered until rare illnesses started appearing in young white gay men's bodies in New York, Los Angeles, and San Francisco in the early 1980s. From here the story becomes familiar: if the majority of the men showing up to doctors' offices had been straight, it is clear there never would have been an epidemic. But instead the Ronald Reagan administration reacted with apathy and inaction, and so a plague befell the nation, stemming from a virus that had already traveled the world. In response, people living with the virus, those who loved them, and those who could not stand idly by stepped up.

When we talk about AIDS history, it often leads back to this moment in the early 1980s in the United States, and the urgencies of that time. But everything before this moment gets lost. I wonder what histories could be uncovered, what actions could be taken, and what discussions could be had if we also took a longer approach to AIDS history?

An Introduction to Church History class I took at seminary began with the question: How did a religion started as a cult of outsiders in the Middle East come to be so closely associated with dominance and white supremacy within the southern United States? In hearing the question, I wondered a similar thing: How has a virus that began in a southeast corner of Cameroon possibly as early as the late nineteenth century come to be so closely associated with white gay men living on the coasts of the United States in the late twentieth century?

Walking away from that class with my own experiences in mind, my first answer to both seems similar, clear, and possibly worthy of further discussion at our table: war, colonialism, and, yes, globalization, along with all the white supremacy, homophobia, and patriarchy that comes with all three.

Prompt 2

Shahani: Taken collectively, your responses foreground the different spatial and temporal forms that AIDS globalization has taken in the past, and how newer manifestations of these forms continue to fatally inform our present and future. These "thick histories" (Stanley) of global AIDS, as your responses have pointed out, operate through the local and global pathologization of Black bodies, through the genocidal nexus of bio- and necropolitics, via the state regulation of dissent, through the recycling of colonial violence, through the multinational pharmaceutical corporations' mediation of drug access and the championing of market logics, and through the control of bodies via their enforced movement and/or the policing of social and national boundaries. Furthermore, despite the "end of the nation" narratives that often accompany globalization's seeming challenge to discrete state sovereignty, your responses usefully highlight the renewed and specific roles that nation-states have played in refusing health care and accountability to people living with HIV and AIDS (the former Soviet Union, China, the United States); they also foreground how the Africanization of AIDS or the use of nations in the Global South as sites for clinical trials recentralize the nation-state even amid globalization's supposed abrading of national paradigms.

If, as your responses have emphatically suggested, global capitalism cannot "get AIDS out of our lives" (Schulman), what modes of political, aesthetic, cultural, or activist resistance can we locate to challenge the insistence that global capitalism is the cure? What are the constraints that inform these challenges? Your responses can draw on the past or elaborate on more contemporary modes of resistance to global AIDS.

Schulman: Ian Bradley-Perrin analyzed a year of HIV coverage in the *New York Times* and noted that the vast majority of the articles were about PrEP. Now, as a wizened observer of the media machine, I know that every article that appears in the *Times* has a vast apparatus of lobbying behind it, and that this slanted focus reveals the hard work of Gilead—a company whose name evokes a long history of promised Protestant utopias. The irony here, of course, is that the massive and endless market for PrEP is a consequence of the commodification of health care in the United States. And as the Trump regime deprives even more of us of our already inadequate coverage, I predict a rise in profits for PrEP. And this model of profitability is the global example, since much international care and prevention is funded by, and therefore controlled by, Western pharmaceuticals and governments.

While I support people using PrEP, its profitability is based on fear of HIV infection. Pre-Trump, with 20 million people added to the realm of vague health insurance under the highly dysfunctional, expensive, but existent Obamacare, we approximated that only one-third of HIV-positive Americans were receiving the standard of care. This leaves approximately two-thirds of HIV-positive Americans in some realm of infectiousness. Since global trends in HIV criminalization reflect and promote an international transformation in ideology of HIV negatives from "people responsible to keep themselves negative" to "people who are potentially criminally wronged," feeding the never-ending stigma around HIV is at an all-time high. Of course, if all citizens of planet Earth had adequate health care, and were all at the current standard of existing care, very few would actually be infectious. If the overwhelming majority of HIV-positive people were allowed to access existing treatments, suppressed viral load would be the norm. In this way, not only would fewer new infections take place but the psychological demand for PrEP would cease. In this way, the enormous market for PrEP is dependent on the general perception that people with HIV are overwhelmingly infectious. And this perception is dependent on HIV-positive people not getting existing medications so that this perception persists.

When Jim Hubbard and I went literally around the world with our film *United in Anger: A History of ACT UP*, the absolutely worst conditions that we encountered were in Russia. We arrived just a few weeks after the inauguration of the new antigay laws, and the arrests of Pussy Riot, signifying a coalition between Russian state and Russian church to degrade women and homosexuals. In Russia we found separate organizations for gay people with HIV and for straight people with HIV, since most infected people there are former or current needle users. The distribution of medications was in disarray because all medicines in Russia are ordered by a government office, and this office was not up to date on HIV medication. So while my friends in New York were taking Quad, a compound, we met people in Russia taking seven to fifteen pills per day. Women with HIV were desperate to get Truvada, so that they could prevent transmission prenatally to their children, but their government wasn't ordering it. A subsequent visit to Taiwan revealed similarly uninformed government ministers making bad policy, where uneducated health authorities essentially outlawed poz-on-poz sex, forcing infected people to avoid the state-run health system altogether in order to avoid detection and surveillance.

Juxtaposing the US example and the Russian example and the Taiwanese example, we see that greed and ignorance serve as doppelgangers in the hands of authorities: be they corporate or governmental, using people with HIV and keeping them untreated and infectious as means to their own power.

Lo: In the Chinese context, early representations of AIDS (in the 1980s) framed the epidemic as a "capitalist disease." Locals played around with the Chinese name of AIDS (愛滋病, *aizibing*), changing the middle character to become (愛資病, *aizibing*), for the two middle Chinese characters are homophones. The latter name literally meant "love capitalism disease," implying that HIV/AIDS was the consequence of favoring Western liberalism and capitalism over socialism. In other words, resisting capitalist influence for a socialist country was believed to be the way to stop HIV/AIDS entering and spreading in the country. After the HIV/AIDS outbreak among injection drug users in Yunnan province in 1989, Chinese authorities responded by criminalizing drug use and drug trafficking, and prohibited positive individuals from entering the country. Furthermore, the 1989 "Law of Infectious Diseases Prevention and Control" required HIV/AIDS-infected individuals to be quarantined, with their names and addresses reported to the government.

Despite the prevailing advocacy of HIV/AIDS interventions in an integrative manner in the international community and national governments, there has been a consistent push to maintain the exceptional status of HIV/AIDS as a unique health challenge in China. A program manager of a HIV/AIDS-related NGO in Beijing commented, "NGOs believe that a stand-alone approach is more suitable for HIV/AIDS responses owing to severe stigma problems in China. Infected individuals cannot receive treatment in normal health care settings due to their positive status." Similarly, a CDC official in Zhejiang province stated in 2017, "I believe a stand-alone program is more suitable for HIV/AIDS interventions in China. An integrated approach is more suitable in countries or societies with less HIV/AIDS stigma. HIV-positive individuals in China go to specialized hospitals for treatments; doctors working in these hospitals have trained to treat HIV/AIDS patients." That HIV/AIDS stigma and discrimination can lead to human rights violations has been highlighted in the 1998 *International Guidelines for HIV/AIDS and Human Rights*, advocating for positive and rights-based responses to HIV/AIDS. However, in an authoritarian state where individuals cannot ask for treatments on the basis of personal and human rights, AIDS exceptionalism has become a means to mitigate stigma and discrimination attached to HIV/AIDS without directly addressing or improving human rights situations in China.

Numerous HIV/AIDS activists have been suppressed through imprisonment, house arrest, or assault in the past years. Dr. Wan Yanhai and Dr. Gao Yaojie were two prominent Chinese HIV/AIDS activists who fled to the United States in 2009 and 2010, respectively, due to pressure and harassment by the Chinese authorities. A graduate of Shanghai Medical University in 1998, Wan was the former health education officer in the Ministry of Health. Despite working in the state apparatus, he was dedicated to advocating for the rights of homosexuals and sex workers to receive HIV/AIDS-related treatments. He was arrested and interrogated for leaking state secrets in 2002 since he exposed an internal official document related to the outbreak of the epidemic caused by private blood banks in Henan province. Following his release after widespread international condemnation of his secret detention, Wan continued to address HIV/AIDS in China through the establishment of the Beijing Aizhixing Institute on Health and Education (also called Love Knowledge Action in English) in the same year, advocating for the rights of queer populations, and providing financial and technical support for other small-scale community-based organizations working on HIV/AIDS in the country. A director of an NGO in Beijing recalled the impact of Wan's departure during an interview in 2011: "The director of Love Knowledge Action is the one who helps us write the financial report for the submission to the Global Fund. We can no longer apply for the Global Fund grants after he left China."

Another figure who made a significant impact on AIDS activism in China was Dr. Gao Yaojie, a retired Chinese gynecologist who first discovered HIV/AIDS in Henan in 1996 while treating a female patient infected with HIV/AIDS via blood transfusion in a local hospital. Since then, Gao has devoted her entire life to HIV/AIDS education and prevention work, giving free treatments to people infected with HIV/AIDS in villages of Henan before the implementation of the "Four Free One Care" policy in China in 2004. Her dedication to HIV/AIDS interventions has profoundly raised the public awareness of HIV/AIDS but at the same time exposed the provincial government-initiated plasma selling in Henan. To cover its mismanagement and malpractice, the local government bribed the infected villagers and farmers. Activists like Gao who were engaging in disclosing the official malpractices were harassed and imprisoned. Henan officials blocked reporters from the China Central Television (CCTV) and *The People's Daily* (a widely circulated Chinese newspaper) who wanted to interview Gao. Monitored by more than fifty cops, three police cars, and numerous journalists, Gao was prevented from having any engagement with the rest of the world and was blocked from leaving China to receive a human rights award in the United

States. Gao was placed under house arrest in February 2007, but her work on HIV/AIDS awareness has acquired visibility and created awareness. Based on the 10,001 letters written by infected individuals and their family members between 1996 and 2004, she published the renowned book *China Plague: 10,000 Letters* with a Hong Kong publisher in December 2009, documenting the unhygienic plasma collection/selling in the black market as well as how HIV/AIDS remained rampant in several Henan villages.

Stanley: It seems we have an avalanche of data and evidence that the state (in its various iterations) is well equipped to deliver death, even under a regime, as Foucault might have it, most concerned with the management of life. To this end, the continued reliance on the state as that which will end, or at least diminish, the brutality of the pandemic traps us in a feedback loop while the body count climbs. Perhaps it is a simple answer, but I would say the last twenty years of HIV/AIDS "work" has primarily been focused on disenfranchising people most directly impacted from transforming the terrain of their lives. This takes many forms, including the more quotidian NGO/nonprofitization of HIV/AIDS, to the more spectacularly brutal forms of incarceration and militarization of communities, mostly of color, in the United States and globally.

I do believe that many people providing direct support are vital in the struggle against HIV/AIDS: for example, people working to create and/or expand syringe exchange programs, and people working on housing and food security. Yet here I am attempting to suggest a structural analysis that sees HIV/AIDS as contingent on racial capitalism. The question then is not if work against HIV/AIDS should include a critique of accumulation and extraction but what forms an anticapitalist HIV/AIDS activism/study might take.

To this end, there is radical work being done to think about, for example, the connection between HIV and settler colonization. One artist growing this conversation is Demian DinéYazhi, a Diné transdisciplinary artist/activist from New Mexico, who is currently living and working in Portland, Oregon. His work also helps us know that the "United States" is an imagined project, maintained through brutal force, that is, the attempted confinement and liquidation of hundreds if not thousands of native nations. One of his graphic works is "POZ since 1492," which, through a reassemblage of visual temporality, reads conquest through and beyond the virus.

Along with artistic production like DinéYazhi's, I am also deeply inspired by localized and often unfunded movements that are working against HIV criminalization in Canada and the United States. This is another space where prison abolition, disability justice, and HIV/AIDS activism are cross-pollinating our movements, making them sharper and hopefully more forceful.

This is perhaps a long way of saying that I think supporting direct action and mutual aid, centered on those most affected, is the best, and perhaps only, way of confronting the ravages of racial global capitalism, of which the pharmaceutical industry is a major player. Yet what I don't think we need is a nostalgic "return" to ACT UP that produces HIV/AIDS only in the past tense. To place AIDS as a relic of history, something to be known only through backward glances, is a deadly erasure of both our current moment and the future of HIV/AIDS.

I think history's power is transformative when written through our current moment in an attempt to imagine more radical and liberatory futures. While much of what ACT UP did was central to many of our political educations (myself included), direct action must be a methodology and not simply a series of events. This "direct action as methodology," I think, creates cultures of resistance as an ongoing practice and the precondition of social life for those held against the wall of normative power.

To be clear, I do believe we need continued and expanded confrontational street-based direct actions that disrupt, to the point of collapse, the smooth space of everyday destruction. I also think we need to imagine what working with those in the hard sciences who have the skills to reverse engineer necessary medications as well as conduct research might look like. Perhaps this is a dreaming project, but I think we must still demand, which is to say build, an anticapitalist science and pharmaceutical underground that understands collective freedom and not individual profit as that which guides it.

Kerr: In order to respond to the prompt, I need to give some context, some background on how I see the history of the AIDS response, and then what I see emerging as what we may call resistance.

A few years ago everything was coming up doula. The Radical Doula blog was growing in popularity; people I knew were starting to work more as abortion and death doulas, and colleges were starting gender doula programs to support students through the process of asserting their gender in school. Amid all this I started to wonder: Is there a role for doulas within the ongoing response to HIV?

Around this time, I had the chance to create a one-day think tank about contemporary HIV issues. I took the opportunity to program a roundtable titled "What Would an HIV Doula Do?" To respond I invited Lodz Joseph, a birth doula who has done AIDS work in Haiti; Michael Crumpler, a friend from seminary who was in his final stages of becoming a chaplain; along with other peers I admired from the world of art, literature, activism, and health care.

Lodz, along with practicing end-of-life doula iele paloumpis, explained to the group what a doula did. While the idea of a doula goes back to ancient Greece and relates to the work of a handmaiden centuries later, foundational to doula work, explained Lodz, is holding space. This can mean anything from having ice chips ready for a dry mouth, to knowing when to call a doctor, to supporting someone as they advocate for themselves in the hospital. For Lodz, who works in Brooklyn, much of the power of a doula comes from performing the mundane. She sees how folks can get caught up in worthy complex global health work yet how often this means they miss basic and overlooked life-saving interventions that can happen within one's own community. As Lodz shared, it's not an either/or situation but an invitation to see what is hiding in plain sight.

Upon hearing Lodz share her thoughts, Michael, in a substance recovery program, living with HIV, with a busy church life, pointed out that there are parallels between doula work and the labor of an AA sponsor, a chaplain, and a trusted friend: all are people in your life who can remind you of who you are in the aftermath of trauma, helping you connect to the innate knowledge you possess as you transition toward possible sobriety, a higher power, or living with HIV. While he and others in the think tank have experience with case workers, buddy systems, and mentors, he saw the possible role of an HIV doula as different from these preexisting supports. Others, like myself, agreed.

Helping us think through the differences, Tamara Oyola-Santiago, having worked in needle exchange, student health, and with various AIDS service organizations in Puerto Rico and the United States, invited us to keep the individual in mind while also considering what an HIV doula would do on a systemic level. As she pointed out, it isn't just people who transition in the face of HIV; so too do institutions. For example, many AIDS Service Organizations (ASOs) started off as small groups of people brought together to address the suffering and death of their friends, with many now large multinational service providers, administrators between "clients" and the state. At the root of Tamara's point was, How do we *doula the system* to create the institutions we need and want? I found this line of questioning helpful because it aided me in seeing how the doula work fit into my thinking around the shifts within the HIV response.

The earliest reactions to the epidemic were from those dying and their intimates. It was friends, lovers, and strangers within the struggle, aiding people as they died, holding space for the living, and demanding action from an apathetic public and murderously silent governments. As the 1980s bled into the 1990s, rates of HIV and death increased, and bonds of response replicated and reformed, creating communities upon communities built on mutuality and care. An awareness emerged: the virus is shared within community, no one gets HIV alone, and so the response should be rooted in relationships.

Eventually, though, with the release of protease inhibitors in the late 1990s, things changed. Management of the crisis became more medicalized, thus professionalized. AIDS went from public to private amid the globalized epidemic. Systems of pharmaceutical distribution were introduced and scaled up around the world, administered in no small part—as Tamara was saying—by ASOs. This, of course, saved and improved millions of lives, and should never be downplayed or taken for granted—and is a task still being worked out as around 40 percent of the global population living with HIV still doesn't have access to medication.

At the same time highly active antiretroviral therapy (HAART) was being prescribed around the world, small-scale community responses in North America (and I am sure elsewhere) quickly became hard to find, having disbanded in localized triumph, dwindled due to loss of funding and attendance, or disappeared altogether. In everyday life for people living with HIV in the United States, bonds that had formed out of a shared relationship to death thinned in the face of divergent realities around survival.

For people with insurance, stable housing, and individualized support, HIV can be a manageable chronic illness, a situation between patient and doctor. For people who have been minoritized and are without economic stability, HIV exacerbates preexisting crises, which often are dealt with less by friends and lovers and more by social workers, and increasingly by the criminal justice system. In these experiences, there is no privacy in living with HIV, but the process of dealing with HIV has largely been privatized. Large multinational foundations such as those started by the Bills (Clinton and Gates) compete with nation-states to auction off the work of HIV to for-profit and nonprofit agencies. Due to the enormity of the ongoing crisis, the intimate ways of dealing with HIV are gone. But what is the impact of how they have been replaced? For some people living in the United States, long term with HIV, meeting up with friends at weekly activist meetings is a memory now replaced with sitting in alienating waiting rooms, living in state-subsidized housing in gentrified neighborhoods feeling like a pariah. For those who seroconverted after the release of HAART, the shifted HIV landscape is keenly felt. A cultural history informs them that for some, a diagnosis once came with a rallying community. With AIDS in the twenty-first century, this is not the norm. The promise of medication with a positive test result comes instead with ever-present stigma, renewed public ignorance, a sense of isolation, and increased surveillance. Amid this shift, the thick trust that once ensured that the HIV response was being done in the best interest of those living with the virus has been upended. The response is now more beholden to nefarious tenants of public health, notably, the containment and monitoring of people living with communicable diseases for the peace of mind of the worried well. Gone are the days where a person's T-cells were measured to keep track of a person's health; now viral load is monitored to track pill adherence and transmission rates.

And this is where my response to the second prompt comes in: amid the privatizing shifts within the AIDS response has also been a long legacy of community organizations that have remained connected to the grassroots in their work, for example groups like AIDS Action Now in Toronto, and VOCAL NYC and Visual AIDS in New York. Joining these groups, and inspired by them, is our What Would an HIV Doula Do? collective.

Progressing from a one-time round-table conversation to a collective that now holds open monthly meetings, hosts events, and partners on programming with other organizations, our work is an intervention into the globalized and privatized climate of AIDS. We are building—with others—a critical mass of community into the AIDS response. We are building thick bonds to replace those that have been thinned. We see ourselves as creating new opportunities and supporting preexisting ones for people living with HIV and those deeply impacted to be in community together around the virus, along with those who are new to the conversation. Through writing, direct action, conversation, art making, and other strategies, we are dragging forward lost conversations and actions around HIV/AIDS, creating spaces for people to share private thoughts and experiences around the virus, and helping people to be less afraid and more proactive. This is what we mean by holding space.

Crucial to our work is questioning how testing is done, abolishing HIV criminalization, pushing back against the whitewashing historicization of the crisis, and responding to whatever comes up within the collective. In this work, we consider how medical, professionalized, and global responses are to be included, working toward having those forces respond to the needs, wants, and demands of HIV-centric communities rather than the other way around. This is what we mean by doula-ing the system, and an answer to what does resistance in the face of a globalized AIDS response look like.

Bradley-Perrin: Many of the responses above point toward the intersection of nation and epidemic. The politics of AIDS for much of the first two centuries was played out politically in these arenas. Schulman's early account of AIDS in the Soviet Union resonates with an ongoing silence in former Soviet states and particularly Russia on the expansion of the epidemic into the present day, and Lo's analysis of AIDS in the current Chinese state. And both Stanley and Kerr have written about the social impacts of racial constructions at the national and international level through history. While historically useful in understanding early political responses, national AIDS politics has always played out on an international stage as a social, economic, and political crisis. These dispatches from our brilliant respondents point toward the history of AIDS as a global political phenomenon. While deeply embedded in national policy, AIDS, from its epidemiological trajectory to its economic network to its political responses, has been for four decades and beyond a fundamental part of international politics, global governance, and transnational resistance. I want to think about two classic texts, one historical and one theoretical: Warren Montag's "Necro-Economics: Adam Smith and Death in the Life of the Universal" and Timothy Haskell's "Capitalism and the Origins of the Humanitarian Sensibility." The first historicizes new economic and cognitive patterns and the second questions the countervailing forces that operate against that new cognition from within that new system.

Montag reads Adam Smith's *The Wealth of Nations* through a biopolitical lens and demonstrates Smith's market system operating on the premise of government-sanctioned death. He states, "The subsistence of a population may, and does in specific circumstances, require the death of a significant number of individuals: to be precise it requires that they be allowed to die so that others may live."[15] Different from the execution, this is a death through forced exposure. The government, in Smith's model, must only intervene to prevent the masses from overtaking the food stores in a famine, in order to allow the market to correct its natural dearth. This return to equilibrium is only achieved through the sacrifice of elements of the population in the name of order: "It is here that the sovereign power must intervene, not necessarily to kill those who refuse to die, but to ensure, through the use of force, that they will be exposed to death and compelled to accept the rationing of life by the market." Montag thus describes alongside the *homo sacre*, who can be killed with impunity, the *necro-economic man*: "he who with impunity may be allowed to die, slowly or quickly, in the name of the rationality and equilibrium of the market."[16]

Timothy Haskell's "Capitalism and the Origins of the Humanitarian Sensibility" historicizes the co-ascendance of the new market form and new cognitive style of humanism that produced an abolitionist movement in Britain at the same time as large-scale, capitalist economies arose. Haskell suggests four preconditions in which problematic social issues move into the realm of moral imperatives: the expansion of the conventional boundaries of moral responsibility, an implication in the evil, a method to stop it, and technologies of action of sufficient ordinariness that a failure to use them would represent the suspension of routine. Haskell writes,

> What, then, did capitalism contribute to the freeing of the slaves? Only a precondition, albeit a vital one: a proliferation of recipe knowledge and consequent expansion of the conventional limits of causal perception and moral responsibility that compelled some exceptionally scrupulous individuals to attack slavery and prepared others to listen and comprehend. The precondition could have been satisfied by other means, yet during the period in question no other force pressed outward on the limits of moral responsibility with the strength of the market.[17]

Pharmaceutical development, manufacturing, and distribution is one crucial vein of this global history, put in particular relief in most of the last two decades. Looking at these two works together in the context of the globalized marketplace of AIDS and its therapeutic response, one that appears to require the death of some for the life of others, the infection of some for the legitimization of preventative medications for others, Haskell's differentiation between the humanitarian impulse and capitalism is prescient. Pharmaceutical grants to AIDS Service Organizations and the randomized control and clinical trials of pharmaceutical production itself demonstrate how capitalism and humanitarianism advance in tandem and serve one another's purposes. Unlike the period of moral expansion that abolitionism represented, one that saw civil society respond to this expansion in a synchronized though noncausal relationship with capitalism, "corporate responsibility" now represents the folding in of humanitarianism with capitalism. It is nothing new to recognize the immense adaptability of the market system and to recognize the adeptness of the market (and the actors that sustain it) at the valuation of all of human action. While Haskell describes a moment when the cognitive behaviors necessitated by the market system produced a counterintuitive drive against slavery in those who adopted those behaviors, capitalism has evolved to integrate the humanitarian impulse into its calculations for market production, embedded in its very development. The necro-economic reality of the market remains, but large-scale resistance to these inevitabilities has been neutralized by bureaucratization of humanitarianism and disciplined through a rigorous field of ethics developments.

The expansion of AIDS Service Organizations, operating on budgets composed of corporate grants and government grants, both of which bring a chilling effect to any political impulses, was first noted by Cindy Patton in *Inventing AIDS*. Susan J. Shaw has since demonstrated in *Governing How We Care* how community health organizations act as neoliberal governance structures of marginalized communities, and we can see how this is only the latest adaptation of the market to humanitarian impulses in more than three centuries of refinement. Resistance hinges on once again expanding the moral boundaries within which we must act but cannot rest itself on the assumptions of the system it seeks to disrupt. As Haskell described, a new way of thinking about the value of others arises from a recalibration of economic behavior: capitalism and the necro-economic, alongside humanitarianism and biopolitics. While Foucault's first description of governmentality described a national phenomenon, it came on the eve of the global AIDS crisis, whose political, economic, scientific, technological, and cultural consequences embodied a new global age of governance when Arjun Appadurai's notion of "the social life of things" took on new networked forms characterized by disjunctures and flows of technology, ideas, media, finance, and ethnography. The types of citizenship claims made at a national level must be understood genealogically as co-occurring with global or universal claims to human rights, and this coexistence has characterized activist responses to AIDS throughout its history.

As historians, scholars, and observers of a global crisis, we must be attuned to this dual political response and the slippage between national and global claims in two key ways: First, we need to examine the way the global governance of health through public health organizations like the World Health Organization, the Global Fund, the International Monetary Fund, and the World Bank have evolved in tandem with national bodies and their national (and exclusive) goals vis-à-vis health of national or global citizens. Here we need to ask how nationalist assumptions and intranational hierarchies are inscribed in global responses to the HIV/AIDS epidemic—attention must be paid to the failure of certain states to respond historically and the role played by the global community in approving or censuring these failures—from the United States, to Russia, to China. Second, we need to use historical thinking to situate the present in the longer tradition of national citizenship–based claims, and global or universal claims to rights. If Haskell is right that concern with the faraway other arises with capitalism, then the national and the global citizen have a long history together. How have the limits of each of these claims shaped the AIDS epidemic? When they arose together, capitalism and humanitarianism were revolutionary. Haskell reminds us that we shouldn't forget that the capitalism itself was the most expansive and enduring revolution of the last thousand years and it was operationalized in the midst of feudalism. So how did this sensibility evolve and develop under the AIDS crisis? These are crucial questions to understand where we as activist-scholars go next.

Notes

1 Stanley, "Blood Lines."
2 Robinson, *Black Marxism*, 2.
3 Gilmore, "Race and Globalization," 261, emphasis added.
4 Melamed, "Racial Capitalism," 78.
5 Melamed, "Racial Capitalism," 79.
6 Melamed, "Racial Capitalism," 79.
7 Cazdyn, *Already Dead*, 117.
8 Gao Qiang, "Speech."
9 Personal communication, 2011. Owing to the sensitivity of HIV/AIDS issues, interviewees in China declined to be named. Unless otherwise noted, the remaining quotations in my comments are from interviews conducted in 2016. My research was supported by Hong Kong University Research Council General Research Fund grant #144913.
10 AIDS Healthcare Foundation, "AHF Files FDA Complaint."
11 Curry, "AHF's Michael Weinstein."
12 Peterson, "Securitizing AIDS." This was brought to my attention by Alexander McClelland and I relied heavily on his notes and analysis of the panel in my description here.
13 Schulman, *Stagestruck*, 143.
14 See Garry et al., "Documentation of an AIDS Virus Infection"; Worobey et al. "'Patient 0.'"
15 Montag, "Necro-Economics," 14.
16 Montag, "Necro-Economics," 17.
17 Haskell, "Origins of the Humanitarian Sensibility," 563.

Bibliography

AIDS Healthcare Foundation. "AHF Files FDA Complaint against Gilead for Truvada PrEP Ads Promoting Off-Label Use." January 19, 2016. https://www .aidshealth.org/2016/01/ahf-files-fda-complaint-gilead-truvada-prep-ads -promoting-off-label-use/.

Appadurai, Arjun. *The Social Life of Things: Commodities in Cultural Perspective.* New York: Cambridge University Press, 1989.

Cazdyn, Eric. *The Already Dead: The New Time of Politics, Culture, and Illness.* Durham, NC: Duke University Press, 2012.

Curry, Tyler. "AHF's Michael Weinstein Gets It Wrong (Again)." *The Advocate,* January 21, 2016. http://www.advocate.com/commentary/2016/1/21/ahfs -michael-weinstein-gets-it-wrong-again.

Dumit, Joseph. *Drugs for Life: How Pharmaceutical Companies Define Our Health.* Durham, NC: Duke University Press, 2012.

Gao, Qiang. "Speech by Executive Vice Minister of Health, Mr. Gao Qiang, at the HIV/AIDS High-Level Meeting of the UN General Assembly." September 22, 2003. http://www.china-un.org/eng/lhghyywj/ldhy/previousga/58/t28511 .htm.

Gao, Yaojie. *China's AIDS Plague: 10,000 Letters.* Hong Kong: Kai Fang Press, 2009.

Garry, R. F., et al. "Documentation of an AIDS Virus Infection in the United States in 1968." *JAMA* 260, no. 14 (1988): 2085–87.

Gilmore, Ruth Wilson. "Race and Globalization." In *Geographies of Global Change: Remapping the World,* edited by R. J. Johnston, Peter J. Taylor, and Michael J. Watts, 261–74. 2nd ed. Malden, MA: Blackwell, 2002.

Haskell, Thomas L. "Capitalism and the Origins of the Humanitarian Sensibility, Part 2." *American Historical Review* 90, no. 3 (1985): 547–66.

Joint United Nations Programme on HIV/AIDS (UNAIDS). *International Guidelines for HIV/AIDS and Human Rights.* 2006. https://www.ohchr.org/Documents /Publications/HIVAIDSGuidelinesen.pdf.

Melamed, Jodi. "Racial Capitalism." *Critical Ethnic Studies* 1, no. 1 (2015): 76–85.

Montag, Warren. "Necro-Economics: Adam Smith and Death in the Life of the Universal." *Radical Philosophy,* no. 134 (2005): 7–17.

Murphy, Tim. "Sex without Fear." *New York Magazine,* July 13, 2014. http://nymag .com/news/features/truvada-hiv-2014–7/.

National Center for AIDS/STD Control and Prevention, Chinese Center for Disease Control and Prevention. "State Council Notice on Strengthening HIV/AIDS Prevention and Control." 2004. http://ncaids.chinacdc.cn/english/Resources /200708/t20070829_1032205.htm.

Patton, Cindy. *Inventing AIDS.* New York: Routledge, 1990.

Peterson, Kristin. "Securitizing AIDS: Migratory Sex Work, Clinical Research, and the US War on Terror in Africa." Paper presented at the Second International Conference for the Social Sciences and Humanities in HIV, Paris, France, 2013.

Robinson, Cedric J. *Black Marxism: The Making of the Black Radical Tradition.* Chapel Hill: University of North Carolina Press, 2000.

Schulman, Sarah. *Stagestruck: Theater, AIDS, and the Marketing of Gay America.* Durham, NC: Duke University Press, 1998.

Shaw, Susan J. *Governing How We Care: Contesting Community and Defining Difference in U.S. Public Health Programs.* Philadelphia: Temple University Press, 2012.

Smith, Adam. *The Wealth of Nations.* Introduction by Robert Reich. New York: Modern Library, 2000.

Stanley, Eric A. "Blood Lines: AIDS, Affective Accumulation, and Viral Labor." Paper presented at the Gender Studies Symposium, Lewis and Clark College, Portland, OR, March 13, 2015.

Worobey, M., et al. "1970s and 'Patient o' HIV-1 Genomes Illuminate Early HIV/AIDS History in North America." *Nature* 539 (2016): 98–101.

TWO THE COSTS OF LIVING: REFLECTIONS ON GLOBAL HEALTH CRISES

Bishnupriya Ghosh

"Goodbye, Mother," writes Clara Maass in a poignant letter penned at the Las Animas Hospital in Havana, Cuba, in August 1901. "I will send you nearly all I earn, so be good to yourself and the two little ones. You know I am the man of the family, but do pray for me."[1] A few days later, Maass, an American contract nurse, would succumb to a virulent strain of yellow fever that she contracted after volunteering as a human subject for an experimental vaccination. She was one of many volunteers for the Walter Reed Yellow Fever Commission's pursuit of the *flavivirus* that wreaked havoc on human hosts in the Cuban archipelago and the American South (figure 2.1). Finding a panacea against this viral infection is something of a scientific landmark in historical annals.[2] The life-saving vaccination was significant not only because it was an obvious public good but also because it allowed the American army to complete the construction of the Panama Canal (1904–14).[3] It assured American control of trade between the Americas. Thus, the commission's human experiments were regarded as righteous sacrifice; special mention is always made of Jesse Lazear, a young scientist whose self-experimentation proved fatal. But less is known about the deaths of contract nurses, rank and file army personnel, and local Cuban volunteers.

I begin here, in another time and another place, in order to reflect on the distributive logic inherent in articulations of health security regimes as a modern form of power over biological existence. While much has been said about biopower and its calculative rationality, in this chapter my focus is on how *crisis* as the governing epistemology of health emergencies habitually reinforces that rationality. Etymologically, the "crisis" hails from the Greek

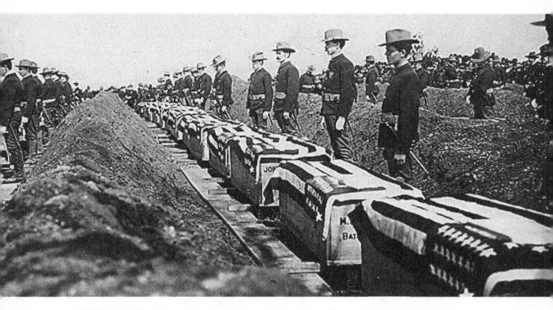

FIGURE 2.1. Military burial during the Spanish-American War, in which 2,500 American soldiers died of yellow fever. Source: Philip S. Hench/Walter Reed Collection, University of Virginia.

krinô, meaning to decide or to judge, and soon the term came to mean a turning point that called for definitive action. In its migration into the Hippocratic school and therein into medical parlance, "crisis" came to mean the turning point in a disease—a critical phase with high stakes. This chapter focuses on the "epidemic" as such a critical phase: an event that opens new pathways into the past (what went wrong?) and the future (what action is the best way forward?). The continuing "long-wave" HIV/AIDS epidemics— events with waves of spread and waves of impact that take a long time to slow down and that have long-term impacts—are my primary loci.[4] But I start with an emerging infectious disease outbreak at the start of the twentieth century to underscore recursive logics salient to HIV/AIDS epidemics, then (in the period known as "early AIDS") and now (in the post-1995 antiretroviral therapy period).

I also question the production of a unitary human subject as the antagonist to microbial hordes in a seemingly eternal species war. I do this not to undermine nonhuman agencies but to interrogate the universalizing abstraction galvanized during health crises: "the human" on whose behalf there must be needful experiments, daring innovation, and even self-sacrifice. My point is not to undermine such efforts, and certainly not where deadly pathogens are concerned. Rather, it is to interrogate how the "public good" as a horizon of action relies on a distributive logic of security, one that divides and separates an abstract public who will reap benefits in the future from disposable congeries who will court death for those benefits to materialize: like the contract nurse who had to man up to feed a large family of German immigrants to the United States, like the recent immigrants to Cuba whom the Spanish Embassy sent as volunteers to Reed's camp, and like the ordinary privates in the US Army barracks who were inducted into heroic sacrifice.[5]

Scholars who celebrate the commission's chutzpah point out that it generated the first consent forms for such experiments. Volunteers received $100 in "American gold" for their participation, and an additional $100 was available for those who developed yellow fever. Those critical of the commission's medical ethics argue that the forms did not indicate the risk of death in adequate terms. Whichever side one chooses, the health emergency features the first materialization of the unequivocally modern power to "make live" and "let die" populational aggregates as legal-medical protocol.[6] As Reed agonized over his young colleague's death, the calculative rationality of health security found new expression as a matter of rights: by allowing volunteers to sign onto the medical experiment, the law legitimated their right to gamble on their lives for economic gain. This legalization of risk framed as individual choice held two costs of the experiment in tension: the first, the incalculable personal loss (physical, emotional, social) in which the health crisis was a protracted experiential condition; and the second, a probabilistically assessed loss (political and economic) in which the health crisis was suspended as aberration, contained in the time and space of the camp. As a state of exception, the camp ensured that the latter (well-calculated) cost would hold the former (experiential) one at bay. The most dangerous part of the experiment (the first phase in 1900) was conducted at an army camp outside the United States, a space over which the US military had sovereign jurisdiction. During the course of the century, we would see many such "camps" materialize around health crises. The US government's willed negligence of the HIV/AIDS epidemic during the Ronald Reagan years, for one, which turned vibrant neighborhoods into deathly ghettos, has been amply chronicled.[7] At global scale, the cost-benefit calculus has played out in the struggle over access to low-cost antiretroviral generics; further, there is excellent scholarship on how the global distribution of resources allocates "surplus life" to some, while others die in clinical trials.[8] Meanwhile, the huge documentation of mourning and melancholia in AIDS media has sharpened the need to change the terms on which we narrate the histories of health crises.[9]

Such histories inspire this chapter on the continuing impact of chilling calculations that appear during health crises every so often so as to organize common futures. The recurrence indicates those calculations are the abiding scaffolds for modern power over life. Recent scholarship on health security has drawn on Michel Foucault's writings (and especially on his lectures in *Security, Territory, Population*, delivered between 1977 and 1978) to make the case. There, Foucault analyzes what the earliest state-run inoculation campaigns reveal about modern governance: a different mode of power operating on vital circulations (blood, plasma, hormones, microbes, toxins, proteins, or lipids) whose maintenance remains unassailably necessary for the generation of goods and people.[10] Foucault distinguished this kind of power from sovereign juridical power that punishes or kills, and disciplinary power that surveys, observes, and corrects. The power to "secure" life *calculates* and *intervenes* in the vital circulations of human life; its locus is not *this* subject of law or *that* docile body but biological existence.

What is important here is Foucault's emphasis on calculation as the basis of sorting, dividing, and segregating populations. A calculative rationality mobilizes the modern technologies of measurement and assessment: consider the calculations necessary to test positive and to remain undetectable; consider the percentile goals for epidemic amelioration in national and global strategic public health plans; consider the fact that the threat of diseases to the gross national product (GNP) is one of the main motors of state intervention into epidemics. The economic modality of this health calculus and its manifold political articulations qualify the liberal fiction of the "public good." Health is not a universal human right but an economically adjudicated enfranchisement at both national and global scales. Hence states and global institutions back big pharma and insurance companies in their parsing and valuation of life in terms of risk aggregates; and state and interstate legal systems continue to protect their interests. In this regard, modern advances in self-testing, prophylaxis, and treatments are also *qualified* achievements whose benefits do not accrue to all. The uneven burdens of clinical labors are but a stark reminder of this enduring economic calculus that girds the valuation of life.[11]

Valuation is well concealed in a liberal fiction of the public good that is invoked everywhere where there is a massive state and international response to emerging infectious diseases. We have been witnessing many such responses, from SARS to Ebola to Zika. The resurgence of deadly pathogens like Marburg, Ebola, and HIV in the 1980s proved to be the tip of the iceberg. Emerging infectious disease emergencies are particularly significant because they intensify and accelerate security regimes. Following Foucault, Stefan Elbe notes in *Virus Alert* (2009) that in these circumstances three distinct modes of power *all* come into play. National security imperatives protect soldiers, civilian populations, and sovereign territories. But since such diseases speedily lay to waste individual lives and livelihoods, human security apparatuses further discipline behaviors, habits, and lifestyles. Working alongside these two security regimes, health security regulates vital circulations, statistically quantifying populations into risk groups according to their vital states and promoting pharmacological intervention. These three security regimes constitute biosecurity interventions that calculate internal borders within populations, separating one social aggregate (high-risk cases such as the elderly) from another (low-risk groups, often prized for reproductive futures). Strong conjugations of the three enforce a rigorous biopolitics of "making live" and "letting die."[12] Where the HIV/AIDS epidemics are concerned, we are now in the fourth decade of fighting these thanatopolitics: a deluge of documentaries and biographies, oral history projects and commemorative exhibits, activist histories and public arts record how we survived the late twentieth-century plague of thirty-four million dead and counting. What better time is there to reflect on landmarks and turning points, periods and eras? In this regard, this volume is most timely in exploring a core concept for historical narration: crisis as an epistemological category that prompts a diagnosis of the past and a blueprint for the future.

In returning to such epistemological matters, one must first question the "global AIDS crisis" as a singular phenomenon as well as the emergent periodization that separates "early AIDs" as the high crisis years (when new incidences were unabated) from the post-1995 years (when the pharmacological solution changed the course of the epidemic). *Of course* the antiretroviral therapies produced a major shift in the conception of this health crisis. To the great relief of my generation, which had lost so many, in the Global North the tide turned from acute to chronic states of infection. Once a collectively lived experience, HIV infection is now a medicalized condition lived in the privacy of the doctor's office. But, as so many scholars have noted, this is hardly the case in the "Global South"—with the caveat that south is not a cartographic projection but an amoeboid geography that includes high-crisis pockets in industrialized contexts.[13] There, in those pockets, the logic of security unmasks its calculative rationality, its distributive logic sometimes in plain sight and sometimes in muted, benign forms.

Such pockets suggest there cannot be a global history of AIDS but a global archaeology attentive to discontinuous space-times of HIV/AIDS epidemics—in the plural. One way to approach such heterogeneous space-times is to interrogate hegemonic disease geographies organized around nation-states. Such geographies are inevitable mainly because sovereign nation-states are *the* global conduits for materializing antiretroviral therapy (ART) rollouts, public health infrastructures, and viral load testing and monitoring procedures; nation-states further govern general health parameters such as nutrition, drinking water, and sanitation. Hence, global institutions such as the World Health Organization (WHO) or the Joint United Nations Programme on HIV/AIDS (UNAIDS) routinely measure the successful epidemic interventions along national indices. And yet, what such assessments obscure are crisis situations, often locally or regionally marked, that are at odds with national ones. I characterize such situations as "high-crisis" pockets that are "discontinuous" with the scale of the national HIV/AIDS epidemic. In this chapter, I offer an illustration from India, a nation once home to the third-largest HIV-infected population but one which is currently applauded for its successful epidemic management AIDS control programs. The "case" of Manipur, a northeastern state in India that borders Myanmar, bucks the national upward swing in epidemic management, and, as we shall see, it is critically significant for what it tells us about the distributive logic of global public health.

Manipur has remained in a perpetual state of exception—under military rule within the sovereign space of the Indian nation-state—for the last sixty years. Even as the national AIDS control programs pour resources (drugs, funds, expertise) into Manipur, the Indian government's draconian emergency measures remain partly responsible for the health crisis. As the political and health emergencies feed into each other, we are confronted with a macabre articulation of the "letting die" that underlies modern health security in democracies, Western or otherwise. What, then, can conditions in this region (which is analogous to Kashmir or Palestine) tell us about the democratic fictions of public health? How do those fictions conceal an underlying logic of debility? Certainly, these extreme cases shore up the norm, but I choose a lesser-known example from the Global South as a methodological move. In part, that move constitutes a refusal to tuck away such an instance into the safe corners of area studies—as just another historical example that enriches the increasingly heterogeneous archives of global AIDS. My intent is to track the governing logic of modern health security from North America to South Asia to West Africa, and therein to provincialize every epidemic situation. Put differently, if one followed a classic colonial account, Manipur is simply a "backward" instance of the crisis in which progressive agendas have not as yet achieved their full potential. In such an account, the Global South is still caught in the waiting rooms of history. Instead, if we think of extreme instances as sudden recursions of a continuous modern global rationality—as evident in early twentieth-century Cuba as it is in late twentieth-century Manipur and early twenty-first-century West Africa—then the task at hand is to write nonlinear discontinuous histories of HIV/AIDS epidemics attuned to global viral emergences.[14]

But before the illustration, a few remarks on crisis as an epistemological category. My reflection on the term by no means suggests that crises are not real, or that the term is not productive. If Reagan invoked the "AIDS crisis" only after the nine-year-old Ryan White died, whole populations decimated by the disease heaved a sigh of relief. It has been decades since then, time enough to reflect on what invoking crisis means for common futures of those living with HIV. Here, Janet Roitman's *Anti-Crisis* provides a strong scholarly foundation for the reflection. Roitman's focus is not on health but on the financial crisis of 2008 and its aftermath. Instead of a blame game of what was fixed and what continues, Roitman points out that, as a turning point, as a catalyst for change, crisis undertakes political work. Drawing on Reinhart Koselleck's theory of crisis, Roitman positions crisis in the second order of knowledge. For example, I may experience ill health and "know" my symptoms *before* the second level of abstracting them as a crisis or turning point in an underlying disease. My perception will spur thought about how this critical phase came to be: What had I missed? Where was I negligent?

This reconstruction of the past, almost inevitably a critique of the past, also galvanizes a new future: I must act differently from now on. Crisis is thus not "intrinsic to the system," says Roitman, but "a distinction that produces meaning."[15] In this sense, crisis is an epistemological cut in previous understandings of how things progress in time. So far, so good: crisis can be immensely productive in establishing a moral demand for a difference between past and present. No business as usual, as we say. It opens a critique of the past laying bare normative practices that brought us to the present pass. If we think about the HIV/AIDS crisis in the United States, the activist mobilization of crisis changed the dimmed futures of the HIV affected. It shored up the social stigma that enabled an epidemic to course through a population without recourse to remedy. In all these ways, crisis as a perceived "event" is enabling critique, and it marks a new time to come.[16] Even when crisis has become an enduring condition, it can be a terrain of action.

But it is often the case that crisis does not change on what terms we narrate the past. To follow the example above: I still know my symptoms in the same way, even though I now gather them up as a crisis. In analyzing the financial crash as historical crisis, Roitman questions whether the recognition of the crash as a crisis *really* changed the terms in which we understand the past and the future. Even though home foreclosures prompted homeowners to organize into self-help groups, for instance, Roitman notes that these gatherings often came up with strategies to stem harm (moving personal funds to safer banks, for instance) but not to change the terms of harm; the question of changing the legal burden from borrower to lender came with legislative bank regulations in the aftermath of the crash, but there were almost no penalties imposed on lenders for irresponsible loans that were part and parcel of the crash.[17]

In this way, crises compel new causalities for the past and future, but that impetus might well produce blind spots around what we continue to take for granted. We may understand the financial crisis. But have we changed the terms sufficiently for it to never happen again? We might ask the same question of the HIV/AIDS epidemics. The struggle for the antiretroviral therapies was epic, and we have moved into times when the scientific-technological panacea—when and where available and accessible—seems to have abated the crisis. But that abatement has not substantially changed the valuation of population aggregates: high-risk groups continue to be targets of intervention rather than actors whose assessments of their futures shape expertise.

Now it is not the case that global institutions like UNAIDS or private foundations like the Bill and Melinda Gates Foundation simply push the antiretroviral therapies without attending to the social demands of the economically vulnerable; indeed, their scalable models strategically account for structural inequities in housing, employment, education, and migration patterns of the global AIDS crisis. Nor is there a sense the crisis is over. In fact, the UNAIDS 2016–2021 *Strategy* warns of a "fragile window of opportunity" for a fast-track to the end of AIDS; anything short of this would make possible a slide backward.[18] Here again, crisis as an enduring condition is the terrain of action. And yet the economic motor that informs population aggregation remains firmly lodged in health security regimes. Babies are always best, they are the future; newly infected drug addicts, not so great. Mothers, working people, tax-paying citizens, and property owners have the right to medical recourse, and can demand it—not so easy for those who live on the edge, migrate constantly for employment, fall off the meds, and are not versed in the protocols of demand. It is too facile to dismiss such inequities as secondary social issues; rather, these segregations embedded in risk assessments are a problem *intrinsic* to modern power over life.

And it takes the extreme case to shore up the norm. Few cases are more extreme than the enduring health crisis in Manipur, a state that borders Myanmar and falls along the busy drug-trafficking routes of the Golden Triangle (Thailand, Laos, Vietnam) through which heroin enters Indian markets. Many Manipuri youth get their first hit as adolescent revelers at Myanmar's Moreh markets, which are as popular for acquiring cheap consumer goods (clothing, electronics, furniture) as they are for illicit trade in drugs and guns.[19] Injecting heroin (the crude No. 4) through homemade devices (a rubber stopper and a needle), a large percentage of the youth that visit Moreh for kicks are quickly addicted—and some are infected.

Manipur has been one of the main targets for the Indian government's rollout of antiretroviral therapies because it has always been and remains one of the states with the highest incidence of HIV/AIDS infections. These include new infections; in this regard, the epidemic is still emergent, and the crisis unabated. In contrast, India is celebrated for the state's successful eradication of new HIV infections: a 57 percent reduction between 2000 (274,000) and 2011 (116,000) from HIV Sentinel Surveillance data. With an estimated 2.1 million living with AIDS, new infections declined from 150,000 in 2005 to 80,000 in 2016. The Indian National AIDS Control Programme (NACP) was launched in 1987, a point at which India had the third-largest population of people living with HIV/AIDS (after South Africa and Nigeria). In the 2017 survey, Manipur recorded the second-highest estimated adult prevalence in India despite state efforts to provide access to testing and antiretroviral therapies (in accordance with the 2010 Indian Supreme Court directive[20]). The state wing of the NACP had set up twelve Anti-Retro Viral treatment centers, eleven linked ART centers, and ten community care centers since the 2000 report.[21] Yet Manipur remained at crisis.

Just as these 2011 reports were appearing, I found myself in Manipur conducting research for a book on HIV/AIDS epidemics. My research was on grassroots organizations that had long provided health care amid acute health crises of these epidemics. The national NACP often drew on the enduring social credit of these outfits to implement its programs among the socially vulnerable. In Manipur, the most vulnerable were the addicted, and a few went on to organize informal networks that still remain foundational to HIV/AIDS healthcare. The success stories among the four or five fledging organizations that tackled the raging epidemic in the mid-1980s are CARE and MNP+ (Manipur Network of Positive People), which distributed generics from Cipla and Ranbaxi, and followed up testing viral loads without formally registering patients. Since there are scant resources for archiving the intervention of such groups in the Global South—no oral histories, no papers, no documentaries—a part of my research agenda was to collect and circulate their achievements at a point when the Indian state garnered the lion's share of credit for handling the HIV/AIDS crisis. This is particularly ironic, if not offensive in this context, because it is the Indian state that is partly responsible for the exacerbation of Manipur's health crisis.

Manipur has remained in a perpetual state of exception since 1958, when India imposed the Armed Forces Special Powers Act (generally known as AFSPA) to eliminate radical secessionist tendencies in the provinces bordering China and Myanmar. On grounds of national security, the Indian Army was granted legal immunity to restore order in the state; much like in Kashmir, the army's abuses are legendary.[22] Within the discourse of national security, Manipur is positioned as a "backward region" of Indigenous "hill tribes"; the cultural corollary makes appearance in the national bourgeoisie anthropological curiosity about Manipuri "folk" ethnicity. Thus, it is small wonder that the many Manipuris see themselves as stranded on an island; on my visit, I was extremely aware of my own status as a mainlander (although the state is topographically contiguous with India). And why not, since the roads into the state are heavily guarded against twenty-some insurgent groups who battle the army for a "free Manipur."

The low-intensity warfare reorganizes every aspect of life, from petroleum shortages to interrupted antiretroviral medicine shipments. In the midst of this ongoing emergency came the HIV/AIDS epidemic. Unlike other Indian states with high infection rates, Manipur's infected communities were and are primarily injectable-drug users (IDU): among 2.38 million, if 8 percent are HIV positive, 72 percent of the infected are drug users.[23] Unable to contain insurgencies in Manipur, military personnel often regard anyone who makes frequent trips to the border with suspicion. Drug users are widely regarded as irresponsible citizens who are potential threats to national security, for they can be economically persuaded to run guns for the insurgents. In the earliest phase of the epidemic in Manipur, the army began to run random checks on Manipuri youth under the AFSPA provisions for arrest without trial on "reasonable suspicion" (figure 2.2). Anyone with needle marks on their arm was unceremoniously thrown in jail *before* testing and housed in the HIV cells. National security measures amped up disciplinary and calculative interventions, so much so that the HIV/AIDS crisis presented an opportunity for cleaning up the border state's drug problem.

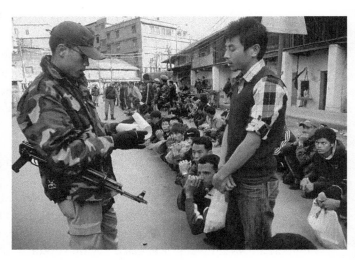

FIGURE 2.2.
News photo of army
roundup, Manipur,
February 20, 2012.
Sinlung North East
India. Source:
www.sinlung.com.

The real problem was that drug users would have to register for regular testing to avail of the therapies. But the "high-risk" group found themselves in a bind. The health crisis had changed nothing about the value the state placed on their health; they were always subjects of benign welfare. On the other side of the aisle, the insurgent groups mirrored the same terms of calculation. Groups that saw themselves as the de facto government of Manipur (the larger groups even have a parallel tax structure) threatened to shoot addicts: in their view, an autonomous Manipur should be a drug-free one. Here, crisis as a second order of knowledge created an epistemological moment to rewrite the past and anticipate the future. For the socially vulnerable, that future became more precarious than ever before, for now they were faced with arrests, imprisonment, and death threats. At a juncture when eight of every ten families had a regular drug user in the household, drug users refused testing and went underground, while HIV infection rates among them jumped from 1–2 percent in 1990 to 50 percent in 1994 to as much as 80.7 percent in 1997.[24]

Thus the opportunity to seize the future only exacerbated existing inequities. This failure has much to do with the unchanging calculative logic of modern governance that shapes health interventions. And it is against this logic that time and again we see another kind of compensatory intervention: activist networks that contacted drug users in secrecy (in gyms, eateries, market hangouts, Narcotic Anonymous meetings); ensured regular clinic visits, compliance with drug regimens, and advice to patients on diet and exercise; and offered social support in forums, camps, screenings, and meetings. In Manipur, CARE and MNP+ gathered social credit because they were affiliated with neither the government nor the insurgents: as self-organizing networks, they remained open-ended, contingent upon their "users," and a parallel health infrastructure in the state.[25] State-run programs secure life as it determines economic productivity and political stability; the costs are unevenly distributed and that distribution is masked through the liberal fiction of the "people of Manipur." The activist health-care networks, however, organize life around another kind of cost: personal and communal losses. The head of MNP+, for instance, started the outfit with five other HIV positive friends, one of whom did not survive the crisis. Here, too, the costs are experientially uneven, but they cannot be split, sorted, and distributed; in short, they are incalculable. When this second "calculus" of personal and communal loss overtakes the first, we witness a shift in the terms in which we narrate crises. The ground of the "health crisis" is no longer eternal microbial-human war but willful politics of making die. The call is for policies and programs that ensure such thanatopolitics has no place in the future of public health. The re-narration of the HIV/AIDS epidemics has achieved just this in all kinds of fabulous ways all over the world. Those achievements are localized, often singular, and the interventions are not always portable. Yet they signal the horizon for what is to be done for communities living with HIV/AIDS.

As we zoom out from Manipur, let me close with a recent iteration of a global health crisis in which deathly calculations once more made their mark: the Ebola outbreak in Guinea, Liberia, and Sierra Leone, from March to September 2014.[26] In the health crisis that followed, a miracle drug came into view. Only three doses stored at Kailahun, Sierra Leone, spurred hopes: Could this be *the* scientific breakthrough on the scale of the antiretroviral therapies? Would science once again save the day? Amid the anticipation, national interest dictated the distribution of the scarce doses. Mainstream media carried news of two Americans airlifted from Sierra Leone to the safety of American shores: a doctor, Kent Brantley, and a health worker, Nancy Writebol, were saved by their access to ZMapp. But legal-medical protocols prevented the same access for African scientist and doctor Sheikh Umar Khan.[27] Defenders of global governance highlighted striking differences between national health-care systems as the reason why Umar Khan was not given one of the three available doses. The administration of ZMapp required the kind of monitoring and supportive care, they maintained, that was inconceivable in the West African epidemic situations. Others decried the cost-benefit calculus foundational to the military-economic foundations of global health security. In this replay, Umar Khan joined Clara Maass in a recursive history. As uncontainable microbial life from those hot zones on the blue planet skip into new human, plant, and animal host populations, the calculation that values some lives over others remains the real cost of crisis as epistemology.

Notes

1 Chaves-Carballo, "Yellow Fever and Human Experimentation," 557.
2 The extensive Philip S. Hench Walter Reed Yellow Fever Collection at the University of Virginia archives the work of the commission. For an overview, see "Yellow Fever Collection 1806–1995."
3 While the credit for the vaccine goes to Walter Reed, who wrote about the experiments in great detail, a Cuban physician, Carlos Finlay, had long argued that the mosquito was the vector for the disease; when the commission decided to test the mosquito theory, Finlay provided the infected mosquitoes.
4 Whiteside, HIV/AIDS, 4.
5 One of the privates, William H. Dean, was X.Y. in Reed's records; he was later honored for his sacrifice (see Kelley, "Private Dean").
6 Foucault, "Society Must Be Defended."
7 President Reagan did not mention AIDS as a health crisis until 1987; by that time twelve thousand Americans had died. As early as 1985, the Centers for Disease Control (CDC) had put together a $33 million preventive plan that was rejected by the White House. But things began to change in October 1987, with the death of the president's friend Rock Hudson. There are many well-known accounts of this silence and its effects. See, for instance, Jefferson, "How AIDS Changed America," and Shilts's exposé, And the Band Played On.
8 See Sunder Rajan's Pharmocracy and Cooper's Life as Surplus. There is also a considerable history of medical apartheid, as elaborated in Washington's Medical Apartheid.
9 There is a massive literature on mourning and melancholia in the AIDS epidemic: notable bookends are Crimp's early "Mourning and Militancy," which was later collected with his other writings in Melancholia and Moralism: Essays on AIDS and Queer Politics; and Woubshet's Calendar of Loss, a book that represents efforts to globalize the literature on mourning.
10 See Foucault, Security, Territory, Population; Lakoff, Unprepared; Elbe, Virus Alert; and Ahuja, Bioinsecurities.
11 Cooper and Waldby elaborate the notion of clinical labor in their coauthored Clinical Labor.
12 Elbe, Virus Alert. These concepts from Foucault, "Society Must Be Defended," have become axiomatic in discussions on race, biopolitics, and globalization.
13 The "Global South" was a term that emerged as early as 1969 but gained momentum after the fall of the Berlin Wall in 1989, which threw the

cartographies of First, Second, and Third Worlds into question. Scholars prefer the geographic descriptor for a number of reasons, not the least of which is to refute the historical trajectories of economic development implicit in the terms *Third World* or *developing world*. *Global South* captures global regions often interconnected by histories of colonialism or neo-imperialism, some of which are "within" the cartographic reaches of North America or Europe, where large-scale inequities in living standards, life expectancies, and resource access persist. For a conceptual argument for the efficacy of the term, see Levander and Mignolo, "Introduction."

14 "Emergence" (from the Latin *emegere*, meaning "to appear") is a capacious term for multileveled occurrences across scales of action, human and nonhuman, that resists linear causality and is therefore difficult to predict.

15 Roitman, *Anti-Crisis*, 93.

16 Roitman, *Anti-Crisis*, 19.

17 Roitman, *Anti-Crisis*, 67–68.

18 *UNAIDS 2016–2021 Strategy*, 3.

19 Moreh is to Imphal what Tijuana is to Los Angeles—a border town with all the trappings of pleasure and danger. As India's gateway to Southeast Asia, the town has been growing in size and importance, fueling talk of beefing up security. See Bhattacharya and Daniel, "India's Wild East Unprepared."

20 The directive instructed the federal and state governments to provide therapies to patients as a "right to life" guaranteed under the Indian Constitution's Article 21. The bill against discrimination based on HIV and AIDS passed in the upper house, the Rajya Sabha, in March 2017.

21 "AIDS Situation Alarming."

22 In 1949 the princely state of Manipur was annexed to the newly independent Republic of India, and secessionist groups sprouted in the region. About a decade later, the Indian Parliament passed the draconian AFSPA—whose extreme provisions derive from a British Ordinance of 1942, designed to quash the historic Quit India Movement—ushering in a perpetual state of emergency in the region. See Tarapot, *Bleeding Manipur*.

23 Bhagat, "In a Vicious Circle."

24 Bhagat, "In a Vicious Circle."

25 I elaborate on the vital health infrastructure in the state in "Staying Alive."

26 The first case is traced to December 2013 and the last to June 2016; the World Health Organization reported 28,616 reported cases of infection.

27 There was a lot of coverage of the two infected Americans, and brief references to the controversy. Maina Kiai, a human rights activist in Kenya, reported that the seeming inequity in dose distribution was discussed on the sidelines of the summit meeting of African leaders held in Washington: "There was a sense of the same pattern," he said, that "the life of an African is less valuable." See Pollack, "Ebola Drug"; and Hayden and Reardon, "Should Experimental Drugs Be Used?"

Bibliography

Ahuja, Neel. *Bioinsecurities: Disease Interventions, Empire, and the Governance of Spaces*. Durham, NC: Duke University Press, 2016.

"AIDS Situation Alarming in Manipur: CM." *Hindustan Times*, December 1, 2012. https://www.hindustantimes.com/india/aids-situation-alarming-in-manipur-cm/story-UZVYTDqKK6Pm6aGhX7spnM.html.

Bhagat, Rasheeda. "In a Vicious Circle." *Frontline* 19, no. 15 (July 20–August 2, 2002). https://frontline.thehindu.com/static/html/fl1915/19150420.htm.

Bhattacharya, Satarupa, and Frank Jack Daniel. "India's Wild East Unprepared for New Myanmar." *Reuters World News*, February 22, 2012. https://www.reuters.com/article/us-india-myanmar-idUSTRE81L03T20120222.

Chaves-Carballo, Enrique. "Clara Maass, Yellow Fever and Human Experimentation." *Military Medicine* 178, no. 5 (2013): 557–62.

Cooper, Melinda. *Life as Surplus: Biotechnology and Capitalism in the Neoliberal Era*. Seattle: University of Washington Press, 2008.

Cooper, Melinda, and Catherine Waldby. *Clinical Labor: Tissue Donors and Research Subjects in the Global Bioeconomy*. Durham, NC: Duke University Press, 2014.

Crimp, Douglas. *Melancholia and Moralism: Essays on AIDS and Queer Politics*. Cambridge, MA: MIT Press, 2002.

Crimp, Douglas. "Mourning and Militancy." *October* 51 (Winter 1989): 3–18.

Elbe, Stefan. *Virus Alert: Security, Governmentality, and the AIDS Pandemic*. New York: Columbia University Press, 2009.

Foucault, Michel. *Security, Territory, Population: Lectures at the Collège de France, 1977–78*. Edited by Michel Senellart. Translated by Graham Burchell. Basingstoke: Palgrave Macmillan, 2007.

Foucault, Michel. *"Society Must Be Defended": Lectures at the Collège de France, 1975–76*. Edited by Mauro Bertani and Alessandro Fontana. Translated by David Macey. New York: Picador, 2003.

Ghosh, Bishnupriya. "Staying Alive: Imphal's HIV/AIDS Digital Video Culture." In *Asian Video Cultures: In the Penumbra of the Global*, edited by Joshua Neves and Bhaskar Sarkar, 288–306. Durham, NC: Duke University Press, 2017.

"A Guide to the Philip S. Hench Walter Reed Yellow Fever Collection 1806–1995." *Virginia Heritage: Guides to Manuscript and Archival Collections in Virginia*. https://ead.lib.virginia.edu/vivaxtf/view?docId=uva-hs/viuh00010.xml.

Hayden, Erika Check, and Sara Reardon. "Should Experimental Drugs Be Used in the Ebola Outbreak?" *Nature*, August 12, 2014.

Jefferson, David. "How AIDS Changed America." *Newsweek*, May 14, 2006.

Kelley, John M. "Private Dean—Apotheosis of Courage." *Grand Rapids Herald*, August 26, 1928. https://search.lib.virginia.edu/catalog/uva-lib:2225669/tei.

Koselleck, Reinhart. *Critique and Crisis: The Enlightenment and the Pathogenesis of Modern Society*. Translated by Thomas McCarthy. Cambridge, MA: MIT Press, 2000.

Lakoff, Andrew. *Unprepared: Global Health in a Time of Emergency*. Oakland: University of California Press, 2017.

Levander, Caroline Field, and Walter Mignolo. "Introduction: The Global South and World Dis/Order." *Global South* 5, no. 1 (2011): 1–11.

National AIDS Control Programme. *HIV Facts and Figures*. 2018. http://naco.gov.in /hiv-facts-figures.

Pollack, Andrew. "Ebola Drug Can Save a Few Lives. But Whose? *New York Times*, August 8, 2014.

Roitman, Janet. *Anti-Crisis*. Durham, NC: Duke University Press, 2014.

Shilts, Randy. *And the Band Played On: Politics, People, and the AIDS Epidemic*. New York: St. Martin's, 1987.

Sunder Rajan, Kaushik. *Pharmocracy: Value, Politics, and Knowledge in Global Biomedicine*. Durham, NC: Duke University Press, 2017.

Tarapot, Phanjoubam. *Bleeding Manipur*. New Delhi: Har-Anand, 2007.

UNAIDS 2016–2021 Strategy: On the Fast-Track to Ends AIDS. 2015. https://www .unaids.org/sites/default/files/media_asset/20151027_UNAIDS_PCB37_15 _18_EN_rev1.pdf.

Washington, Harriet A. *Medical Apartheid: The Dark History of Medical Experimentation on Black Americans from Colonial Times to the Present*. New York: Anchor Books, 2008.

Whiteside, Alan. *HIV/AIDS: A Very Short Introduction*. Oxford: Oxford University Press, 2008.

Woubshet, Dagmawi. *The Calendar of Loss: Race, Sexuality, and Mourning in the Early Era of AIDS*. Baltimore: Johns Hopkins University Press, 2015.

THREE AIDS, WOMEN OF COLOR FEMINISMS, QUEER AND TRANS OF COLOR CRITIQUES, AND THE CRISES OF KNOWLEDGE PRODUCTION

Jih-Fei Cheng

On October 28, 2018, during game 5 of the World Series at Dodger Stadium, a group of protesters from the TransLatin@ Coalition, founded by immigrant and AIDS activist Bamby Salcedo, unfurled a 20 x 15 foot blue, pink, and white transgender pride flag. The phrase TRANS PEOPLE DESERVE TO LIVE was emblazoned across it, most immediately referencing the Donald Trump administration's aims to dismantle protections for trans, intersex, nonbinary, and gender nonconforming peoples. This visual tactic also reflected the historical Women's Committee of New York City's AIDS Coalition to Unleash Power (ACT UP), which, on May 8, 1988, protested the public silence on the impact of AIDS upon women by unleashing several large banners during a Mets game at Shea Stadium. The banners displayed phrases such as DON'T BALK AT SAFE SEX, AIDS KILLS WOMEN, and MEN! USE CONDOMS.[1]

Today's social movements, such as #BlackLivesMatter, #MeToo, and AIDS activism, come from long histories of women of color feminist and radical traditions that challenge white supremacist, masculinist, capitalist, militarized, and authoritarian rule. These movements have also been adapted by liberal and mainstream politics at the cost of intersectional and radical traditions. That is, these liberal, or even conservative, adaptations of intersectional and radical movements shift focus away from the women of color and queer and trans people of color that founded these movements. Instead, they refocus white experiences and reaffirm our institutions and their racist, patriarchal, hetero- and gender-normative, class, and ableist conditions of exclusionary power. This includes #AllLivesMatter as well as the growing attention to white women and men in both #MeToo and AIDS movements. The deflection away from those who suffer the most under structural violences ultimately strengthens rather than transforms our institutions of power.

In reverberating the past actions of ACT UP's Women's Committee, the TransLatin@ Coalition drew a historical through-line between AIDS activism and the intersectional politics of #BlackLivesMatter, #MeToo, #NoDAPL, and #IdleNoMore, whose campaigns for justice are explicitly led and/or organized around women of color feminisms and queer and trans of color critiques.[2] By highlighting these genealogies of intellectual and political leadership, we find how women of color feminisms, which gave rise to queer and trans of color critiques, have been foundational to much longer radical traditions extending back to resistance against settlers, organizing for the abolition of slavery and prisons, demanding civil rights, as well as other earlier and varying forms of insurgency against white supremacy and heteropatriarchy.[3] Today's radical movements recognize how the interlocking oppressions of Native dispossession, histories of enslavement, massive resource extraction, the policing of borders and public space, war, sexual violence, the enforcement of the gender binary, and AIDS are fundamentally linked. By taking stock of the interventions made by women of color feminisms and queer and trans of color theories and practices, or praxes, I ask: How and when do our institutions of knowledge production recapitulate the structures of violence that comprise the global AIDS pandemic? How are the crises in knowledge production addressed by women of color feminisms and queer and trans of color critiques within and across institutions of power, including academia?

Women of color feminisms and queer and trans of color critiques generate networks of solidarity across institutions by analyzing and shifting the terms of power. Thus, they understand that we cannot begin with AIDS as the object of study within our institutions or as the central object of critique in our social movements. Otherwise, women of color and queer and trans peoples of color will always need to be added, as afterthoughts, to the popular narrative that AIDS and its activism have been about and by white men. Rather, we must seriously consider how women of color and queer and trans people of color praxes engage our institutions, and how these praxes critique and organize against the local and globalized crises that place all of us, but particularly them, at the greatest risk for violences—including AIDS—that are perpetuated by our institutions of knowledge. Thus, if we turn to scholarship embedded in histories of organizing that centers women of color and queer and trans people of color, we find roadmaps for accounting *and* countering the multiple crises that facilitate the AIDS pandemic, including that of knowledge production within academia.

Intersections: Between Insurgency and Institutions

I teach Cathy J. Cohen's 1997 article "Punks, Bulldaggers, and Welfare Queens: The Radical Potential of Queer Politics?" in introductory courses in the Department of Feminist, Gender, and Sexuality Studies at Scripps College, which was founded in Claremont, California, in 1926 during the Jim Crow era, as a white-serving women's liberal arts college.[4] Scripps College was built on Tongva Indigenous lands using the settler colonialist Mission Revival style of design that the school conceives as "uncommon beauty, a tribute to the founder's vision that the College's architecture and landscape should reflect and influence taste and judgment."[5] While feminist and queer studies have become somewhat requisite among US women's liberal arts colleges, many of these schools were founded by white suffragists who, as the Black feminist, journalist, and antilynching activist Ida B. Wells documented, campaigned on an anti-Black platform to demand white women's right to vote before all others in order to protect white heteropatriarchal families and homes against "great dark faced mobs."[6] Therein lies the liberal paradox embedded in the academic institutionalization of feminist and queer politics. "Punks" persists as a women of color feminist interventional pedagogical tool against the disciplinary and exclusionary practices of knowledge production.

Within the US educational system, people of color—particularly Black, Indigenous, Latinx, and certain Asian peoples—remain low in representation. Meanwhile, the funding and emphasis on science, technology, engineering, and math (STEM) continues to increase. In 2002, a commission letter written by the Western Association of Schools and Colleges (WASC) noted that Scripps College had fallen far short of its goal of "achieving greater levels of diversity. . . . Scripps has been successful in recruiting a diverse staff. However, student diversity has shown little change over the last four years, and faculty diversity remains a challenge."[7] For its fall 2016 census, Scripps enrollment data shows that, of its student population, only 37 percent are of color while 5 percent are international students.[8] Almost two decades after the WASC report, and over ninety years of institutional history, Scripps College remains hampered by a stark lack of racial/ethnic diversity, especially among students and faculty.

Meanwhile, Scripps College reflects the growing trend toward emphasizing a science curriculum, with biology/life sciences as its top-ranking major.[9]

The rigorous and time-sensitive curricular demands placed on science majors means that Scripps students have very limited options when selecting courses that would integrate their learning in science with the liberal arts. As such, issues and scholarship on race/ethnicity, gender, and sexuality remain institutionally segregated from matters of science, which are thought to be objective and ahistorical. The few interdisciplinary courses that bring together the sciences and their historical or sociopolitical contexts, then, become additive rather than foundational to education. These courses are rendered optional, oftentimes fulfilling general education "diversity" requirements that are taken in the student's junior or senior year after all science major/minor requirements have been prioritized.

In the fall of 2015—my first semester teaching at Scripps College—students of color across the Claremont Colleges Consortium staged walkouts, rallies, and marches as part of the international "Blackout" to protest anti-Black racism in school systems and other institutions. During the 2016–17 academic year, our queer and trans of color communities at the Claremont Colleges lost two student activist leaders. One of these students—a young Black woman and daughter of immigrant parents—was in my Introduction to Queer Studies course. She was, and is, a powerful leader who led others in coalition-building work that ranged from addressing institutional racism to anti-Zionist activism. She was a science major in her junior year who finally found some time in her curricular schedule to study the ways women of color feminisms and queer and trans of color critiques could be applied to her lab research on HIV antibodies. We had met during my office hours to discuss her work. We also sat on campus-wide committees tasked to address social and economic inequities and initiate structural changes. She was a residential adviser, and she passed away in her dorm room.[10]

Tatissa Zunguze.

Tatissa's leadership and coalitional organizing—staged against her multiple encounters with structural and everyday violence—were guided by genealogies of women of color feminisms, specifically Black feminist and queer thought that she read in class but which also reflected her experiences. Black feminist, queer, and trans intellectual projects continue to serve as antiracist and anti-colonial pedagogical tools precisely because of their historical interjections into systems of oppression, including white feminist scholarship and other white-centered and/or heteropatriarchal canons of higher education. Black cis-women, nonbinary, gender nonconforming, intersex, trans, and/or queer faculty, students, staff, and coalitional community members continue to demand engagements with Black feminist, trans, and queer studies to confront the mundane racism and institutional oppositions that form our stubbornly and continually white-dominated US educational settings.

In "Punks," Cohen questions the radical potential for queer politics because its settling into institutions elides the operations of power by "reinforc[ing] simple dichotomies between heterosexual and everything 'queer.'"[11] "Punks" foregrounds Black feminist interventions into queer politics by calling attention to the then-recent resignation of three Black board members from the first and largest AIDS service organization of its time, Gay Men's Health Crisis (GMHC), over its alleged racism. In turn, Cohen calls for a "new politics" where the "*nonnormative* and *marginal* position of punks, bulldaggers, and welfare queens, for example, is the basis for progressive transformative coalition work."[12] It is through the "intersection of oppression and resistance" of these nonnormative and marginal positions, Cohen submits, that multi-issued, coalitional organizing could manifest the radical potential of queer politics.[13] Cohen states,

> Both the needle exchange and prison projects pursued through the auspices of ACT UP New York point to the possibilities and difficulties involved in principled transformative coalition work. In each project individuals from numerous identities—heterosexual, gay, poor, wealthy, white, black, Latino—came together to challenge dominant constructions of who should be allowed and who deserved care. No particular identity exclusively determined the shared political commitments of these activists; instead their similar positions, as marginalized subjects relative to the state—made clear through the government's lack of response to AIDS—formed the basis of this political unity.[14]

Because, until the mid-1990s, effective antiretroviral medications that could maintain the health of those living with HIV did not exist, the mounting toll of deaths during the early years of the AIDS pandemic pointed to the "interlocking systems of oppression" and structural violence borne from the dismantling of the US welfare state, including health care, hospitals, and housing, and the diversion of funds toward the arms buildup and military imperialism. Yet Cohen also emphasizes the crucial role of Black and intersectional feminisms as key to the radical and transformative potential of queer politics and cites Kimberlé Crenshaw, Barbara Ransby, Angela Y. Davis, Cheryl Clarke, Audre Lorde, and the Combahee River Collective, among others.[15] She illuminates the operations of power that have persisted before (and now after) AIDS was widely seen as a "death sentence" by pointing to the historical regulation of women of color who continue to be rendered perverse and criminal as "single mothers, teen mothers, and, primarily women of color dependent on state assistance."[16]

As Roderick A. Ferguson has shown in *Aberrations in Black*, his theorization of the field of "queer of color critique," the stigmatization and demonization of these nonnormative and marginal Black and other people of color subjects through sociological documents, such as the 1965 Moynihan Report, led to the dismantling of the welfare state. Furthermore, Ferguson contends in *The Reorder of Things* that the liberal implementation of "diversity" initiatives in higher education reflects the management of Black and other radical social movements through the simultaneous inclusion of ethnic, gender, and sexuality studies and the continued marginalization of people of color in higher education. Put simply, the proliferation of the AIDS pandemic is historically and persistently tied to the institutionalization of Black feminist and queer studies alongside the ongoing structural violence that Black and other people of color, and especially Black cis-women, nonbinary, gender nonconforming, trans, intersex, and queer peoples, experience as liminal subjects across the institutions of scholarship, art, media, and politics. Yet, in spite of these crises in knowledge production, Black feminist, queer, and trans studies continue to operate as modes of insurgency within and beyond academia, including the realm of popular culture.

For instance, drawing upon the work of Alexandra Juhasz, Cohen, and others involved in AIDS activism and scholarship, I have assessed how there is a trend among recent critically acclaimed popular films addressing AIDS activist historiography whereby people of color have nearly disappeared from the historical record.[17] I contend that this is because the white men who direct and appear in these films are invested in telling a story about political progress since the earlier years of the AIDS crisis. Rather than examine the root causes for AIDS as embedded in histories of colonialism, racism, patriarchy, and socioeconomic inequality that block access for US people of color and the Global South, David France, the director of the feature-length documentary film *How to Survive a Plague* (2012), tells an incomplete, even false, story meant to convince audiences that biomedical interventions generated and distributed by corporate pharmaceuticals, like preexposure prophylaxis (PrEP), will solve the pandemic.[18] However, this narrative of biomedical progress comes at the cost of jettisoning analysis about how the AIDS pandemic is historically and continually formed through structural inequalities experienced by nonwhite peoples who are denied biomedical access.

Moreover, much of the historical video footage adapted into films like *How to Survive a Plague* is extracted from earlier AIDS activist films and the personal archives amassed through a large network of video artists.[19] These archives were donated to institutions like the New York Public Library. Film directors, like France, access these public archives and use the footage. As I intend to show in future writing, for his film, France left out images of the extensive activist leadership and on-camera discussions by Black women, people of color, and white coalitional members that relay their experiences and interventions into the AIDS crisis despite their marginalization by white-dominated institutions and mainstream media.[20]

Black and other people of color artists, activists, and scholars who point to the dearth of people of color representations in public forums for AIDS cultural productions are met with vehement resistance. They must fight through the ongoing and simultaneous conditions of exploitation and neglect in order to have their contributions and needs acknowledged. As of this writing, the Tacoma Action Collective continues to protest the book and touring exhibition *Art AIDS America* for nearly banishing artists of color, especially Black artists.[21] Tourmaline (formerly known as Reina Gossett), a Black trans activist and artist, codirected with Sasha Wortzel the film short *Happy Birthday, Marsha!* (2017), which focuses on the influence and activism of Marsha P. Johnson, who was "HIV positive, a sex worker, and an incredible performer and member of the group Hot Peaches." Johnson also cofounded the Street Transvestites Action Revolutionaries (STAR) with Sylvia Rivera.[22] Yet Gossett has had to contend with the aforementioned France, who stands accused of appropriating much of Gossett's labor and research on Johnson's life while amassing funding and a media platform that far exceeds Gossett's.[23] Eventually, France's feature-length film version, *The Life and Death of Marsha P. Johnson* (2017), was distributed via Netflix's video-on-demand.

Prompted by such systemic erasures, Visual AIDS commissioned Erin Christovale and Vivian Crockett to co-curate "Alternate Endings, Radical Beginnings"—a "video program [that] prioritized Black narratives within the ongoing AIDS epidemic" for the 2017 annual "Day with(out) Art." "Alternate Endings, Radical Beginnings" includes video shorts by Gossett, Mykki Blanco, Cheryl Dunye, Ellen Spiro, Thomas Allen Harris, Kia LaBeija, Tiona Nekkia McClodden, and Brontez Purnell. Each of these works transforms time and memory by reimagining and recalling the presence of Black cis-women, nonbinary, gender nonconforming, intersex, and trans peoples precisely at the moments and sites where they were excluded or forgotten to exist. Dunye's earlier film, *The Watermelon Woman* (1997), was a watershed for the New Queer Cinema movement. The experimental film yields critical insight into how the memories of Black feminist and queer women fall out of official archives. Public memory, then, must be recast to assert Black queer women's pasts, presences, and futures. In each of the works and conditions cited above, Black cis-women, nonbinary, gender nonconforming, trans, and queer people speak out on their own behalf but also on behalf of a queer radical imagination that seeks liberation for all. This form of Black feminist thinking and action is rooted in the Black radical tradition.[24]

Writing more recently, Cohen recognizes the powerful and collectivized vision and work of "young black women who identify as queer" that have built a "leaderful movement with cis and trans women taking positions of power," including Black Lives Matter. She contends,

> Young people who have taken classes on black queer studies and black feminist theory through ethnic studies, African American studies and gender and sexuality departments are using the lessons taught in those classes to inform the organizing practices they are deploying on behalf of and in partnership with black people who may never see the inside of our classrooms. These young activists, who blend the politics of the academy and the politics of liberation, daily make black queer studies relevant to a changing world.[25]

In response to Tatissa's passing, Black queer and trans students across the Claremont Colleges Consortium gathered their pain and anger and transformed it into direct action. During the spring of 2017, Claremont McKenna College brought pro-police speaker Heather MacDonald to campus. MacDonald has advocated for the use of police against the Black Lives Matter movements. Overnight, in the tradition of nonviolent protest, Black queer and trans students organized and led other students to block access to the venue. They stood front and center while white students and other students of color strategically positioned themselves as a buffer between Black students and campus security, who did not intervene when hecklers not only shouted and taunted but took to shoving the nonviolent protesters. Students chanted "Black lives matter" and "Black lives—they matter here." They cited solidarity with immigrants faced with the militarization of the US-Mexico border as well as Palestinians living under Zionist occupation. These students of color transformed their grief into a deep well of care and coalition building. As a result, the event was effectively shut down. They continue to build movements led by Black queer and trans intellectuals, writers, and artists. They teach me the radical potential of queer politics.

Ironically (or not), there are those who presumably identify as anti-racists who describe such nonviolent protest tactics and aforementioned chants, which echo AIDS activists who adopted these strategies from earlier social movements, including Black-led social movements, as seemingly incoherent and "meaningless slogans."[26] There are even those who would, in stark self-contradiction, laud the Black-led civil rights movement as decidedly nonviolent while, in the same breath, describing these student protesters as "violent." The presumption is that white supremacists could be called to their senses because they are, at the bottom of their hearts, benevolent even if misguided people. Yet there is no history that shows that white people have been willing to dismantle white supremacy without the combined approach of civil rights protest and Black militancy.[27] On many occasions, I have heard decriers of Black protest urge, instead, that Black activists conduct research and write articles—as if they have not and are not already doing so.

We bear witness to intense racial profiling, Black imprisonment and murder, border patrolling and detention of immigrants and refugees in concentration camps, hyperprivatization of all social safety nets, and ballooning college tuition and educational debt. Meanwhile, Donald Trump has attempted to dismantle public arts and scholarship, including the National Endowment for the Arts and the National Endowment for the Humanities. Inclusion into "civil society" means the institutionalization of Black feminisms and the concurrent silencing of Black cis-women, nonbinary, gender nonconforming, trans, and queer peoples. Yet all people from all sectors of society benefit from the historical advancements made by Black feminists. Meanwhile, the "alt right" is ramping up attacks against students of color and ethnic, feminist, trans, and queer studies scholars by claiming that expressions of white supremacy amount to "freedom of speech" and "academic freedom" when, in fact, proclaiming the right to terrorize Black subjects and other people of color enacts the opposite. Allowing and including white supremacy in our parades for "free speech" disassembles the public sphere and tears down freedom itself, including academic freedom.

Women of Color Feminisms Navigating Knowledge Crises

What if, then, we as non-Black and/or non-Indigenous people of color and white people take up women of color feminisms to ask questions such as: How would we understand the AIDS pandemic differently if we consider it the outcome of histories of settler colonialism, Native displacement, massive resource extraction, and antiblackness? How might we understand this, specifically, from the experiences of Black and Indigenous cis-women, nonbinary, gender nonconforming, trans, intersex, and queer peoples in the midst of the enduring AIDS pandemic? How might women of color feminisms form a foundation for challenging the liberal inclusion of white nationalist discourse and action in academe?

Citing the radical tradition of Black feminisms as central to his approach to the study of antiblackness and AIDS, Adam Geary explains that a "materialist epidemiology and its Marxist inheritance allows me to connect the health research that I read with materialist traditions in Black, feminist, queer, and cultural studies, especially those connected, if in complex ways, to the Marxist tradition. These critical, radical traditions are essential for elaborating the histories of struggle, violence, and domination that have made an AIDS epidemic possible and structured its development."[28] The week before Tatissa's passing, we had read Geary's work in class. She shared with me her excitement at the potential of engaging in a materialist epidemiology of AIDS that keeps at its core Black feminist, queer, and trans analyses.

People of color—especially women of color, students, staff, faculty, and community leaders—cannot be expected to tirelessly research, write, produce culture, and organize against enduring racism, heteropatriarchy, and AIDS while others appropriate or even disparage such work. As non-Black and/or non-Native faculty, staff, students, artists, and participants in social movements, we must teach and learn from Cohen's article as a genealogy of Black and other women of color feminisms that makes the radical potential of queer, trans, and AIDS studies and activism possible. How to engage intersectional feminisms and their continued critical importance to social movements while addressing the insistently low yet highly crucial representation of women of color, and other people of color, in scholarship, the classroom, and the pandemic is something we must continually ask and push ourselves to do.

To this end, I close with a few pedagogical questions that I take up in the classroom, which could be applied across the disciplines.

When teaching feminism, queer theory, or AIDS, it matters how we bring the relationship between these things into view. Does the course engage women of color feminisms and/or AIDS in a sustained way? If so, does the course leave unquestioned the epidemiological narrative of "Patient Zero," wherein white gay men constitute the source and the solution to AIDS? How, if at all, does the course address women of color feminisms and their radical traditions as the theoretical and political foundations for ethnic, queer, and trans studies as well as the AIDS social movement and scholarship? How do we understand women of color feminisms and queer and trans of color critiques as they operate within and across institutions of power, as well as within and across nation-states and geopolitical formations, to address multiple forms of globalized crises, including AIDS? Finally, how is AIDS a part of colonial histories of science as they are produced on and through the bodies of racialized subjects who are deemed gender nonconforming and/or sexually aberrant?[29]

Furthermore, to address the crises in knowledge production, we must take stock of the barriers women of color and queer and trans people of color must continually leap over to get into and remain in our classrooms. In addition to recasting our disciplinary and curricular foundations, we must transform our institutions from within by confronting how our institutions fundamentally erode "free speech," "academic freedom," and the public sphere by maintaining barriers to access while fortifying white heteropatriarchal voices and violences. A materialist epidemiology of AIDS would account for why people of color, particularly Black, Native, and Latinx peoples, continue to be underenrolled and unable to survive US higher education. Meanwhile, women of color, as well as queer and trans people of color, are sexually assaulted at higher rates and are at greater risk for HIV infection on US college campuses.[30] Yet people of color, particularly Black peoples, including Black women and trans peoples, are intensely racially profiled and experience police violence on and off campuses. They are more greatly criminalized for HIV transmission and spend more time in prisons, where the rates of HIV infection are disproportionate to the general population.[31]

Finally, we must take stock of what inhibits each of us from making the necessary connections offered by intersectional feminism. As noted in Julia Jordan-Zachery's contribution to this volume, the public discourse on Black women, their sexualities, and HIV/AIDS are often media-driven. The "Ass" and "Strong Black Women" scripts predominate mainstream media and often exert shame and undue pressures upon Black women to engage in personal behavior change while diverting attention from direct address of structural concerns. During #MeToo founder Tarana Burke's talk for a plenary session at the 2018 HIV Biomedical Prevention Summit, Burke foregrounded the shame she experienced regarding her sister, who was HIV -positive, a sex worker, used drugs, and passed in 1987. In writing about Burke's talk, HIV prevention and treatment activist, and former executive director of Queers for Economic Justice, Kenyon Farrow, describes how the widespread shame of HIV/AIDS, and the stark power imbalances within institutions and organizations where sexual harassment and assaults occur, have prevented more people who are involved in social justice, art, and scholarly work from making the necessary connections between sexual trauma and the AIDS pandemic.[32] This is why intersectional feminisms are so crucial and potentially enabling to those of us working to bridge knowledge gaps while participating in movements that are often rendered distinct. Without diagnosing and shifting the terms of power across movements and institutions—as intersectional feminisms can uniquely do—we find that our activist, creative, and intellectual work reproduces the crises in knowledge while replicating the structures of violence.

Those of us with institutional power must decide whether to heed the call of women of color feminist and queer and trans of color counterstrategies— not simply to apply intersectional, queer, and trans analyses but to think and act with those who remain the most marginalized from our institutions, including those spaces that produce AIDS knowledge, politics, and policies. Where I have participated in symposia, conferences, and exhibitions explicitly addressing AIDS, it is often the case that people of color and the Global South in general, but especially women of color and trans people of color, are not represented or are severely underrepresented. That is also the case within this volume, AIDS *and the Distribution of Crises*, wherein women of color feminisms are drawn upon for critical thinking and yet the impact of AIDS upon women of color and trans people of color are not frequently enough the topic of study. This is a problem that is endemic to many kinds of institutional discourses—academic, epidemiological, public health, policy, and more—on AIDS, which then greatly impacts the broader public view. By observing and turning to the roadmaps of how women of color feminisms and queer and trans of color critiques mobilize intersectional thinking and coalitional organizing within and across institutions—even as these voices are minoritized within these institutions—we gain insight into how histories of power are interrogated in the present.

During the fall of 2018, as I struggled to complete revisions to this piece of writing in response to the incisive comments provided by the external reviewers and press editors, I found myself stifled and panicking about how to counter growing fascism while supporting those students who are most vulnerable to structural violence. Is writing and publishing drawing me away from attending to students who lack the resources and family care to sustain their livelihood during frightening times? Yes. What is also crucial to recall is that AIDS activism has always been a social movement embedded simultaneously in extensive coalitional organizing, direct action, and artistic and scholarly forms.[33] As Cohen and others who have taken up women of color feminisms remind us, AIDS activism crossed institutional and disciplinary boundaries as well as social justice movements to address historical amnesia and our crises in knowledge production. These pedagogical interventions move much faster than our institutional knowledge forms, including our timelines for conferences, exhibitions, and published writing.[34] In this sense, what is written here is a much delayed reaction to the ways in which women of color feminist and queer and trans of color praxes circulate within and beyond institutions. Yet, in asking these questions about the relationship between women of color feminisms, queer and trans of color critiques, and AIDS politics, we continue to present within our institutions the already existing roadmaps that address the urgent need to attend to histories of power that are neither linear or progressive but operate through sudden shifts, recursions, and yet always breakable patterns that open the possibilities toward radical futures.

Notes

Adapted from Jih-Fei Cheng, "AIDS, Black Feminisms, and the Institutionalization of Queer Politics," GLQ 25, no. 1 (2019): 169–77. © 2019 Duke University Press. My heartfelt gratitude goes to Tatissa Zunguze and all the students who have foregrounded Black feminisms in the struggles for social and economic justice; to Cathy J. Cohen for creating a living document through which to manifest the intellectual, cultural, and political interventions of Black, feminist, and queer studies; to the editors of GLQ, Alexandra Juhasz, Nishant Shahani, C. Riley Snorton, and Abigail Nubla-Kung, for their extensive feedback and support in this writing; and, finally, to my dear friend and comrade Nic John Ramos, who organized the "Punks" commemorative panel at the 2017 Annual Meeting of the American Studies Association.

1   Wolfe, "Shea Stadium Women's Action."
2   Garza, Cullors, and Tometi, "Herstory"; Burke, "MeToo Founder"; TallBear, "Badass (Indigenous) Women".
3   Robinson, Black Marxism; Haley, No Mercy Here; Reddy, "Neoliberalism Then and Now."
4   This section title was inspired by the language introduced in a proposal for a faculty workshop, titled "Queer/Trans* of Color Critique in a Liberal Arts Context," authored by Ren-yo Hwang (Mount Holyoke College) and Treva Ellison (Dartmouth College), and awarded by the Alliance to Advance Liberal Arts Colleges for the 2018–19 academic year. Co-conveners included Kyla Wazana Tompkins (Pomona College), Jih-Fei Cheng (Scripps College), and Jennifer DeClue (Smith College).

5   Scripps College, "About Scripps College."

6   Wells, *Crusade for Justice*, 151–52.

7   Scripps College, "IDEA Initiative."

8   Scripps College, "At a Glance."

9   Scripps College, "At a Glance."

10 Bramlett, "Loss of Student"; Zunguze Family, "In Memoriam."

11 Cohen, "Punks," 438.

12 Cohen, "Punks," 438.

13 Cohen, "Punks," 440.

14 Cohen, "Punks," 460.

15 Cohen, "Punks," 441–42.

16 Cohen, "Punks," 455.

17 Cheng, "How to Survive."

18 Shahani, "How to Survive the Whitewashing."

19 Cheng, "How to Survive."

20 Juhasz, *AIDS TV*. My forthcoming monograph includes a chapter that examines
    the contemporary adaptation of video activist footage from the earlier years
    of the AIDS crisis, including footage from the documentary film *Voices from
    the Front* (1992) by the Testing the Limits Collective. Drawing upon the
    scholarship and activism of Evelynn Hammonds, I analyze how the footage of
    Voices continues to reveal AIDS activists' intentional efforts to foreground Black
    feminisms and the crucial leadership of Black and other women of color.

21 Tacoma Action Collective, "STOP ERASING BLACK PEOPLE."

22 Gossett, "Reina Gossett on Transgender Storytelling."

23 Weiss, "'The Death and Life of Marsha P. Johnson.'"

24 Combahee River Collective, "Combahee River Collective Statement";
    Robinson, *Black Marxism*; Kelley, *Freedom Dreams*; Moten, *In the Break*;
    McLane-Davison, "Lifting"; Taylor, *How We Get Free*.

25 Cohen, "Foreword," xiii.

26 Casil, "Don't Expect Nothing."

27 Singh, *Black Is a Country*.

28 Geary, *Antiblack Racism*, 23.

29 For examples of scholarship that take up this question, see, among others,
    TallBear, *Native American DNA*; Snorton, *Black on Both Sides*; and Chen,
    Animacies.

30 End Rape on Campus, "Survivor of Color."

31 Positive Women's Network, "Fact Sheet"; Center for HIV Law and Policy, *HIV
    Criminalization*.

32 Farrow, "#MeToo Movement Founder." For research and writing on the topic
    of queer and trans people of color and childhood sexual assault, see Swadhin,
    "Mirror Memoirs."

33 Juhasz, *AIDS TV*.

34 I thank one of our Duke University Press anonymous confidential readers for
    this keen observation.

Bibliography

Bramlett, Matthew. "Loss of Student Leaves College Community in Mourning." *Claremont Courier*, March 9, 2017. https://www.claremont-courier.com/articles /news/t22468-student.

Burke, Tarana. "#MeToo Founder Tarana Burke on the Rigorous Work That Still Lies Ahead." *Variety*, September 25, 2018. https://variety.com/2018/biz /features/tarana-burke-metoo-one-year-later-1202954797/.

Casil, Amy Sterling. "Don't Expect Nothing in Return from Scripps College: They Just Want Your Money." *Medium*, April 23, 2017. https://medium.com/real-in -other-words/dont-expect-nothing-in-return-from-scripps-college-they-just -want-your-money-79699d345897.

Center for HIV Law and Policy. *HIV Criminalization in the United States: A Sourcebook on State and Federal HIV Criminal Law and Practice*. 3rd ed. New York: Center for HIV Law and Policy, 2017. http://www.hivlawandpolicy.org /sourcebook.

Chen, Mel Y. *Animacies: Biopolitics, Racial Mattering, and Queer Affect*. Perverse Modernities. Durham, NC: Duke University Press, 2012.

Cheng, Jih-Fei. "How to Survive: AIDS and Its Afterlives in Popular Media." *Women's Studies Quarterly* 44, nos. 1/2 (2016): 73–92.

Cohen, Cathy J. "Foreword." In *No Tea, No Shade: New Writings in Black Queer Studies*, edited by E. Patrick Johnson, xi–xiv. Durham, NC: Duke University Press, 2016.

Cohen, Cathy J. "Punks, Bulldaggers, and Welfare Queens: The Radical Potential of Queer Politics?" *GLQ: A Journal of Lesbian and Gay Studies* 3, no. 4 (1997): 437–65.

Cohen, Cathy J., and Sarah J. Jackson. "Ask a Feminist: A Conversation with Cathy J. Cohen on Black Lives Matter, Feminism, and Contemporary Activism." *Signs: Journal of Women in Culture and Society* 41, no. 4 (2016): 775–92.

Combahee River Collective. "Combahee River Collective Statement." 1977. http:// circuitous.org/scraps/combahee.html.

Dunye, Cheryl, dir. *The Watermelon Woman*. New York: First Run Features, 1997. VHS.

End Rape on Campus. "Survivor of Color Prevalence Rates." Accessed November 17, 2018. https://endrapeoncampus.org/new-page-3/.

Farrow, Kenyon. "#MeToo Movement Founder Tarana Burke Opens the Biomedical HIV Prevention Summit—and a Conversation about Sexual Violence and Harassment." TheBody, December 6, 2018. https://www.thebody .com/content/81518/metoo-movement-founder-tarana-burke-opens-the-biom .html?ic=tbhwnbox&fbclid=IwAR2nDNnhavgjtoPPk4iHto8wFEBWVAj -GudNzgt_amp4Q5yGZvEfzcr2a18.

Ferguson, Roderick A. *Aberrations in Black: Toward a Queer of Color Critique*. Minneapolis: University of Minnesota Press, 2004.

Ferguson, Roderick A. *The Reorder of Things: The University and Its Pedagogies of Minority Difference*. Minneapolis: University of Minnesota Press, 2012.

France, David, dir. *How to Survive a Plague*. New York: Sundance Selects, 2012. DVD.

France, David, dir. *The Life and Death of Marsha P. Johnson*. Los Gatos, CA: Netflix, 2017.

Garza, Alicia, Patrisse Cullors, and Opal Tometi. "Herstory." Accessed November 17, 2018. https://blacklivesmatter.com/about/herstory/.

Geary, Adam M. *Antiblack Racism and the AIDS Epidemic: State Intimacies*. New York: Palgrave Macmillan, 2014.

Gossett, Reina. "Reina Gossett on Transgender Storytelling, David France, and the Netflix Marsha P. Johnson Documentary." *Teen Vogue*, October 11, 2017. https://www.teenvogue.com/story/reina-gossett-marsha-p-johnson-op-ed.

Haley, Sarah. *No Mercy Here: Gender, Punishment, and the Making of Jim Crow Modernity*. Chapel Hill: University of North Carolina Press, 2016.

Juhasz, Alexandra. *AIDS TV: Identity, Community, and Alternative Video*. Durham, NC: Duke University Press, 1995.

Kelley, Robin D. G. *Freedom Dreams: The Black Radical Imagination*. Boston: Beacon, 2003.

McLane-Davison, Denise. "Lifting: Black Feminist Leadership in the Fight against HIV/AIDS." *Journal of Women and Social Work* 31, no. 1 (2016): 55–69.

Moten, Fred. *In the Break: The Aesthetics of the Black Radical Tradition*. Minneapolis: University of Minnesota Press, 2003.

Positive Women's Network. "Fact Sheet: Criminalization as Violence against Women Living with HIV." Accessed November 17, 2018. https://www.pwn-usa.org/doa2016/factsheet-doa2016/.

Reddy, Chandan. "Neoliberalism Then and Now: Race, Sexuality, and the Black Radical Tradition." *GLQ: A Journal of Gay and Lesbian Studies* 25, no. 1 (2019): 150–55.

Robinson, Cedric J. *Black Marxism: The Making of a Black Radical Tradition*. London: Zed, 1983.

Scripps College. "About Scripps College." Accessed March 17, 2018. http://catalog.scrippscollege.edu/content.php?catoid=9&navoid=628.

Scripps College. "At a Glance." Accessed March 17, 2018. http://www.scrippscollege.edu/about/glance.

Scripps College. "IDEA Initiative at Scripps College." Accessed November 17, 2018. http://www.scrippscollege.edu/diversity/about/institutional-capacity-building.

Shahani, Nishant. "How to Survive the Whitewashing of AIDS: Global Pasts, Transnational Futures." *QED: A Journal in GLTBQ Worldmaking* 3, no. 1 (2016): 1–33.

Singh, Nikhil Pal. *Black Is a Country: Race and the Unfinished Struggle for Democracy*. Cambridge, MA: Harvard University Press, 2004.

Snorton, C. Riley. *Black on Both Sides: A Racial History of Trans Identity*. Minneapolis: University of Minnesota Press, 2017.

Swadhin, Amita. "Mirror Memoirs." Accessed December 12, 2018. https://mirrormemoirs.com.

Tacoma Action Collective. "Stop Erasing Black People." Accessed March 1, 2017. http://stoperasingblackpeoplenow.tumblr.com.

TallBear, Kimberly. "Badass (Indigenous) Women Caretake Relations: #NoDAPL, #IdleNoMore, #BlackLivesMatter." Hot Spots, *Fieldsights*, December 22, 2016. https://culanth.org/fieldsights/badass-indigenous-women-caretake-relations-no-dapl-idle-no-more-black-lives-matter.

TallBear, Kimberly. *Native American DNA: Tribal Belonging and the False Promise of Genetic Science*. Minneapolis: University of Minnesota Press, 2013.

Taylor, Keeanga-Yamahtta. *How We Get Free: Black Feminism and the Combahee River Collective*. Chicago: Haymarket Books, 2017.

Visual AIDS. "Alternate Endings, Radical Beginnings." December 2017. https://visualaids.org/projects/alternate-endings-radical-beginnings.

Weiss, Suzannah. "'The Death and Life of Marsha P. Johnson' Creator Accused of Stealing Work from Filmmaker Reina Gossett." *Teen Vogue*, October 8, 2017. https://www.teenvogue.com/story/marsha-p-johnson-documentary-david-france-reina-gossett-stealing-accusations.

Wells, Ida B. *Crusade for Justice: The Autobiography of Ida B. Wells*. Edited by Alfreda M. Duster. Chicago: University of Chicago Press, 1991.

Wolfe, Maxine. "Shea Stadium Women's Action." Actupny.org. https://actupny.org/diva/CBstory-shea.html

Zunguze Family. "In Memoriam: Tatissa Zunguze SC '18 Remembered for Scripps Leadership, Passion for Social Justice." *Student Life*, April 14, 2017. http://tsl.news/news/6706/.

FOUR SAFE, SOULFUL SEX: HIV/AIDS TALK

Julia S. Jordan-Zachery

Editors' Note

As a reprint of a chapter from her book *Shadow Bodies: Black Women, Ideology, Representation, and Politics* (Rutgers University Press, 2017), Julia S. Jordan-Zachery's contribution to this volume asks and responds to a crucial and confounding question regarding Black women's experiences with the AIDS pandemic:

> "Is it a crisis if it is not seen?"

To recall, Black women were immediately invisibilized by the popular representational emphasis on white (gay) men when the "Patient Zero" myth took hold to shape the public imagination of AIDS. According to the myth, AIDS only emerged and mattered when a cluster of North American white gay men's sexual activity and disease transmission could be seemingly traced back to the French Canadian flight attendant Gaëtan Dugas around 1981. As mentioned several times throughout this volume, that myth has long since been debunked. Activists, artists, and scholars continue to upend this narrative. However, its grip on the public imagination has manifested in public health policies that continue to trace HIV transmission based upon fixed identities and presumed behaviors rather than structural forms of violence. This includes the emphasis on proving high rates of HIV infection and cumulative AIDS diagnoses among a given population. Meanwhile, the historical and persistent barriers that Black women continue to face among all US institutions, which leaves their experiences and lives unaccounted for, are left unexamined. Without analyzing and addressing these forms of structural violence, the miscategorizations, misrepresentations, and misrecognitions of Black women amid the AIDS pandemic will persist.

Jordan-Zachery's research in health policy leads her to address what she calls "shadow bodies"—Black women whose experiences with structural violence are subtended by histories of racialization, gendering, and sexualization as well as the limitations that proscribe the already marginalized arenas for Black women's public discourse. In particular, she examines the cultural representations of Black women in literature and music. In the chapter that appears in this volume, Jordan-Zachery focuses on how AIDS is addressed by contemporary Black congresswomen, *Essence* and *Ebony* magazines, and Black women bloggers. She considers how the long-standing "scripts" about the bodies and lives of Black women, developed since the era of enslavement and maintained throughout the postslavery era, continue to elide from progressive political agendas the compounding issues faced by Black women who remain the most vulnerable to structural violence—that is, Black lesbians, Black trans women, Black women who have engaged in sex work, and Black women who have been incarcerated, to name a few "shadow bodies."

As Jordan-Zachery theorizes in an earlier chapter of *Shadow Bodies*, two commonly rehearsed "scripts" circumscribe Black women's bodies and experiences:

> [The *Ass* script] is actually a compilation of three subscripts—the *physical ass*, a *piece of ass* (sexual relations), and, borrowing from Ralph Ellison (1995), the *ass question*—which focuses on issues of democracy and belongingness. The second script is one of the *Strong Black Woman*—that is externally and internally ascribed onto Black women's bodies, and over time has resulted in the muting or silencing of Black women. Similar to the *Ass* script, there are three (at least) subscripts that constitute this larger *Strong Black Woman* script: *physical strength*, *sacrificial/nurturing*, and *spiritual/supernatural*. These metascripts are used to show how Black women, via the discourses used by Black women, become shadow bodies.[1]

Jordan-Zachery's analyses take stock of the cultural prohibitions set against the articulations of Black women's bodies and knowledge. To understand the longer historical trajectory of these scripts, and their operations across multiple sites of Black women's health and political issues, one must read *Shadow Bodies*. The book's attentiveness to how these scripts function in various fora for Black women's political discourse and policy initiatives underscores how AIDS has been, erroneously and fatalistically, separated from other arenas of Black women's lives, such as housing and education. Jordan-Zachery's chapter featured in this volume prompts our readers to consider how epidemiology, public discourse, and health policy fail to apply the intersectional feminist analyses necessary in order to effectively end the AIDS pandemic. In turn, Jordan-Zachery reveals and challenges how the "Patient Zero" narrative itself is an enduring colonial, white supremacist, patriarchal, and classist script that fuels our cultural representations and public health policies. Meanwhile, that "Patient Zero" script depends entirely on the persistence of the *Ass* and *Strong Black Woman* scripts, which devalue, invisibilize, and silence Black women while also denying their foundational, complex, and ongoing cultural, intellectual, and activist work to end all forms of structural violence, including the AIDS pandemic.

Years ago, I organized an undergraduate course that focused on race, gender, and public policy. I opted to focus on women of color who were affected and impacted by HIV and AIDS. There was a plethora of materials to teach, relatively speaking. But I noticed that there were indeed some gaps. I observed that there were few works that centered on Black women's voices and their lived experiences. Furthermore, there was not much research on AIDS service organizations, particularly those serving communities of color.

Now, as a researcher who focuses on Black women and public policy, I am not particularly surprised by these gaps in the literature. Black feminists, such as Nikol Alexander-Floyd among others, have poignantly written about the absence of Black women in scholarly research. But HIV and AIDS and blackness are particularly vexing, as Cathy J. Cohen points out.[2] There is a type of silence in relation to Black women, HIV, and AIDS. Why do Black women disappear and what are the consequences of such disappearances? These are important questions to consider as we grapple with the notion of crisis (which is as much socially constructed as it is epidemiologically defined) as it relates to HIV and AIDS. Data tells us that Black women are disproportionately affected and impacted by HIV and AIDS and that the spread of the disease is concentrated in communities of color in the United States.[3]

However, is it a crisis if it is not seen? Black women have long talked about our disappearance from society—indeed much has been written on the topic of Black women's invisibility in relation to HIV and AIDS and other social issues. Black feminist theory has sought to counter the narratives of invisibility by bringing Black women from the margins to the center.[4] But who determines the center? In the face of #BlackLivesMatter, we see the assertion of #Sayhername, which is a call to insert Black girls and women into the narratives of Black death that result from state-sanctioned violence. Yes, Black women in the United States are actively participating in the political economy through voting and protest. Yet somehow we are simultaneously disappearing. While it is important to study the mechanics of this disappearance, we need to come back to the question of who gets to be in the center. Specifically, we need to explore how Black women work to bring other Black women from the margin to the center. This chapter explores who gets abandoned in Black women's framing of HIV and AIDS and shows how Black women abandoned other Black women, failing to bring them into the center, through their use of discreet silences.[5]

Much has been written on the silence around HIV/AIDS. This silence has been discussed by journalists and academics alike, with the goal of "breaking the silence" to facilitate the necessary steps to stem the spread of the disease. It is implied that although we are now more than thirty years into the disease, the initial framing still dominates our current thinking. Some of the theorizing suggests that the silence results from the fact that AIDS is still considered a "gay man's disease."[6] Others propose that Black folk and the Black church in particular are silent around HIV/AIDS because of its intimate relationship to morality.[7] While we discuss the silences, what is often not discussed is who among Black women are produced as shadow bodies and what this means for Black gender justice.[8] I argue that the scripts ascribed to Black women's bodies are the templates used to define and understand an issue and that such definitions embody power structures within the Black women's community.[9] In this case there are at least three scripts that influence how Black women speak of Black women who are impacted and affected by HIV and AIDS. There is the *Ass* script, which is actually a compilation of three subscripts— the *physical ass*, a *piece of ass* (sexual relations), and, borrowing from Ralph Ellison (1995), the *ass question*—which focuses on issues of democracy and belongingness. The second script is one of the *Strong Black Woman*—that is externally and internally ascribed onto Black women's bodies, and over time has resulted in the muting or silencing of Black women. Similar to the *Ass* script, there are three (at least) subscripts that constitute this larger *Strong*

Black Woman script: *physical strength, sacrificial/nurturing,* and *spiritual/ supernatural.* These metascripts are used to show how Black women, via the discourses used by Black women, become shadow bodies.[10]

In this chapter I show how such power structures are represented in the talk and silence related to HIV/AIDS and its intersection with Black womanhood to show how shadow bodies are produced. In exploring how some women are abandoned, my focus is on the following:

> Understanding and analyzing the framing employed by Black congresswomen, Black female bloggers, and *Essence* and *Ebony* magazines. Specifically, I ask: how is intersectionality integrated into the HIV/AIDS frames?
>
> Understanding the suggestions made by these women for addressing these issues, I ask how and if the talk is contextualized by Black women's social location and the relationship between structural violence and the spread of HIV/AIDS.

The analysis of the talk brought to the forefront the following frames: (a) celebratory/recognition and (b) human disaster. The frames used to offer suggestions on how to address HIV/AIDS include (a) take care of yourself and (b) education. These general frames incorporate subthemes used by Black female elected officials, *Essence* and *Ebony*, and Black female bloggers. The overarching themes capture how some Black women are rendered shadow bodies and as just abandoned. By centering the above, I am able to then identify and analyze which categories of difference are employed in the talk and if there are silences. As such, I am able to better understand how Black women make sense of HIV/AIDS and its intersection with Black womanhood. By focusing on who is included and excluded in the talk, on what types of actions are advocated for, and what types of actions are excluded from the talk, I am better able to understand intragroup Black women's politics.

The silences in Black congresswomen's, *Essence* and *Ebony*, and Black female bloggers' talk is evident in (a) who is left out, for example Black lesbians; (b) what issues are not discussed, for example structural violence and class; and (c) what types of actions are advocated for—personal responsibility versus public political action. To explain Black women's susceptibility to HIV and later AIDS, researchers argue that Black women's experiences with structural violence bring to the forefront the barriers they confront that increase not only their vulnerability and exposure to the virus but also the barriers and challenges they face in seeking treatment and recognition. The intersectionality of racial discrimination, poverty, racial segregation, high incarceration rates, low-sex ratios, fractured gender identity, gender roles,

stigma, and high levels of illicit drug use results in Black women's disproportionate exposure to HIV and later AIDS.[11] Yet Black women in their talk on
HIV and AIDS do not talk about these issues. To show how these are indeed
discreet silences, I analyze the frames used in the talk. It is only by seeing
what is talked about that one can better see the absence of some frames and
bodies.

Who and What Do We See? Framing HIV/AIDS and Its Intersection with Black Womanhood

Among Black elected officials, HIV/AIDS was discussed on the floor 396
times. Within the pages of *Essence* and *Ebony* magazines, there were a total
128 stories (52 and 76, respectively) on HIV/AIDS, and Black female bloggers had 113 blog posts on the topic. There are two main frames, explored
below, used in the talk on HIV/AIDS: celebratory/recognition and human
disaster. These frames show how discreet silences are used, consciously or
unconsciously, within Black women's talk.

CELEBRATORY/RECOGNITION FRAME

Among Black female elected officials, *Essence* and *Ebony* magazines, and
Black female bloggers, the celebratory frame was the most deployed frame
in their talk on HIV/AIDS. As I explored this dominantly used frame, I asked
what type of cultural and political productions result from such framing. I
present three typical celebratory/recognition sub-frames from elected officials, *Essence* and *Ebony* magazines, and bloggers. What cuts across this
overarching frame, regardless of its structure, in these public spaces of talk
is the deflection of attention from social-structural factors that are critical
in understanding the spread of the virus among Blacks in general and Black
women specifically.

A typical celebratory/recognition frame used among congressional
members looks like this, from Congresswoman Carrie Meek, who served on
behalf of Florida's Seventeenth Congressional District in the US House of
Representatives from 1993 to 2003:

> We must never forget the contributions of those who have gone be-
> fore us. Today as we recognize the 20th Anniversary of the discovery of
> AIDS, I commend the 12 National Organizations from across the coun-
> try, who have come together to launch a national campaign to provide
> health care, treatment, and prevention education and information to

millions of Americans impacted by this epidemic . . . AIDS Action Committee of Massachusetts, AIDS Project Los Angeles, The Balm in Gilead, Broadway Cares, Gay Men's Health Crisis, The National Association of People with AIDS, National Minority AIDS Council, The NAMES Project Foundation, San Francisco AIDS Foundation, and the Whitman-Walker Clinic are all to be commended for coming together in this unique partnership to launch a national public affairs campaign to provide health care, treatment, and prevention education and information to millions of Americans.[12]

Given their social standing as elected officials, the information provided by Meek and other congresswomen serves as legitimized discourse framers that can impose meaning upon and orient attention to particular experiences. Meek's statement of support not only recognizes the organizations but also draws attention to a number of issues in an attempt to address the epidemic. Primarily, her talk centers on awareness and treatment. Embedded in this frame is a silence about how to prevent HIV/AIDS by addressing poverty, incarceration, and housing segregation, for example. In essence, Meek does not offer transformational talk (this is the silence) that challenges HIV/AIDS beyond the personal responsibility approach.

Black women bloggers also center the work of celebrities within the recognition frame. A post by Brown Sista (Sheryl Lee Ralph) offers an example of the celebrity/recognition frame used by bloggers. Brown Sista informs us about the activities of biker babes when she writes:

Actresses Gabrielle Union (Bad Boys 2) and Essence Atkins (Half and Half) will join the all-star celebrity line up for the NABB's Miami International Bikefest 2006 to be held Labor Day weekend in Miami, Florida. Presented by the National Association of Black Bikers (NABB), the Miami International Bikefest will be hosted by BET and radio personality Big Tigger and will bring together Hollywood celebrities, entertainers and athletes for the must-attend charity event August 31—September 3, 2006 in Miami. Joined by TV host Melyssa Ford and R&B Artist Tank, Union and Atkins will support the Miami International Bikefest and the Miami International AIDS Ride; the premier charity event for motorcycle enthusiasts and those attracted to the biking lifestyle. . . . A portion of the event proceeds will go towards donations to Big Tigger's Street Corner Foundation for their work in building public awareness of HIV/AIDS and New Horizons Community Mental Health Center for their work in mental health and substance abuse care. (August 16, 2006)[13]

The work of Ralph, Alicia Keys (Black Girl Gives Back), other celebrities, and their organizations was also prominent in bloggers' recognition frames. In these blog posts it appears that the celebrity is the primary subject in the story and HIV/AIDS is secondary—this can also be read as a form of discreet silence. As such, these posts might be considered more as "gossip" posts. This is an example of what I discussed in the introduction to *Shadow Bodies*. On the surface there seems to be quite a bit of talk on HIV and AIDS; however, the talk fails to critically address HIV or AIDS.

Among bloggers, another recognition frame focused on World AIDS Day and National Women & Girls HIV/AIDS Awareness Day, and the resulting campaigns/activities of this day. Consider posts by Afrobella, whose entries were titled, for example, "Are You Rocking Red Pumps Today?" Afrobella tells her readers:

> Bellas, I can't even really *wear* heels, but today on Afrobella I'm proud to represent and rock these fly Alexander McQueen red pumps online all day! Today is National Women & Girls HIV/AIDS Awareness Day. One year ago, Karyn and Luvvie founded The Red Pump Project—an enthusiastic non profit organization which has tirelessly worked to raise awareness both online, and with a series of awesome events around the country. Today marks the celebration of the 500 in 50: Rock the Red Pump campaign—where fellow bloggers are encouraged to be part of the movement and show solidarity by featuring a Red Pump badge on their blog. And to write about what National Women & Girls HIV/AIDS Awareness Day means to them.[14]

Posts such as the examples shared above prioritize concerns and normalize some behaviors—charity becomes the norm. Consequently, this talk can make invisible other concerns and alternate forms of action. Activities or programs such as "Rock the Red Pumps" represent a rather abstract and depersonalized way of addressing the issue of HIV/AIDS. Such an approach is similar to the "pinking" of products used in campaigns designed to raise breast cancer awareness. It is suggested that such campaigns are simply marketing ploys.[15] Pinking, similar to Rock the Red and other such campaigns, tends to focus on buying products (as a means of helping those in need). Furthermore, as Verta Taylor and Marieke Van Willigen argue, the self-help movement that characterized the breast cancer movement of the 1990s fostered a movement that promotes internal reflection and personal transformation as opposed to external or structural change.[16] Like pinking, rocking the red pump seems suitable for encouraging a volunteer citizen while making HIV/AIDS "chic" as it is linked more to celebrities than "regular" people. It promotes the status quo of our approach to HIV/AIDS, which encourages charity and not politics. What this suggests is a form of silence where HIV and AIDS are not linked to structural factors that require political action to foster and demand change. The personal approach, specifically the consumer approach, renders silent the role of government policy in addressing AIDS. Consequently, the US federal government can continue its long-standing policy of no national AIDS policy outside the Ryan White Act.

Similarly, *Essence* and *Ebony* magazines recognized the actions of celebrities in their talk on HIV/AIDS. In 2001, Cori Murray saluted "20 of the most outstanding sisters leading the war on HIV/AIDS."[17] Included in the list of women who were recognized were legislators, community pillars, facilitators, and the fact keeper. Also recognized was Nella P. Mupier (Miss Prairie View A&M University Queen) for her HIV/AIDS activism.[18] Sports figures and celebrities, such as Magic Johnson, Montel Williams, and Alicia Keys, were also recognized for their HIV/AIDS activism.[19] Such frames more often than not took the following form: "In the last few years, the Jamie Foxx Foundation has supported causes related to orphanages in Haiti, HIV/AIDS in Africa through Save Africa's Children, and victims of Hurricane Katrina."[20] Again, we see that charity as opposed to activism is promoted within this type of framing.

The deployment of a celebratory frame as a means of discussing HIV/AIDS can be inspiring and can encourage others to become involved in the fight against HIV/AIDS even if only in the form of charitable giving. However, while Black women are talking about HIV/AIDS, there is a silence. A celebratory frame fails to highlight how women live daily with AIDS and puts some distance between non-HIV-positive and HIV-positive women. These women become invisible, a form of discreet silence, as society never has to "see" them and as such never has to see their struggles as real. The result of this silence, in part, is reflected in how the Black community specifically and the wider society in general makes demands for the protection of this segment of the body politic. While the work of celebrities is highlighted in the talk, the HIV/AIDS status of these individuals remains private. In comparison, the talk on celebrity and mental illness, and to some extent domestic violence, speaks directly to celebrity experiences. This contributes to the silence. While HIV/AIDS appears to be in the public arena, the disease itself remains in the private realm. Consequently, Black women who are HIV positive and those living with AIDS become shadows when this celebratory frame is used because of the limited talk. Additionally, such a frame does very little to center the relationship between structural factors such as poverty, oppressive structures such as sexism, and the spread of HIV/AIDS among Black women.

HUMAN DISASTER FRAME

Beyond the celebratory frame, Black women also employ a human disaster frame in their talk on HIV/AIDS. A human disaster frame is one that includes discussion on the number of victims, the impact on the individual and their family and society, and the prevalence of the illness. I borrow this frame, in part, from prior research that coded HIV/AIDS discourses.[21] As we analyze this frame, we must ask: How does it work to encourage an inclusive social action? Below I offer three representative examples of this frame. These examples highlight the similarity in the talk of this issue among congress-women, *Essence* and *Ebony*, and bloggers.

Congresswoman Maxine Waters, in discussing the spread of the disease and the changing face of HIV/AIDS, opined: "What do we find when we look at the African American community? We find, of course, that it is the leading cause of death for African Americans between the ages of 25 and 44. What do we find when we look at African-American women? We find that in the new AIDS cases, we are 30 percent of that population. We also find that we are infected 16 times more than white women."[22]

In *Essence* and *Ebony* magazines, the human disaster frame assumed the format of the following example: "Black females are diagnosed with HIV at 20 times the rate of White females and more than four times the rate of Hispanic females. Among Black females, roughly 78 percent of the HIV diagnoses were attributed to high-risk heterosexual contact. Intravenous drug use accounted for 19 percent."[23]

A post by Brown Girl Gumbo is illustrative of the human disaster frame used among bloggers. She writes: "According to the Centers for Disease Control, we African-Americans face the most severe burden of HIV in the United States. At the end of 2007, we accounted for almost half (46 percent) of people living with a diagnosis of HIV infection in the 37 states and 5 US dependent areas with long-term, confidential, name-based HIV reporting."[24] Beyond such reporting, Black women were often not explicitly discussed among bloggers.

The human disaster frame is often presented in a neutral and value-free manner. A human disaster frame, which relies on statistics, is frequently thought of as reflecting objective reality. The notion of an objective reality is used to offer the recipients of this frame a "realistic" depiction of HIV/AIDS and infected individuals. However, what remains hidden is the subjective decision of frame selection. Such a frame, while speaking to Black women's susceptibility, does not address risk factors—including those at the micro- and macrolevels. As such, it might be easier for some to dismiss this frame, as they do not see themselves as being susceptible to the virus. Additionally, this seemingly neutral and value-free frame can hide the realities of the women behind these statistics. Consequently, alternative framing that might make HIV and AIDS real and visible is ignored—therein lies another form of silence.

While the human disaster frame is used in Black women's talk on HIV/ AIDS to inform the listener/reader of the spread of HIV/AIDS, it is employed in a rather restricted manner. Such framing tends not to include talk of the realities of women living with HIV/AIDS and the impact on their families. For example, there are no stories in *Essence* and *Ebony* that profile women who are living daily with HIV/AIDS. However, there exist stories of women who have "triumphed" over domestic violence. In AIDS stories we tend not to see Black women portrayed as "patients," "survivors," or HIV-positive political actors. Thus, HIV/AIDS remains in the abstract realm. We have to ask: How does this human disaster frame work to transform HIV/AIDS from a personal problem into a social issue with consequences for the larger Black community?

Manifest in the framing of HIV/AIDS and its intersection with Black womanhood as a social problem are both the *Ass* and *Strong Black Woman* scripts. The use of these scripts, often implicitly, leads to a type of misrecognition and possibly a denial of the intersecting factors that contribute to the spread of the disease among Black women. Consequently, to borrow from Elmer E. Schattschneider, many of the controversial factors, such as sexism, are organized out of politics.[25] This is evident in the two frames discussed above. Neither the "celebratory" frame nor the "human disaster" frame, in terms of their content, speaks to the multiplicity of identities of Black women who are affected by the disease. Alberto Melucci argues that "collective identity is an interactive and shared definition produced by several individuals (or groups as a more complex level) and concerned with the orientation of action and fields of opportunities and constraints in which the action take place."[26] The *Ass* and *Strong Black Woman* scripts prescribe opportunities and constructions for actions. In the case of HIV/AIDS, these scripts do not permit Black women to engage, in a substantive manner, with the multiplicity of Black womanhood as they serve to delimit the understanding of community by determining who is talked about and why.

Missing in the Stories on HIV/AIDS:
Black Women and Their Lived Realities

In this section, I consider how diverse Black women are represented in the HIV/AIDS talk. More specifically, I analyze how gender, class, and sexual identity, in the vein of Black feminism, are utilized in the talk. The tension between making visible Black women's experience with HIV/AIDS and also making them invisible becomes apparent in the structuring of the talk. Although the women spoke of Black women and HIV/AIDS, generally the talk did not address the structural factors often cited as contributing to the spread of the disease among Black women.

Consider this response that appeared in *Ebony* magazine. A letter writer asked, "Why have African-American women become the fastest-growing group of new HIV/AIDS cases?" Dr. Lorraine Cole responded:

> It is a result of unprotected sex with an infected partner. Biologically, women are more susceptible to contracting the virus than men and, subsequently, contract the disease at twice the rate as men. Women often believe they are in a monogamous relationship when they are not. A further complication is that many infected individuals do not know their HIV status and don't get early treatment or take precautions when engaging in sexual behavior. Also, one out of every three Black women does not have health insurance to access routine care, that means health problems that place some women at greater risk for contracting HIV are undetected.[27]

A primary focus on the response is on intimate relationships and as such her focus remains in the private realm and at the individual level. In her response, Dr. Cole speaks fleetingly of the issue of Black women's access to health care. However, she does not address gender roles and a host of other factors that contribute to the spread of the virus among Black women; this is a form of discreet silence, the unwillingness to discuss Black gender politics. These factors, cited by researchers such as Adaora A. Adimora and Victor J. Schoenbach and Eric R. Wright and Tiffany N. Martin, are often left out in the talk by Black women.[28] Although some Black women make HIV/AIDS visible in their talk, they are also making some Black women's experiences with the disease invisible—those who are susceptible to the disease as a result of gender politics, those who are lesbian and/or bisexual for example, and those for whom poverty enhances their susceptibility to the virus—thus casting them as shadows at best in the public understanding of the disease. It is important to consider what is left out of the talk as it helps us analyze and explain how some Black women become shadow bodies. Below, I present examples of how this type of shadowing occurs. I start with the issue of gender.

One might argue that Black women's talk on HIV/AIDS does center gender. In their use of the human disaster frame, Black women do rely on statistics that speak to the rate of infection among Black women and other groups. While statistics are useful in telling stories of the extent of the disease among Black women, they do not speak to the relationship between the spread of HIV/AIDS and gender. Gender—roles, practices, and resulting sexual scripts—is also a part of the contextual factors that influence Black women's exposure to HIV and AIDS. In terms of the gendering of AIDS, Margaret Weeks, Merrill Singer, Maryland Grier, and Jean J. Schensul inform us that "gender definitions and relations embody multidimensional ideals and interactions among women and men, including those associated with desires, preferences, and practices. They also express and embody relationships of power and dominance, assign value to kinds of sexual behaviors and relationships, and impose codes for 'traditional,' acceptable and forbidden roles and behaviors."[29]

Gender norms and resulting sexual scripts further perpetuate women's inequitable position, relative to men's, but such a frame is absent in the talk among Black women. There is a value of including such a frame in the talk on HIV/AIDS. Sexual scripts, as argued by William Simon and John Gagnon, include cultural, interpersonal, and intrapersonal scripts that are used to inform and influence the individual's sexual decisions.[30] The relative permanence of these scripts transcends time. Black women's reliance on existing gender norms and their ensuing sexual scripts can result in: sexually passivity engaging in unprotected sex, and/or in their inconsistent or nonuse of condoms because they see such behavior as normative or outside of the domain of the "good" woman.[31] Black women did little to address and/or challenge gender roles, practices, and sexual scripts in their HIV/AIDS talk, and therefore failed to address gender equity and justice for Black women. Such failure is but one manifestation of discreet silences and reflects on how the subscript of the *ass question*, which looks at Black gender politics, influences collective action or inaction in this case. Given the failure of the larger Black community to critically engage in gender politics, the Black women who inform this study focus on the act of sex and not gender inequality that influences how women engage in sex acts.[32] Furthermore, in their understanding of the spread of HIV/AIDS, they render silent a potential cultural approach to addressing and understanding this public health crisis.

In *Essence* magazine there was one article that explicitly discussed the issue of gender bias and its impact on Black women. It states:

> Men get more attention and more intensive treatment. At my clinic, I see women go into the doctor's office and come out in five minutes; men go in and come out in an hour. I think the doctors pay more attention to men because it was originally considered a man's disease. And they don't listen to Black women. They put us in a box—either you're a prostitute or a drug addict. Once they put you in a box, they stop listening to what your needs are, prescribe some drugs and send you on your way. I'm lucky I have a female doctor who listens. She understands that I'm a woman and that I have different needs. Still, it's real scary. I see Black women getting pushed against the wall and not being taken care of.[33]

Dunn, Perry and Wiltz utilize a Black feminist stance, particularly in her treatment of the intersection of race and gender and the lived realities of Black women. In their article, Dunn, Perry and Wiltz seek to empower readers by addressing the powerless position of women, relative to men, and how such a position complicates their treatment in general. They actively engage the limiting quality of the *ass question* subscript. However, in her talk there is an implicit assumption that this is a universal experience among women, and so, for example, class does not influence the nature of treatment received by Black women. (I discuss this form of silence below.)

The silence on the relationship between gender and the spread of HIV/AIDS continues even among the "new" media (i.e., blog posts). Bloggers did not address Black sexual politics, gender roles and expectations, and the relationship to the spread of the virus among Black women. There were minimum posts that challenge the notion that Black women are the "new face" of AIDS. As argued by Brown Sista:

> As a Black woman, I'm so sick and tired of every time there is a media story about HIV/AIDS, a Black woman is featured predominately front and center. For example, Black In America, which was watched by nearly 5 million people in CNN's two-day airing, dedicated nearly the entire HIV/AIDS segment enforcing the poster person to be a Black female, but there are numerous other examples. Making a Black female the face of HIV/AIDS is a radical form of racism at its highest level and more proof that there is a conspiracy to keep Black women without love. This image of Black women creates more negative stereotypes that Black women are diseased and along with being loud, fat, bitches and hos, who are

overbearing, booty-bouncing, undesirable she-men, no wonder Black women are the least married; sadly unbeknown, Black Women Need Love, Too! The trickery to take the stigma of HIV/AIDS from being a White male homosexual disease to being a Black female heterosexual disease is consistent with racism in America. I cannot allow this type of deliberate prejudice to continue, especially since this is a big fallacy and here's why . . . : HIV/AIDS is NOT a female disease! Black women have NEVER encompassed the highest number of HIV/AIDS cases—the quote was "Black women are the FASTEST growing group of HIV/AIDS," which is no longer true, meaning Black women were growing in numbers fastest, but are not the most. Then why are Black women positioned predominately everywhere when this virus is discussed? The answer is RACISM and MISOGYNY at its finest. (August 13, 2008)

Gina The Blogmother continues this critique with her assertion that "AIDS Is NOT a 'Black Disease.'" She tells readers that she "questions his [Phil Wilson, founder and CEO of Black AIDS Institute] marketing methods" in terms of linking HIV/AIDS to Black folk. This marketing approach, she posits, was shortsighted because of "the damage that will likely follow if people are able to write off AIDS as a problem for 'that other group of people.'" She sees the problems as encompassing "a loss of funding, compassion and drug research." Why? Because, to paraphrase, Black folk are treated as second-class citizens.[34]

It is worth mentioning that another challenge (again, minimally employed) focused on the mainstream media's depiction of Black women and HIV/AIDS. *The Sauda Voice* blog made such a challenge when the blogger posted, "For the past several years, black women have comprised the largest number of new HIV-AIDS cases in America. *Didn't know?* I'm not surprised. Little to no attention has been paid to this growing epidemic by the mainstream media (MSM). Is it because the devastation is primarily affecting people of color? Perhaps, but one can only speculate at this point."[35]

Brown Sista and *The Sauda Voice*, in the vein of the Combahee River Collective and other Black critical scholars, are challenging the use of the social construction of Black womanhood in the organization of society. By challenging the racialization of HIV/AIDS, they highlight the possible damage—from both hypervisibility and invisibility—that can result from these often employed constructions. It is posts such as these, the notes between the silences, that hint at Black feminist practice. However, the posts simultaneously ignore how gender influences Black women's vulnerability to the virus. Thus, Black women who are HIV positive and those with AIDS are simultaneously visible and not visible; they are there but not there. This is the process that renders them shadow bodies in politics.

With respect to HIV/AIDS and its relation to social class, there are also limited, and often indirect, references appearing in Black women's talk. Throughout the 113 blog posts, there was one explicit reference to social class made in a blog titled *A Lady's Perspective*. In this post, she states,

> The HIV/AIDS epidemic in African American communities is a continuing public health crisis for the United States. At the end of 2006 there were an estimated 1.1 million people living with HIV infection, of which almost half (46 percent) were black/African American. While blacks represent approximately 12 percent of the U.S. population, they continue to account for a higher proportion of cases at all stages of HIV/AIDS— from infection with HIV to death with AIDS—compared with members of other races and ethnicities. The reasons are not directly related to race or ethnicity, but rather some of the barriers faced by many African Americans. These barriers can include poverty (being poor), and stigma (negative attitudes, beliefs, and actions directed at people living with HIV/AIDS or people who do things that might put them at risk for HIV).[36]

Ignoring the relationship between economic status and susceptibility to HIV/AIDS can limit our response to the spread of the virus. While it is important to recognize that the virus is not bounded by economic class, in our desire to be universal we must remain mindful that there is a relationship between the prevalence of HIV/AIDS and individuals of a lower economic bracket.[37] Additionally, we also have to recognize that an individual's economic resources influence how she can live with HIV and AIDS in terms of access to care for example.[38]

Black congresswomen very rarely explicitly integrated poverty and class in their talk—that is, specific use of the terms. Instead, access to health care appears to serve as the proxy to discuss issues of class and poverty and HIV/AIDS. Congresswoman Maxine Waters articulated one such frame when she stated, "The Ryan White CARE Act is critical for minorities who often lack access to traditional health care and support services. About half of all Ryan White Care Act clients are black, and that proportion is much higher in some care settings."[39]

What was often missing from this frame is an explicit understanding and/or questioning of how the lack of access to care influences Black women's vulnerability to and experiences with HIV/AIDS. This silence I interpret as a manifestation of the *spiritual/supernatural strength* subscript ascribed to Black women's bodies. This script, which is part of the *Strong Black Woman* metascript, suggests that Black women somehow are able to cope regardless of the structural violence levied against them. Thus, Black women who are affected by HIV/AIDS, because its understanding is coupled with a narrative of transcendence, cannot be talked about as they challenge the narrative of progress and respectability that is often relied upon by many in the Black community.[40]

Over the ten-year period covered in this study, there were three explicit references to economic class and its relationship to HIV/AIDS within the pages of *Essence* and *Ebony*. In the article "An HIV Cure?" it was asserted:

Community Outreach in the United States, HIV/AIDS treatment dollars are available, and most people who need care get it. But what of the groups that show increasing infection rates—namely women of color and young gay Black men? "Many factors have led to the upsurge, including poverty, drug abuse, lack of education and jobs," says Arboleda. Activists are lobbying to ensure that appropriate education and treatment reach people of color.[41]

Another reference to class stated, "Along with ending the silence, experts say prevention efforts must address socioeconomic factors, such as poverty, that discourage Black women from getting diagnosed and seeking treatment. 'The epidemic disproportionately affects people who are poor,' says Dr. Gayle. 'They have poor access to information, poor access to health care and services.'"[42]

The above two quotations focused on issues of poverty. However, the third reference was different in comparison. The third referenced the intersection of class and HIV/AIDS by centering middle-class Black women. Accordingly, it stated:

Unfortunately, many Sisters make that same mistake, experts say. "Part of the problem reaching middle-class Black women who have achieved a certain level of success is that they think AIDS is for other women of color," says Dr. Cargill. "They think if he's a nice guy with a nice car and lives in a nice neighborhood, he couldn't possibly be infected with HIV. But HIV doesn't care if he has a Rolex watch or if he went to the premier college in the land. It's about risk behavior."[43]

Given the minimum references to the relationship between class and the spread of HIV/AIDS, I assume that *Essence* and *Ebony* sought to show the universality of the spread of the disease regardless of economic class. The unwillingness to talk about the relationship between economic class and HIV/AIDS must be read in this context of Black women's politics. Such politics often responds to the negative construction of Black womanhood and engages in actions to not perpetuate already existing negative constructions. However, in failing to explore the relationship between HIV/AIDS and economic class, these women might not be taking advantage of the possibility of connecting HIV/AIDS to already existing issues that tend to be mainstays on the Black political agenda—issues such as access to housing and education, for example. The failure to link AIDS to such issues is but another form of silence.

With regard to HIV/AIDS, researchers confirm a systematic relationship between HIV/AIDS incidence and prevalence to economic deprivation.[44] Poverty and its resulting manifestations such as unequal access to education, employment, and livable wages (due in part to racial and gender segregation and access to jobs); limited access to health clinics; and heightened exposure to violence influences women's ability to make decisions over their lives and their abilities to negotiate power in their relationships at both micro- and macrolevels. At the microlevel, a 2005 report by the Centers for Disease Control and Prevention (CDC) shows that HIV-positive Black women (in North Carolina) who were financially dependent on their partners tended to engage in risky sexual behavior because they were unable to negotiate condom use (in part).[45] Consequently, the approach most often taken to address HIV/AIDS—prevention through behavioral modification and education— continues to be challenged. Failure to speak on Black women's economic situation might prove difficult in convincing some women to change their sexual behaviors. Poverty, at the macrolevel, also limits HIV-positive Black women's ability to negotiate their care. Simply put, income influences access to health care. In a 1998 study, Samuel A. Bozzette and colleagues stated that HIV-positive adults in the United States, relative to the general population, are one-fifth more likely to lack health insurance. Additionally, these individuals are three times as likely to be insured by Medicaid and nine times as likely to have Medicare coverage. Women, in comparison to men, are more likely to be covered by Medicaid—61 percent women, 39 percent men.[46] A 2010 report on minority women's health indicates that "African-American women are less likely to receive health care. When they do get care, they are more likely to get it late."[47] Financial barriers are one of the major factors that limit Black women's access to health care. Financial restrictions include, for example, health-care costs for out-of-pocket expenses and medications.

Some women are also often financially limited in their ability to afford transportation to seek care.[48]

When Black women fail to systematically and critically engage the interrelatedness of class and HIV/AIDS, this can be the result of a "controlled morality," discussed by scholars such as E. Frances White.[49] Given African Americans' commitment to "respectability politics," there is an attempt by many within the community to control the public presentation of blackness and Black womanhood specifically.[50] Discussing Black womanhood in relation to class and its intersection with HIV/AIDS falls outside the types of control of the representation of Black people that organize respectability politics. As I argue in the concluding chapter of *Shadow Bodies*, to bring such women out of the shadows would suggest that Black womanhood is "flawed" and as such the Black community has failed. It has failed in the sense that the Black community has not lived up to its notions of strength and respectability—which is also connected with the *Ass* metascript.

The issue of sexual identity also represents another discreet silence in Black women's talk. Heterosexuality, although not prominently talked about, was privileged in the discourses. The discourses centered the spread of HIV/AIDS via heterosexual sex and the failure to use condoms. This can been seen when Representative Juanita Millender-McDonald asserted, "Among minority women, the most prevalent modes of contracting HIV are injecting drug use, 37 percent, and heterosexual contact, almost 38 percent. . . . In the inner-city community, there are often greater perceived notions that sex is not as good if a condom is used. Frequently women do not encourage their sexual partners to use condoms for fear of retribution."[51] Congresswoman Eva Clayton also centered heterosexuality when she stated, "Rates of infection continue to grow among adolescents and among women, with heterosexual contact as their primary mode of transmission."[52]

Black lesbians were rendered completely invisible in the discourses of Black female congressional members. The HIV/AIDS and sexuality frames focused on the Black male homosexual. While such terms were not widely used (only one reference), Representative Diane Watson mentioned the phenomenon related to "men on the down low": "There has been a lot of discussion about many facts and a lot of individuals and communities really heap a lot of blame on men who are considered on the 'down low.' . . . Some people feel that the down low is contributing to these statistics. But the truth is, we just do not know."[53] The dominant sexual identity frame tended to be employed in the "celebratory" frame discussed above. In this frame the work of gay organizations was highlighted and celebrated. However, there was very little discussion about either the needs of transgender or lesbian individuals who are HIV positive, particularly Black transgender and lesbian peoples, or the extent and the impact of the disease among these populations. These subjects are in essence the shadow bodies of this discourse.

Sexual identity, unlike economic class, did receive a bit more attention by Black female bloggers. Bloggers tended to focus on the issue of men who have sex with men. To a lesser extent a few bloggers discussed the issue of prison sex and its implications once the men are released. More often than not, women were projected as the prey/victims of these men. Consider Brown Sista's post, which says:

> Best-selling novelist Terri McMillan shares her emotionally-charged testimony on the controversial BET News documentary, "The Down Low Exposed," premiering March 28 at 10 p.m. ET/PT. "I think that what [BET is] doing should be applauded because I think more than anything there are women out there that are victims," the author of "Waiting to Exhale" said during the one-hour news special—a probing look into the world of men with wives or girlfriends who also secretly engage in sex with other men. "I think we need to hold men accountable for their actions," McMillan added, in what she said is her final public interview on the subject. Last year, her marriage to Jonathan Plummer publicly unraveled with a nasty divorce as a result of his admission to a secret gay life. "I think that he should be charged with attempted murder for risking my life without my knowledge or consent," the chick-lit diva said in the documentary. Helmed by Park Hill Entertainment President Shirley Neal, "Exposed" examines this divisive subject from a variety of angles including prison sex and its impact on the spread of HIV/AIDS; the Black church; the impact of HIV and AIDS on women infected by men who hid their homosexuality; and the crucial importance of being tested for the disease. (March 27, 2006)

Such posts sought to expose the secrecy around men who have sex with men but who do not consider themselves gay.

This type of talk, prevalent over the time period of this study, is reflected in a 2009 post in which Brown Sugar writes, "Sex in prison is normative."[54] She then goes on to talk about men on the "down low." On December 10, 2007, Brown Sugar explicitly links prison sex and the HIV/AIDS epidemic. As stated, "Many men contract HIV and other diseases in prison. And we know what those numbers are like for black males. They get out and voila we've got ourselves an epidemic."[55]

In *Ebony* and *Essence*, the framing of the intersection of sexuality and HIV/AIDS focused on how women contract the disease from homosexual or bisexual men. For instance, Nikitta Foston writes:

> Contributing to the alarming rate of infection are a variety of factors, including unprotected sex, sex with multiple partners, needle sharing among intravenous drug users, and the growing population of "down-low Brothers"—men who do not consider themselves gay or bisexual, but engage in sex with both men and women. The return of previously incarcerated men into our communities also affects the rate of infection among Black women. "We have a huge population of African-American males who go into prison HIV-negative and come out HIV-positive," says Thornton. "When these men get out, they come back to our daughters, our mothers and our sisters. They don't go back to men because they don't consider themselves gay."[56]

Gwendolyn Goldsby Grant asserts, "Statistics show that nationwide Black women have the highest rate of reported AIDS cases among any racial or gender group. And we're getting the virus largely from having unprotected sex with bisexual men and drug users."[57]

Beyond the so-called men on the down-low phenomenon and how women have sex with these men unknowingly, there was one story that explicitly discussed homosexuality, with a particular focus on lesbians. Readers were informed, "Homophobia kills. It would be bad enough if it killed only lesbians and gay men. But the impact it has on the battle against AIDS in Black communities is devastating." Wilson further states,

> A contributing factor is the veil of secrecy and the disgrace surrounding homosexuality in the Black community. "If we really are going to be serious about helping to end HIV infections and building a proud and strong Black community, we are going to have to begin by making it clear that there can't be any space for discriminating against gays and lesbians," says A. Cornelius Baker, executive director of the Whitman-Walker Clinic, an influential non-profit lesbian and gay community health organization based in Washington, D.C.[58]

Across the diverse platforms that I used to analyze talk on HIV/AIDS (and for that matter the other two public issues), this was the only instance that explicitly discussed protecting homosexual individuals (most of the talk focused on how to protect oneself from homosexuals—particularly men "on the down low").

Once again, Black lesbians and transgender individuals are not included in the talk. There is a silence with regard to this population. In explaining the absence of women who have sex with women and self-identified lesbians, Nancy Goldstein argues that it is "impossible to construct an HIV-infected person with a complex identity from within the confines of the CDC-regulated AIDS discourse."[59] She further argues, "Although the CDC surveillance definitions play a significant role in obscuring the rate or cause of HIV infection among women who have sex with women, the construction of risk categories, and hence, responsibility for lesbian invisibility in the AIDS epidemic, also lies with other sectors of the scientific community"[60]

While she focuses on the scientific community, I would argue that "everyday" individuals and those in some relative position of power to frame discourses on HIV/AIDS also contribute to the invisibility of some who are affected and infected by the disease. I posit that such exclusion is a result of Black women's protectionist politics, which is an outgrowth of the scripts ascribed to Black women's bodies. Thus, Black lesbian women, for example, are not seen as epitomizing the "good" elements of Black womanhood. Consequently, they are not included in the agenda—which is a manifestation of the *piece of ass* and the *ass question* subscript. While this protectionist approach (i.e., not displaying perceived "negative" images of Black women) can be read as liberatory, it can also be read as oppressive. A protectionist politics limits who we can advocate on behalf of and it fails to open spaces that can facilitate a more transformative and inclusive integration of intersectionality.

Living with AIDS: Suggestions on How to Confront the Disease

Two frames, couched under the umbrella of behavioral modification, dominated Black women's approaches to addressing HIV/AIDS. Black congresswomen, Black female bloggers, and *Essence* and *Ebony*, as a means of fighting the spread of HIV/AIDS, instructed their listeners and readers to know their status and that of their partners. Additionally, women were instructed to "take care" of themselves—either in terms of seeking medical attention when seeing their primary care physicians or in terms of their intimate relationships. Another element of the behavioral modification approach involved the promotion of condom use and the call for women, in particular, to "wake up" and learn about the dangers of HIV and AIDS. This I refer to as the "education frame." Beyond the education frame, and among Black elected officials only, there were policy demands made for increased funding of the Ryan White Care Act. The policy demands also included specific requests for how such funding would benefit communities of color. While I highlight the use of these frames, it is not to suggest that they were frequently or abundantly employed in the talk on how to confront HIV/AIDS among Black women.

Particularly evident in Black women's talk was the marked absence or limited references to structural factors as contributing to the spread of HIV/AIDS—this shows the discreet silences deployed by the women. Below, I present the "Take care of yourself" frame followed by the "Education" frame. These frames suggest the types of political action engaged in and encouraged. They also speak to notions of citizenship, who is included and how and who is excluded, and the role of the state as it relates to HIV and AIDS.

TAKE CARE OF YOURSELF: KNOW HIS AND YOUR STATUS

As part of the larger behavioral modification frame, Black women are instructed to "take responsibility for their bodies."[61] Such instruction may be read as a response to the *piece of ass* subscript and the notion of the hypersexual/irresponsible Black sexual being. However, the framing of the policy responses, in the manner of take personal care, tends to ignore sexual power relations within the Black community. According to a 2004 *Ebony* article, taking responsibility for their bodies involves Black women screening their "sexual partners carefully. If he doesn't want to be honest about his sexual history, then he should be history. And latex condoms are a must when you are sexually involved."[62] Readers were also cautioned about the factors they use to evaluate their sexual partners.

> But it's not just the insidious nature of AIDS that gets us in trouble, observes Wyatt. Most of us simply use the wrong criteria to evaluate our partners. "Women are looking at jobs and clothes and appearance and what the person says and how much money he makes," she says. Those may be appropriate criteria for deciding whether to have dinner with someone, but they're hardly worth considering when it comes to deciding whether to have unprotected sex. Instead, says Wyatt, you should ask: *Is this person a player? Has he been in prison? Does he use drugs? Is he sleeping with more than one person? Does he have my well-being at heart?* And most important: *Has he been tested recently, and does he practice safe sex?* Keep in mind that one in 50 Black men is HIV-positive or has full-blown AIDS. "Once the virus becomes prevalent in a community, as it is in ours, your risk of bumping into it becomes much higher," says Helene Gayle, M.D., M.P.H., senior adviser for HIV/AIDS with the Bill & Melinda Gates

Foundation in Seattle. As a result, she says, Black women need to evaluate their sexual partners much more carefully.[63]

While in this article Jeannine Amber discusses the prevalence of the virus, she fails to address the factors (beyond behaviors) that influence the spread of the disease among Black women. This approach to dealing with HIV/AIDS relies heavily on a language of self-help and individual behavior, a trend that runs throughout the suggestions on how to address HIV/AIDS. Ignored are those women who cannot readily protect themselves—the women who are not strong enough or who are treated as a *physical ass* or a *piece of ass*. These women become problematic because they challenge Black racial advancement in the sense that they do not fit the model of the "strong" Black woman. Also, they are damaged and consequently cannot be used in the racial uplift project, thus the silence.

EDUCATION IS KEY: A MEANS OF PROTECTION

As suggested in the naming of this frame, its primary purpose is to provide general education to readers. Such information draws attention to how HIV is contracted and how it could be prevented. The education frame varied across the three areas of talk but covered related topics. For example, there was the focus on how one can contract HIV and testing options. Below, I offer a few illustrative examples of the education frame.

This quote, taken from blogger Is It Just Me, highlights one aspect of the education frame, which focused on protecting one self. Is It Just Me writes:

My humble opinion says, why not fight the urge for sudden instant physical gratification and see if the person is really worth giving so much of yourself to? Trust and believe I know it's hard, but it's a far cry better than doing something of minimal value and not having anything of merit to show for it than waiting. It's sad that people are more willing to shed their clothes than to share their true selves. . . . Blog fam, we're already a community broken and this behavior trend plays a key role in why. Yes, I realize other races probably have this issue to[o], but I'm speaking on *my* community. With the HIV rate skyrocketing, it's one more reason to slow your roll.[64]

This approach encourages women to look after their sexual health in general. A similar approach was taken in *Essence* and *Ebony* magazines, which often inform readers:

But thanks to faster and more convenient methods of testing, you and your partner can now go to the doctor and get results in as little as

20 minutes. To get your partner on board, Know HIV/AIDS, a national campaign to raise awareness of the disease, suggests this: Tell your partner you want to talk about testing so that the two of you can be closer and worry less. Emphasize that sex will be less stressful once you both know your status. Then together go over the information below so that you know what your alternatives are.[65]

The article then lists and discusses various types of testing options, such as rapid testing. As a final example of the education frame, I offer the following: "Dr. Yolanda H. Wimberly, assistant professor of clinical pediatrics for Grady Health Systems and Morehouse School of Medicine in Atlanta, says schools, churches and parents must assume a larger role in educating young people about AIDS and other sexually transmitted diseases like bacterial vaginosis, trichomonas, Chlamydia, herpes, syphilis and gonorrhea."[66] Black congresswomen such as Watson often stated, "We must continue to educate/ prevent and care for our members who have been affected by [this] atrocious epidemic and continue to fight against HIV/AIDS."[67] Representative Maxine Waters, in articulating the actions of the Congressional Black Caucus, asserted that the organization "has and continue to assume a leadership role in addressing the issue through AIDS education and other actions. We are increasing our efforts to insist on personal responsibility, mandatory testing, outreach and education, advocating for increased funding, more legislation."[68] Representative Waters's approach is one of educate, prevent, and increase access. Embedded in this frame (implicitly and explicitly) are notions of behavioral modification as a means of limiting the spread of the infection. It centers, minimally, on addressing structural issues that heighten Black women's susceptibility to HIV/AIDS. Furthermore, such a frame limits the role of government in addressing the spread of the virus to simply offering education, and does nothing to call on the government to pursue gender or race equity policies or other policies designed to challenge systemic inequality.

It should be of no surprise to learn that Black female bloggers, in general, tend to promote and encourage an individualistic response, one of personal responsibility, to HIV/AIDS. When HIV/AIDS is framed in a manner that does not recognize the intersection of HIV/AIDS and multiple systems of oppression, then it is more difficult to challenge these systems. The majority of the blog posts did not offer specific suggestions for addressing HIV/AIDS. This is a result of the "laundry list" approach where HIV/AIDS is referenced as another ailment, among several, that plagues the Black community. Or, it could be the result of the bloggers, in a rather neutral manner, simply citing the impact and extent of HIV/AIDS in the Black community. Whatever the rationale, bloggers tended to encourage support of various charities and for individuals to engage in sexually healthy practices as means for confronting HIV/AIDS.

Support for various charities and encouraging readers to purchase various products was a somewhat typical call to action. Readers were informed, by Ari (on Brown Sista's blog):

> A couple days ago I decided to go to Dillard's and visit the Mac counter for new cosmetics I hadn't tried yet. During my visit I picked up an amazing lip gloss by Viva Glam called Tinted Lipglass. There are three distinctive shades to choose from depending on your personality and style. It's long-lasting effect will keep you wanting more. Despite its great color and shine, all proceeds of Viva Glam lipstick and lipglass is donated to M-A-C Aids Fund. This fund supports men, women, and children living with HIV and AIDS. This gloss is so rich and stunning you're bound to fall in love. (August 12, 2009)

As suggested in this post, not only will you get a great lipstick but your purchase would be put to a greater good. The *I Like Her Style!* blog also encouraged their readers to shop at the Body Shop in order to support various HIV/AIDS charities. The blogger suggested to readers that they make such purchases their "good deed for the day and look great doing it!"[69] This approach seems to fit the model of the woman as consumer and by extension consumerism as "activism." Consequently, other forms of activism and organizing remain invisible.

There was one blogger who went beyond the personal sexual healthy frame and consumer activism. In 2008, blogger A Lady's Perspective wrote:

> "Leadership-Stop AIDS. Keep the Promise" is this year's theme. People living with HIV and AIDS (PLHIV) and their supporters are the driving force in the fight against the disease. They have taken the lead in asking questions and getting global leaders and governments fully involved in the fight, but the struggle continues. Without PLHIV leadership, universal access to prevention, treatment and care will remain a dream. To achieve the goal, everyone must do his/her part in the fight. Governments must get involved and keep the promises they made. Community leaders must encourage its members to take leadership roles in sharing information. Individuals must get tested, know their rights to prevention and treatment, and take action against stigma and discrimination, because HIV/AIDS does not discriminate.[70]

She made a similar call to governments, community leaders, and individuals in 2009. Although this post does not explicitly address the intersection of HIV/AIDS and multiple systems of oppression, it does hint at recognizing that individual-level behavior alone cannot stop the spread of the disease.

The only post that suggests a Black feminist politics recognizes the organization Women Alive. This post, contributed by Kim Anthony for *Black Gives Back*, states:

> Another "story" that is close to Cookie Johnson's heart is the plight of the women served by the evening's beneficiaries, Women Alive. Created in 1990 by a group of women living with HIV/AIDS who recognized the need to provide a more specialized gender specific AIDS service organization for women, Women Alive reaches nearly 150 HIV+ clients and their families, and over 1,000 individuals through their outreach endeavors, out-patient clinics, health fairs, home visits, posters, brochures, and role model stories.[71]

In the words of Michele Tracy Berger, the policy suggestions offered by Black women fail to recognize "the multifaceted response to injustice that galvanize women" to act in response to HIV/AIDS and its relation to structural and systemic oppression.[72] Not only do the policy suggestions fail in the manner suggested by Berger, but they also fail because they do not recognize the modalities of Black womanhood. The pervasive silence around structural violence and HIV/AIDS in Black women's talk leaves us to wonder who is this group muting and why. The "activism" around Black women and HIV/AIDS among Black congresswomen, Black female bloggers, and *Essence* and *Ebony* magazines erases the broader social structures that impact the lived realities of diverse Black women who are affected with HIV/AIDS. Such Black women seem to have no political efficacy. Their political efficacy is stymied, as there is a perception that such women cannot be "innocent" and used in the project of racial uplift—they are too closely aligned with the negative aspects of the *Ass* script and fail to satisfy the requirements necessitated by the *Strong Black Woman* script. Consequently, Black HIV-positive women cannot be used to organize activism and political change among Black women and the larger Black community.

Conclusion

As articulated by Berger, "the degree to which women have been affected by the disease is inseparable from the historical scars of inequality in American society."[73] Black women are susceptible to HIV and later AIDS as a result of a number of factors, including gender inequality, race/racism, age, poverty, marital status, geographic location, and work-related issues. Singularly and combined, these factors play a vital role in increasing women's vulnerability to the disease.[74] Overwhelmingly, these women tend to be poor, solo parents, and residents of urban communities.[75]

However, in the face of the growing AIDS epidemic among African American women and the relationship between the virus and the legacy of inequality, they have been rendered both invisible and hypervisible. In discussing the invisibility and hypervisibility of African American women who are affected by and infected with HIV/AIDS, Evelynn Hammonds says:

> African-American women with AIDS are constantly represented with respect to drug-use—either their own or their partners. They are largely poor or working-class. They are single mothers. Media portrayals of these people with AIDS allude to the specter of drug abuse and controlled sexuality coupled with welfare "dependency" and irresponsibility. Such allusions undermine any representations of African-American women with AIDS that would allow them to be embraced by the larger public.[76]

The Black response to AIDS, because of its conscious or unconscious reliance on negative images of women and its inability to incorporate gender into its freedom struggle, has also contributed to the neglect of HIV-positive Black women.[77] Consequently, many Black women find themselves abandoned.

Part of being made invisible and at the same time hypervisible means that these women are often denied access to care and their plight does not make it to the public agenda—they go unrecognized and unrepresented. While it appears that they are being talked about, in essence they are not being talked about—thus rendering them shadow bodies in the framing of HIV and AIDS. Relying on a negative construction, which results from scripts ascribed to the Black feminine body, of Black womanhood, HIV-positive African American women are viewed as sexually and morally impure and as vectors in the spread of the disease. AIDS-related discourses, both inside and outside the Black community, tend to construct these women in a rather negative light. Public health officials and government decision makers' response to AIDS and its relation to race, class, and gender is generally one of neglect. According to Bill Rodriguez, there was a systematic failure to recognize the relationship between the disease and "poverty, economic hardship, or sexual oppression."[78] Additionally, the social construction of HIV/AIDS as resulting from deviant behavior and the fact that it appears to disproportionately affect marginalized members of society have resulted in a state of complacency in governments' response and general neglect.

In addition to the challenges of gender inequality in the Black community, the avoidance of an AIDS discussion is, according to H. L. Dalton, "less a response to AIDS, the medical phenomenon, than a reaction to the myriad social issues that surround the disease and give it meaning. More fundamentally, it is the predictable outgrowth of the problematic, mutual fear and mutual disrespect, a sense of otherness and a pervasive neglect that rarely feels benign."[79]

The discourse of HIV/AIDS captures much of what Frantz Fanon describes in *Black Skin, White Masks*. In this work, Fanon demonstrates the enormous power of the discursive and political effects of responses to the Black body. Running through much of the construction of HIV/AIDS discourse is the concern over the Black female body. The Black female body remains a site of contestation in our discussions of HIV/AIDS not only in Africa but also in the United States. Patricia McFadden, in characterizing the body of research on HIV/AIDS and Africa, asserts that "everyone is researching and analyzing the drama that is unfolding on the bodies and in the lives and deaths of Africans, but of special interest is the besieged body and life/death struggle of the black woman and the black girl."[80] She captures the silences I discussed above and, while she speaks of the silence as it relates to Africa, I argue that the same can be said of US discourses.

Cohen says that, "A more accurate characterization of the political positioning of most black Americans is that of a qualified linked-fate, whereby not every black person in crisis is seen as equally essential to the survival of the community, as an equally representative proxy of our own individual interests."[81] Hegemonic discourse, birthed from the scripts ascribed to Black women's bodies, results in Black women who are positive or who have AIDS as being disqualified for inclusion into the understanding of the survival of the larger Black community. They are not useful to sell commodities (the *physical ass*), they are not useful as sexual partners (*piece of ass*), and as such they are treated as the troubling *ass question*. The result is that there is a tendency to focus on individual-level sexual and cultural practices of Black women. Consequently, individuals constructed as outside the "norm" find themselves the recipients of moralizing rhetoric and policies. Much of the response to HIV/AIDS has been heavily concentrated in normalizing sexuality, promoting heterosexual behavior, and changing women's behavior. Sandra D. Lane and others challenge this conceptualization of HIV/AIDS and the resulting response. They suggest that the "individual-level risk factors" approach ignores structural violence and the resulting spread of HIV/AIDS among racially marginalized groups.[82] Using this understanding of structural violence, researchers posit that to better understand and address the spread of HIV/AIDS among Black women, we should look at macrolevel risk factors that include disproportionate incarceration rates of African American men, residential segregation, gang turf, constraints on access to sexually transmitted disease services, and commercial sales of douching products, among others.

While extant research highlights the relationship between structural violence and HIV/AIDS, the public discourse of Black congresswomen, *Essence* and *Ebony*, and Black female bloggers seems to ignore such understandings. To incorporate such an understanding into their talk would require that these Black women challenge the "original" construction of HIV and AIDS. Additionally, they need to confront how the understanding of the Black female body is intimately used in the dominant narratives of HIV/AIDS—a narrative of deviance that predated the spread of HIV/AIDS. Beyond confronting such usage, Black women also need to investigate how their talk is influenced by the larger project of "respectability," which in part is a response to the scripts ascribed to Black women's bodies, the *Ass* and *Strong Black Woman* scripts. The devastating impact of HIV/AIDS provides us with a unique, albeit sad, opportunity to address the systems of oppression resulting from gender, race, and class relations and practices. It allows us to critically think about who is allowed in the "center."

Notes

Adapted from Julia S. Jordan-Zachery, "Safe, Soulful Sex: HIV/AIDS Talk," in *Shadow Bodies: Black Women, Ideology, Representation, and Politics* (New Brunswick, NJ: Rutgers University Press, 2013), 76–100. © 2017. Reprinted by permission of Rutgers University Press. The chapter title is taken from Grant, "Safe, Soulful Sex."

1 Jordan-Zachery, *Shadow Bodies*, 31.
2 Cohen, *Boundaries of Blackness.*
3 Centers for Disease Control, "HIV and African Americans."
4 hooks, *Feminist Theory.*
5 Discreet silences are used as a means for avoiding the mention of sensitive subjects, resulting from issues of tactfulness, confidentiality, or taboo topics; see Huckin, "Textual Silence."
6 See Hammonds, "Missing Persons."
7 See Cohen, *Boundaries of Blackness.*

8 Shadows suggest the absence of light; however, there can be no shadows unless there is light. This captures the positionality of Black women who are affected by HIV/AIDS in the talk of Black women. The notion that these women are shadow bodies does not suggest that they are completely absent but that they exist in a space in-between—a space of both proximity and separation. Some Black women are rendered *shadows* of other members in the Black community as they are often vaguely represented.

9 Scripts serve as mechanisms used to express beliefs and values that define our roles in the world and how we should "play" these roles. Scripts are learned patterns of framing and interpreting not only an individual's behavior but also the behavior of others.

10 Jordan-Zachery, *Shadow Bodies*, 31.

11 See Adimora and Schoenbach, "Contextual Factors," Adimora and Schoenbach, "Social Context"; Connors, "Sex, Drugs"; Feist-Price and Wright, "African American Women"; Krieger, "Embodying Inequality"; Logan et al., "Women, Sex, and HIV"; Pequegnat et al., "Considering Women's Contextual and Cultural Issues"; Whitehead, "Urban Low-Income"; E. M. Wright, "Deep from within the Well"; E. R. Wright and Martin, "Social Organization of HIV/AIDS Care."

12 "AIDS Epidemic."

13 The Brown Sista blog (http://brownsista.com) is no longer available online.

14 Afrobella, "Are You Rocking Red Pumps Today?"

15 See Singer, "Welcome, Fans."

16 Taylor and Van Willigen, "Women's Self-Help."

17 Murray, "Yours in the Struggle," 82.

18 "Black College Queens."

19 "Champions for a Cause"; Cole, "Alicia Bares Her Soul."

20 Gordy et al., "Do Right Men 2006."

21 See Bardhan, "Transnational AIDS-HIV"; and Princeton Survey Research Associates, "Covering the Epidemic."

22 "Combating HIV/AIDS."

23 Monroe, "Personal Journeys."

24 "World AIDS Day."

25 Schattschneider, *Semisovereign People*.

26 Melucci, "The Process," 44.

27 "5 Questions For: Dr. Lorraine Cole."

28 Adimora and Schoenbach, "Contextual Factors," Adimora and Schoenbach, "Social Context"; E. R. Wright and Martin, "Social Organization of HIV/AIDS Care."

29 Weeks et al., "Gender Relations," 341.

30 Simon and Gagnon, "Sexual Scripts."

31 Bowleg, Lucas, and Tschann, "'The Ball'"; Hynie et al., "Relational Sexual Scripts"; Jones, "Sex Scripts"; Maticka-Tyndale, "Sexual Scripts"; Pulerwitz et al., "Relationship Power."

32 See Alexander-Floyd, *Gender*; Wallace, *Black Macho*.

33 Dunn, Perry, and Wiltz, "Coping."

34 Gina The Blogmother, "AIDS Is NOT a 'Black Disease.'"

35 "Sauda Voice Recommends."

36 A Lady's Perspective, "National Black HIV/AIDS Awareness Day."

37 See Plowden, Fletcher, and Miller, "Factors Influencing HIV-Risk Behaviors."

38 See Watkins-Hayes, "Social and Economic Context."

39 "Ryan White AIDS Care Act."

40 Cohen, *Boundaries of Blackness*; Hammonds, "Missing Persons."

41 Smith, "An HIV Cure?"

42 Starling, "Why AIDS Is a Growing Threat," 136.

43 Starling, "Why AIDS Is a Growing Threat," 136.

44 Farmer, *Pathologies of Power*; Fife and Mode, "AIDS Incidence"; Fife and Mode, "AIDS Prevalence"; Parker, Easton, and Klein, "Structural Barriers"; Plowden, Fletcher, and Miller, "Factors Influencing HIV-Risk Behaviors"; Simon et al., "Income and AIDS Rates"; Zierler et al., "Economic Deprivation."

45 Centers for Disease Control and Prevention. "HIV Transmission."

46 Bozzette et al., "Care of HIV-Infected Adults."

47 Madlock Gatison, *Health Communication*, xvi.

48 National Alliance of State and Territorial AIDS Directors, "Black* Women and HIV/AIDS."

49 White, "Africa on My Mind."

50 Higginbotham, *Righteous Discontent*.

51 "Women's Health Issues."

52 "HIV/AIDS" (Clayton).

53 "Supporting the Goals."

54 Brown Sugar, "Down Low Men."

55 Brown Sugar, "70% of Out of Wedlock Birth Rates."

56 Foston, "Why AIDS Is Becoming a Black Woman's Disease," 174.

57 Grant, "Safe, Soulful Sex."

58 Wilson, "The Wall."

59 Goldstein, "Lesbians and the Medical Profession," 90.

60 Goldstein, "Lesbians and the Medical Profession," 91.

61 Hughes, "Sisters."

62 "HIV."

63 Amber, "Why Don't You Use a Condom?"

64 Is It Just Me, untitled blog post.

65 Carter, "Know Your Status," 99.

66 Bullock, "Explosive Health Crisis."

67 "Supporting the Goals."

68 "HIV/AIDS" (Waters).

69 "Viva Glam!"

70 A Lady's Perspective, "World AIDS Day 2008."

71 Anthony, "CJ by Cookie Johnson."

72 Berger, *Workable Sisterhood*, 187.

73 Berger, *Workable Sisterhood*, 7.
74 See Albertyn, "Contesting Democracy"; Quinn, "AIDS"; Schiller, Crystal, and Lewellen, "Risky Business."
75 Connors, "Sex, Drugs"; Schable, Chu, and Diaz, "Characteristics."
76 Hammonds, "Missing Persons," 11.
77 Cohen, *Boundaries of Blackness*.
78 Rodriguez, "Biomedical Models," 35.
79 Dalton, "AIDS in Blackface," 205.
80 McFadden, "HIV and AIDS," 23.
81 Cohen, *Boundaries of Blackness*, xi.
82 Lane et al., "Structural Violence."

Bibliography

Adimora, Adaora A., and Victor J. Schoenbach. "Contextual Factors and the Black-White Disparity in Heterosexual HIV Transmission." *Epidemiology* 13, no. 6 (2002): 707–12.

Adimora, Adaora A., and Victor J. Schoenbach. "Social Context, Sexual Networks, and Racial Disparities in Rates of Sexually Transmitted Infections." *Journal of Infectious Diseases* 191, no. S1 (2005): S115–22.

Afrobella. "Are You Rocking Red Pumps Today?" *Afrobella* (blog), March 10, 2010. http://www.afrobella.com/2010/03/10/are-you-rocking-red-pumps-today/.

"AIDS Epidemic." 147 Cong. Rec. E1035. Statement of Rep. Carrie Meek, June 6, 2001. http://thomas.loc.gov.

Albertyn, Catherine. "Contesting Democracy: HIV/AIDS and the Achievement of Gender Equality in South Africa." *Feminist Studies* 29, no. 3 (2003): 595–615.

Alexander-Floyd, Nikol G. *Gender, Race, and Nationalism in Contemporary Black Politics*. New York: Palgrave Macmillan, 2007.

Amber, Jeannine. "Why Don't You Use a Condom?" *Essence* 33, no. 4 (August 2002): 118.

Anthony, Kim. "CJ by Cookie Johnson: A Champagne Celebration with a Cause." *Black Gives Back* (blog), October 24, 2010. http://www.blackgivesback.com /2010/10/cj-by-cookie-johnson-champagne.html#.XSjYsehKg2w.

Bardhan, Nilanjana. "Transnational AIDS-HIV News Narratives: A Critical Exploration of Overarching Frames." *Mass Communication and Society* 4, no. 3 (2001): 283–309.

Berger, Michele Tracy. *Workable Sisterhood: The Political Journey of Stigmatized Women with HIV/AIDS*. Princeton, NJ: Princeton University Press, 2004.

"Black College Queens." *Ebony* 61, no. 6 (2006): 138.

Bowleg, Lisa, Kenya J. Lucas, and Jeanne M. Tschann. "'The Ball Was Always in His Court': An Exploratory Analysis of Relationship Scripts, Sexual Scripts, and Condom Use among African American Women." *Psychology of Women Quarterly* 28, no. 1 (2004): 70–82.

Bozzette, Samuel A., et al. "The Care of HIV-Infected Adults in the United States." *New England Journal of Medicine* 339, no. 26 (1998): 1897–904.

Brown Sugar. "70% Out of Wedlock Birth Rages, Half of all HIV/AIDS Cases— Why?" December 10, 2007. https://brownsugar28.blogspot.com/search?q =many+men+contract.

Brown Sugar. "Why Down Low Men Aren't the Problem." *Fitness, Fashion, Food, & Fornicating* (blog), January 3, 2009. http://brownsugar28.blogspot.com/2009 /01/why-down-low-men-arent-problem.html.

Bullock, Lorinda. "The Explosive Health Crisis That No One Talks About." *Ebony* 59, no. 2 (2003): 136.

Carter, Zakia. "Know Your Status." *Essence* 35, no. 8 (December 2004): 99–100.

Centers for Disease Control and Prevention. "HIV and African Americans." N.d. Last updated March 19, 2019. https://www.cdc.gov/hiv/group/racialethnic /africanamericans/index.html.

Centers for Disease Control and Prevention. "HIV Transmission among Black Women—North Carolina, 2004." February 4, 2005. http://www.cdc.gov /mmwr/preview/mmwrhtml/mm5404a2.htm.

"Champions for a Cause." *Ebony* 58, no. 12 (October 2003): 92.

Cohen, Cathy J. *The Boundaries of Blackness: AIDS and the Breakdown of Black Politics.* Chicago: University of Chicago Press, 1999.

Cole, Harriette. "Alicia Bares Her Soul." *Ebony* 63, no. 1 (2007): 68.

"Combating HIV/AIDS in the Black Community." 145 Cong. Rec. H9180. Statement of Rep. Maxine Waters, September 30, 1999. http://thomas.loc.gov.

Connors, Margaret. "Sex, Drugs and Structural Violence: Unraveling the Epidemic among Poor Women of Color in the United States." In *Women, Poverty, and AIDS: Sex, Drugs, and Structural Violence,* edited by Paul Farmer, Margaret Connors, and Janie Simmons, 91–123. Monroe, ME: Common Courage Press, 1996.

Dalton, H. L. "AIDS in Blackface." *Daedalus* 118, no. 3 (1989): 205–27.

Dunn, Kate, Monia Perry, and Teresa Wiltz. "Coping (AIDS: The Second Wave)." *Essence* 28 (September 1997): 130.

Ellison, Ralph. *Invisible Man.* New York: Random House, 1995.

Fanon, Frantz. *Black Skin, White Masks.* New York: Grove, 1967.

Farmer, Paul. *Pathologies of Power: Health, Human Rights, and the New War on the Poor.* Berkeley: University of California Press, 2005.

Feist-Price, Sonja, and Lynda Brown Wright. "African American Women Living with HIV/AIDS." *Women and Therapy* 26, nos. 1–2 (2003): 27–44.

Fife, D., and C. Mode. "AIDS Incidence and Income." *Journal of Acquired Immune Deficiency Syndromes* 5, no. 11 (1992): 1105–10.

Fife, D., and C. Mode. "AIDS Prevalence by Income Group in Philadelphia." *Journal of Acquired Immune Deficiency Syndromes and Human Retrovirology* 5, no. 11 (1992): 1111–15.

"5 Questions For: Dr. Lorraine Cole." *Ebony* 60, no. 12 (2005): 26.

Foston, Nikitta. "Why AIDS Is Becoming a Black Woman's Disease and What We Can Do about It." *Ebony* 58, no. 1 (November 2002): 174–78.

Gina The Blogmother. "AIDS Is NOT a 'Black Disease' and Those Promoting That Foolishness (CNN) Have a VERY. SHORT. MEMORY!" *What about Our Daughters* (blog), August 5, 2008. http://whataboutourdaughters.squarespace.com/waod /2008/8/5/aids-is-not-a-black-disease-and-those-promoting-that-foolish.html.

Goldstein, Nancy. "Lesbians and the Medical Profession: HIV/AIDS and the Pursuit of Visibility." In *The Gender Politics of HIV/AIDS in Women: Perspectives on the Pandemic in the United States*, edited by Nancy Goldstein and Jennifer L. Manlowe, 86–112. New York: New York University Press, 1997.

Gordy, Cynthia, Nazenet Habtezghi, La Shieka Purvis Hunter, Zulaika Jumaralli, Cori Murray, Margaret Williams, and Wendy L. Wilson. "Do Right Men 2006." *Essence* 37, no. 4 (August 2006): 141.

Grant, Gwendolyn Goldsby. "Safe, Soulful Sex." *Essence* 31, no. 1 (May 2000): 66.

Hammonds, Evelynn. "Missing Persons: African American Women, AIDS and the History of Disease." *Radical America* 24, no. 2 (1992): 7–23.

Higginbotham, Evelyn Brooks. *Righteous Discontent: The Women's Movement in the Black Baptist Church, 1880–1920*. Cambridge, MA: Harvard University Press, 1993.

"HIV." *Ebony* 59 (March 2004): 140.

"HIV/AIDS." 147 Cong. Rec. H3839–40. Statement of Rep. Eva Clayton, July 10, 2001. http://thomas.loc.gov.

"HIV/AIDS." 152 Cong. Rec. H7504. Statement of Rep. Maxine Waters, September 27, 2006. http://thomas.loc.gov.

hooks, bell. *Feminist Theory: From Margin to Center*. 2nd ed. Cambridge, MA: South End Press Classics, 2000.

Huckin, Thomas. "Textual Silence and the Discourse of Homelessness." *Discourse and Society* 13, no. 3 (2002): 347–72.

Hughes, Zondra. "Why Sisters Are the No. 1 Victims of HIV: And How You Can Avoid It." *Ebony* 59, no. 9 (2004): 64.

Hynie, Michaela, John E. Lydon, Sylvana Côté, and Seth Wiener. "Relational Sexual Scripts and Women's Condom Use: The Importance of Internalized Norms." *Journal of Sex Research* 35, no. 4 (1998): 370–80.

Is It Just Me? Untitled blog post, August 28, 2008. https://mentallyspeaking .blogspot.com/2008/.

Jones, Rachel. "Sex Scripts and Power: A Framework to Explain Urban Women's HIV Sexual Risk with Male Partners." *Nursing Clinics of North America* 41, no. 3 (2006): 425–36.

Jordan-Zachery, Julia. *Shadow Bodies: Black Women, Ideology, Representation, and Politics*. New Brunswick, NJ: Rutgers University Press, 2017.

Krieger, Nancy. "Embodying Inequality: A Review of Concepts, Measures, and Methods for Studying Health Consequences of Discrimination." *International Journal of Health Services* 29, no. 2 (1999): 295–352.

A Lady's Perspective. "National Black HIV/AIDS Awareness Day." *A Lady's Perspective* (blog), February 7, 2010. https://aladysperspective.blogspot.com /search?q=national+black+HIV.

A Lady's Perspective. "World AIDS Day 2008." *A Lady's Perspective* (blog), December 1, 2008. http://aladysperspective.blogspot.com/2008/11/world-aids-day-2008.html?m=0.

Lane, Sandra D., Robert A. Rubinstein, Robert H. Keefe, Noah Webster, Donald A. Cibula, Alan Rosenthal, and Jesse Dowdell. "Structural Violence and Racial Disparity in HIV Transmission." *Journal of Health Care for the Poor and Underserved* 15, no. 3 (2004): 319–35.

Logan, T. K., Jennifer Cole, Carl Leukefeld, and Nancy Eisenberg. "Women, Sex, and HIV: Social and Contextual Factors, Meta-Analysis of Published Interventions, and Implications for Practice and Research." *Psychological Bulletin* 128, no. 6 (2002): 851–85.

Madlock Gatison, Annette. *Health Communication and Breast Cancer among Black Women: Culture, Identity, Spirituality, and Strength*. Lanham, MD: Lexington Books, 2016.

Maticka-Tyndale, Eleanor. "Sexual Scripts and AIDS Prevention: Variations in Adherence to Safer-Sex Guidelines by Heterosexual Adolescents." *Journal of Sex Research* 28, no. 1 (1991): 45–66.

McFadden, Patricia. "HIV and AIDS: Behind the Iconic Re-presentations of Gender, Race and Class in Southern Africa." Paper presented at the Learning from Our Lives: Women, Girls and HIV/AIDS in Africa and the Africa Diaspora Conference, Spelman College, Atlanta, GA, June 2004.

Melucci, Alberto. "The Process of Collective Identity." In *Social Movements and Culture*, edited by Bert Klandermans and Hank Johnston, 41–63. Minneapolis: University of Minnesota Press, 1995.

Monroe, Sylvester. "Personal Journeys of Women with HIV/AIDS: In Observance of the 19th World AIDS Day, Four Women Share What They've Learned while Living with HIV." *Ebony* 62, no. 2 (2006): 154.

Murray, Cori. M. "Yours in the Struggle." *Essence* 32, no. 6 (October 2001): 82, 188.

National Alliance of State and Territorial AIDS Directors. "Black* Women and HIV/AIDS: Findings from Southeast Regional Consumer and Provider Focus Group Interviews." *Black Women Issue Brief No. 2*, March 2010. https://www.nastad.org/resource/black-women-issue-briefs-1-2.

Parker, Richard, Delia Easton, and Charles Klein. "Structural Barriers and Facilitators in HIV Prevention: A Review of International Research." *AIDS* 14 (2000): S22–32.

Pequegnat, Willo, Ellen Stover, Lillian Comas-Díaz, Gail Elizabeth Wyatt, and Dorothy Chin. "Considering Women's Contextual and Cultural Issues in HIV/STD Prevention Research." *Cultural Diversity and Ethnic Minority Psychology* 5, no. 3 (1999): 287–91.

Plowden, Keith O., Audwin Fletcher, and Lawrence J. Miller. "Factors Influencing HIV-Risk Behaviors among HIV-Positive Urban African Americans." *Journal of the Association of Nurses in AIDS Care* 16, no. 1 (2005): 21–28.

Princeton Survey Research Associates. "Covering the Epidemic: AIDS in the News Media, 1985–1996." *Columbia Journalism Review* 35 (July/August 1996): 1–12.

Pulerwitz, J., H. Amaro, W. De Jong, S. L. Gortmaker, and R. Rudd. "Relationship Power, Condom Use and HIV Risk among Women in the USA." *AIDS Care* 14, no. 6 (2002): 789–800.

Quinn, S. C. "AIDS and the African-American Woman: The Triple Burden of Race, Class, and Gender." *Health Education Quarterly* 20, no. 3 (1993): 305–20.

Rodriguez, Bill. "Biomedical Models of HIV and Women." In *The Gender Politics of HIV/AIDS in Women: Perspectives on the Pandemic in the United States*, edited by Nancy Goldstein and Jennifer L. Manlowe, 25–42. New York: New York University Press, 1997.

"Ryan White AIDS Care Act." 151 Cong. Rec. H21592. Statement of Rep. Maxine Waters, September 28, 2005. http://thomas.loc.gov.

"Sauda Voice Recommends: All of Us." *The Sauda Voice* (blog), July 2, 2009. http:// thesaudavoice.typepad.com/the_sauda_voice/page/85/.

Schable, Barbara, Susan Y. Chu, and Theresa Diaz. "Characteristics of Women 50 Years of Age or Older with Heterosexually Acquired AIDS." *American Journal of Public Health* 86, no. 11 (1996): 1616–18.

Schattschneider, Elmer E. *The Semisovereign People: A Realist's View of Democracy in America*. New York: Harcourt Brace Jovanovich, 1960.

Schiller, N. G., S. Crystal, and D. Lewellen. "Risky Business: The Cultural Construction of AIDS Risk Groups." *Social Science and Medicine* 38, no. 10 (1994): 1337–46.

Simon, Paul A., Dale J. Hu, Theresa R. Diaz, and Peter Kerndt. "Income and AIDS Rates in Los Angeles County." *AIDS* 9, no. 3 (1995): 281–84.

Simon, William, and John Gagnon. "Sexual Scripts: Permanence and Change." *Archives of Sexual Behavior* 15, no. 2 (1986): 97–120.

Singer, Natasha. "Welcome, Fans, to the Pinking of America." *New York Times*, October 15, 2011.

Smith, Tammie. "An HIV Cure?" *Essence* 32, no. 6 (October 2001): 80.

Starling, Kelly. "Why AIDS Is a Growing Threat to Black Woman." *Ebony* 55, no. 6 (April 2000): 136–40.

"Supporting the Goals and Ideals of Domestic Violence Awareness Month." 151 Cong. Rec. H8372. Statement of Rep. Diane Watson, September 27, 2005. http://thomas.loc.gov.

Taylor, Verta, and Marieke Van Willigen. "Women's Self-Help and the Reconstruction of Gender: The Postpartum Support and Breast Cancer Movements." *Mobilization* 1, no. 2 (1996): 123–42.

"Viva Glam!" *I Like Her Style* (blog), September 25, 2006. http://stealstyle .blogspot.com/2006/09/viva-glam.html?q=good+deed+for+the+day.

Wallace, Michele. *Black Macho and the Myth of the Superwoman*. New York: Dial, 1979.

Watkins-Hayes, Celeste. "The Social and Economic Context of Black Women Living with HIV/AIDS in the US: Implications for Research." In *Sex, Power and Taboo: Gender and HIV in the Caribbean and Beyond*, edited by Dorothy Roberts, 33–66. Miami: Ian Randle, 2008.

Weeks, Margaret, Merrill Singer, Maryland Grier, and Jean J. Schensul. "Gender Relations, Sexuality and AIDS Risk among African American and Latina Women." In *Gender and Health: An International Perspective*, edited by Carolyn F. Sargent and Caroline Brettell, 338–70. Upper Saddle River, NJ: Prentice Hall, 1996.

White, E. Francis. "Africa on My Mind: Gender, Counter Discourse and African-American Nationalism." *Journal of Women's History* 2, no. 1 (1990): 73–97.

Whitehead, T. "Urban Low-Income African American Men, HIV/AIDS, and Gender Identity." *Medical Anthropology Quarterly* 11, no. 4 (1997): 411–47.

Wilson, P. "The Wall." *Essence* 29 (December 1998): 62.

"Women's Health Issues." 143 Cong. Rec. H1966. Statement of Rep. Juanita Millender-McDonald, April 29, 1997. http://thomas.loc.gov.

"World AIDS Day." *Brown Girl Gumbo* (blog), December 1, 2010. http://www .browngirlgumbo.com/?s=world+aids+day.

Wright, Ednita M. "Deep from within the Well: Voices of African American Women Living with HIV/AIDS." In *African American Women and HIV/AIDS Critical Responses*, edited by Dorie J. Gilbert and Ednita M. Wright, 29–50. Westport, CT: Praeger, 2003.

Wright, Eric R., and Tiffany N. Martin. "The Social Organization of HIV/AIDS Care in Treatment Programmes for Adults with Serious Mental Illness." *AIDS Care* 15, no. 6 (2003): 763–74.

Zierler, S., N. Krieger, Y. Tang, W. Coady, E. Siegfried, A. Demaria, and J. Auerbach. "Economic Deprivation and AIDS Incidence in Massachusetts." *American Journal of Public Health* 90, no. 7 (2000): 1064–73.

FIVE AIDS HISTORIES OTHERWISE: THE CASE OF HAITIANS IN MONTREAL

Viviane Namaste

How do we tell the history of AIDS, locally and globally? What frameworks are privileged in our understandings of the epidemic, and how do these shape our responses in the current moment? What might be the benefit of rethinking conventional histories of HIV/AIDS at both scholarly and political levels? This chapter explores these questions, interrogating in particular how historical narratives of AIDS in the United States have influenced what we know about the epidemic, and how we know it.

To state that AIDS history has been prominent in the public sphere in recent years would be an understatement. The circulation of documentary films such as Jim Hubbard and Sarah Schulman's *United in Anger* (2012), David France's *How to Survive a Plague* (2012), and David Weissman's *We Were Here* (2010) all testify to a marked interest in the early years of the epidemic in the United States. Academic scholars have also turned their attention to US AIDS history, as evidenced in the research of Lucas Hilderbrand and Deborah Gould.[1] The ACT UP Oral History Project, located in New York, offers numerous interviews with activists and organizers in the 1980s and 1990s, including gay men and feminists.[2] In the Canadian context, a federally funded research project led by Alexis Shotwell and Gary Kinsman provides ample documentation of AIDS history, with a focus on activists in Toronto, Montreal, Ottawa, Halifax, and Vancouver.[3] In the local context of Montreal, a recent theater piece explores the history and impact of AIDS activism. Titled *Propositions for the AIDS Museum*, this work was originally staged in 2014 at the Théâtre des Écuries, with a revised version presented at the Théâtre La Chapelle in April 2017.[4] In France, two monographs establish the central role of the activist group ACT UP (Paris) in the country's specific history with AIDS.[5] These different examples are cited here as evidence of a sustained interest in AIDS history in recent years. The development and production of these works is not recent, as it takes years, even decades, to produce an academic book, a documentary film, or a theater piece. That said, the circulation of these works in the public sphere clearly indicates that there remains a broad political investment and social interest in the history of HIV/AIDS, many involving historiographies of the pandemic and its activism that have come to light only in recent years. Cultural, community and scholarly investigations of the epidemic turn their attention to history in an effort to learn from the past.

While there are some important differences among the content of the different examples cited above, it would not be an overstatement to declare that investigations of AIDS history in North America bring two issues in particular to light. In the first instance, this work shines a spotlight on activism and community organizing, asking for a collective reflection on the lessons to be learned from this history. And in the second instance, the research and cultural productions underline the tremendous role and leadership played by the United States. Indeed, these two different elements are fundamentally linked: explorations of AIDS activist history highlight the contributions of gay communities to collective mobilizing. Of course, these elements are related to a much broader cultural narrative in which the history of AIDS is said to have been first located in US gay male communities.

This chapter puts into question the ways in which the simple adoption of such a US framework occludes local histories of AIDS in North America, including local histories *within* the United States. Through a consideration of AIDS in Montreal's Haitian communities in the early 1980s, I examine how the local history of AIDS in that city was at odds with the conventional narrative that AIDS was first located in white gay male communities. This chapter emerges from a research project I have conducted since 2013 on the history of AIDS in Montreal's Haitian community. Through interviews and archival research, I seek to document both the impact of this epidemic locally as well as the response of Montreal's Haitian community. While space constraints prevent me from presenting this full project in detail, I will bring forth three different elements to help make my point about the importance of considering local data in order to displace conventional US framings of the history of AIDS. These three elements are (1) local epidemiological statistics that attest to the impact of AIDS in Montreal's Haitian communities, (2) clinical observations of AIDS among Haitians, and (3) Haitian AIDS organizing that is often eclipsed in our historical tellings of the epidemic. I conclude with some theoretical and methodological reflections on how to gather different histories of the epidemic, in order to complicate our understandings of the issues.

What's in a Number? Epidemiological Statistics and Local History

The historical telling of the AIDS epidemic that locates it as one emerging from US gay male communities appeals to a public health document, specifically the June 5, 1981, publication of the *Morbidity and Mortality Weekly Report* (MMWR).[6] This publication noted the presence of strange, opportunistic infections among young US gay men, individuals who would normally be assumed to be healthy. This document is cited as one of the central sources in the history of AIDS, consolidating the link between gay men and the epidemic. The framing of AIDS in relation to gay men in the epidemiological literature in turn informed what researchers came to see. Subsequent epidemiological studies focused on gay men in particular, with a notable example being an epidemiological cluster study that sought to trace the origin of this strange phenomenon among urban US gay men.[7]

This narrative has become the predominant one in how we understand the history of the epidemic, particularly in North America. In both the United States and Canada, media articles in 2011 announced the thirty-year anniversary of AIDS, and explicitly stated its undeniable link with communities generalized as gay men.[8] Yet an examination of the local context in Montreal would trouble this historical telling. A consideration of early clinical and epidemiological data in the Canadian context offers a different history of the AIDS epidemic and raises the question of how and why certain knowledge frameworks (notably from the United States) are often applied globally.[9]

In March 1983, the Canadian Red Cross issued a public declaration that requested individuals in certain risk groups—notably gay men, drug users, Haitians, hemophiliacs, and the sexual partners of these people—abstain from giving blood.[10] The statement followed the position of the American Red Cross, and as such was a simple adoption of its logic and framework to the Canadian context. Haitians in Montreal objected to this position, noting in particular that it was unacceptable to name all Haitians as at risk for the disease when its definitive modes of transmission were not yet known (in 1983 a causal agent had yet to be identified) and when the situation was of an infectious disease that was nonhereditary. The relations between Montreal's Haitian community and the Canadian Red Cross raised the important question of data: the agency based itself on the position of the American Red Cross, which itself appealed to epidemiological data from the Centers for Disease Control. These American figures established that 4 percent of diagnosed AIDS cases in the United States were attributed to Haitians.[11]

An appeal to this US data in the Canadian context raised the obvious question: what of the situation in Canada? Haitians had been migrating to Montreal since the 1960s, fleeing the repressive Duvalier regime, and by the early 1980s, there were approximately thirty thousand to forty thousand individuals of Haitian origin living in Montreal.[12] Early clinical observations of AIDS were seen among Haitians in Montreal. The minutes of a meeting between representatives of the Canadian Red Cross and the Haitian community in early 1983 provide an indication that the situation in Canada affected Haitian communities in particular: "Les statistiques canadiennes (confirmées par le Dr. Clayton) présentent 29 cas, dont 37 pour cent sont des Haïtiens" (The Canadian statistics, confirmed by Dr. Clayton, present 29 cases, of which 37 percent are Haitians).[13] In citing these figures, it is not my intent to endorse the Canadian Red Cross declaration or its management of the dossier. Rather, this data offers an indication and a point of entry into understanding that the epidemic in Canada was not the same as that in the United States. Moreover, I am aware of the profound limitations in citing epidemiological data as the definitive knowledge of AIDS: recorded cases were often only of deaths or people in very advanced stages of the illness, and many opportunistic infections were not included among the official criteria for inclusion in an AIDS diagnosis.[14] These methodological limits notwithstanding, early Canadian data clearly confirm that Haitians were profoundly affected by the epidemic. Indeed, if one considers the local context of Montreal (in the early 1980s and even today, most Haitian migrants to Canada established themselves in Montreal), the data is significant.[15] An article in a medical journal from March 1983, for instance, quotes Dr. Morisset, who maintains that "sur 16 cas reconnus à Montréal, neuf des victimes sont haïtiennes" (of the 16 cases recognized in Montreal, nine of the victims are Haitians).[16] These numbers are striking: nine of sixteen diagnosed cases in Montreal were attributed to Haitians. Put another way, early epidemiological data indicated that Haitians comprised 56 percent of the local epidemic. In the early years of AIDS in Montreal, the epidemic was Haitian.

It is not my intention to claim that Haitians were the *only* group affected, nor even to state that they were *more* impacted by this disease than other groups, such as white gay men in particular or gay men in general. But it is my intention to springboard from these raw numbers to inquire as to the limits of simply adopting a common narrative of the history of AIDS in North America in which it primarily touched gay men. The local context of Montreal suggests that if we take for granted the conventional framework for writing history, we risk neglecting entire populations of people and their experience with this disease. And of course, it is not coincidental that the historical telling of an epidemic in which white male bodies are at the center is, to say the least, not the best model for understanding the complex relations between Black bodies, migration, and infectious disease.

Different Clinical Experiences of AIDS

The association of AIDS with gay men as the primary way to make sense of the epidemic had implications beyond epidemiology. Clinical observations were themselves influenced by the initial data related to white US gay men and the opportunistic infections they experienced, most notably Pneumocystis carinii pneumonia (PCP) and Kaposi's sarcoma. Indeed, the opportunistic infection Kaposi's sarcoma, a form of skin cancer usually observed among men of certain Mediterranean regions, was a site of profound clinical research in the field. US epidemiological surveillance included specific attention to Kaposi's sarcoma in tracing the phenomenon of AIDS.[17] Within medical journals, numerous studies were published exploring Kaposi's sarcoma and/or the links between this form of cancer and gay men.[18] This epidemiological and clinical research was disseminated in US community contexts, as evidenced by a *New York Native* article outlining the latest developments with respect to Kaposi's sarcoma in August 1981, or a pamphlet distributed in 1982 by the Kaposi's Sarcoma Committee of Houston titled *Kaposi's Sarcoma, Opportunistic Infections and the Urban Gay Lifestyle: Towards a Healthier Gay Lifestyle; What You Need to Know to Ensure Your Good Health.*[19]

The importance of Kaposi's sarcoma to understanding the epidemic was also taken up internationally in clinical research in the field. French researchers, for instance, examined this phenomenon outside the United States.[20] And a working group on AIDS in Haiti, established in May 1982, included Kaposi's sarcoma in its title: Groupe haïtien d'étude de sarcome de Kaposi et des infections opportunistes (G.H.E.S.K.I.O., Haitian Group for the Study of Kaposi's Sarcoma and Opportunistic Infections).[21]

In short, early US epidemiological surveillance involved very specific attention to Kaposi's sarcoma among gay men to trace the phenomenon of AIDS. This in turn influenced how doctors and scholars studied the epidemic: the kinds of bodies they considered to be afflicted, or at risk, and the kinds of bodies that then entered into research itself. Epidemiology thus profoundly impacted clinical practice.[22] In the context of the United States, but also globally, AIDS clinical research continues to be marked by an epidemiological narrative preoccupied with Kaposi's sarcoma and, therefore, the experiences, bodies, and lives of (white) US gay men.

The privileging of Kaposi's sarcoma in clinical and epidemiological research in the early 1980s focused attention on certain kinds of bodies and certain experiences with the epidemic. While this generated knowledge that was fundamental to better understanding the epidemic for some white US gay men, it simultaneously obscured the clinical realities of AIDS for others. Clinical research on opportunistic infections conducted in Montreal during this time, and organized with regard to race, shows the limits of investigating AIDS with a primary focus on Kaposi's sarcoma.[23] As the data presented in table 5.1 makes clear, an examination of opportunistic infections with regard to race yields the important conclusion, at least for the context of Montreal at the time, that the clinical manifestations of AIDS were markedly different among Haitians than among those categorized as gay men as reviewed in the clinical literature. Whereas Kaposi's sarcoma was understood as one of the primary signs of what was first termed Gay-Related Immune Deficiency (GRID), before the condition was renamed AIDS, this specific infection appeared to manifest itself much less frequently in Haitians living in Montreal. In contrast, Haitians dealt significantly with toxoplasmosis, an infection less observed among white Québécois. My point here is simple: the symbolic weight and global reach of the US clinical definition and surveillance of AIDS, particularly in the early years of the disease, prevented an adequate clinical observation of the phenomenon. The opportunistic infections that manifested themselves among white gay men with access to health care in the United States were extrapolated to define the disease more broadly, such that the experiences of Haitian migrants were eclipsed.

Diseases Diagnosed by Race

Researchers outside the United States noted the limits of the US clinical definition of AIDS, notably with regard to tuberculosis. Jean William Pape, a noted specialist on AIDS in Haiti, underlines the different clinical experiences of the disease according to region.

> Aux États-Unis la tuberculose n'est pas reconnue comme une infection opportuniste sévère répondant aux critères de la définition du SIDA.

Table 5.1 Diseases diagnosed by race in Montreal, 1985

OPPORTUNISTIC INFECTION	WHITE	HAITIAN	BLACK NON-HAITIAN	ASIAN
Kaposi's sarcoma	22	2	2	0
PCP	44	25	11	1
Candida esophagitis	21	12	1	0
Toxoplasmosis	5	16	1	0
CMV	6	4	1	0
Herpes	13	12	1	0
Cryptoccal meningitis	3	1	0	0
Atypical tuberculosis	11	1	0	0
Lymphoma (central nervous system)	2	0	0	0
Cryptosporidiosis	5	3	0	0

Source: Lamontagne, SIDA, 82 (cumulative epidemiological data up to December 13, 1985, taken from Comité SIDA-Québec)

Cependant en Haïti et au Zaïre, 30% à 40% des patients SIDA font une tuberculose, soit précocement (il peut s'agit de la première manifestation) soit plus tardivement. Tous les aspects de la tuberculose peuvent être observés mais les lésions extra-pulmonaires ou des disséminées sont plus fréquentes que dans la tuberculose classique.[24]

[In the United States, tuberculosis is not recognized as a severe opportunistic infection responding to the criteria of an AIDS definition. However, in Haiti and in Zaire, 30 to 40 percent of AIDS patients experience tuberculosis, either prematurely (it could be the first manifestation) or in a late fashion. All aspects of tuberculosis can be observed but extra-pulmonary or scattered lesions are more frequent than in classic tuberculosis.]

Pape's comment illustrates the larger point I am making: the imposition of a US clinical definition of disease excluded certain bodies, notably Black ones, from inclusion in global research. The clinical history of AIDS, in the United States and globally, is wed to the opportunistic infection of Kaposi's sarcoma. Yet this history only brings certain bodies into view. Critical reflection on how we write history, then, can help us imagine different experiences of the AIDS epidemic and as such complicate our understanding of this disease.

To date, I have considered how certain forms of knowledge and of writing history circumscribe what and how we know about AIDS. A generalization of US epidemiological statistics across North America gives the mistaken impression that AIDS first hit white gay male communities. While that may or may not be true for certain locations in the United States, the local context of Montreal is more complicated.[25] Furthermore, the limits of generalizable epidemiological findings on AIDS were extended into the clinical realm. Since the clinical manifestations of AIDS were different among Haitians than among the white US gay men observed in early studies, this meant that Black men and women living with AIDS were simply not counted—or at least not counted in the same way. Having examined some of the constraints of epidemiological and clinical knowledge on the history of AIDS in North America, I turn now to questions of community organizing. Just as Haitians were erased in certain articulations of epidemiological and clinical knowledge about AIDS, we can witness the neglect of collective mobilization within Haitian communities as an integral part of contemporary reflections on AIDS history.

Activism and Community Mobilization

The plethora of scholarly studies and cultural documents on AIDS activism in the United States focus their attention primarily on forms of community mobilization and direct action, most notably through the work of the AIDS Coalition to Unleash Power (ACT UP).[26] To be sure, attention to this group is important: ACT UP helped redefine relations between people with HIV/AIDS and the medical establishment; put tremendous pressure on local, state, and federal governments to develop a coordinated response to the epidemic; and impacted access to and availability of medication, whether experimental or otherwise.[27] The contributions of ACT UP have been significant indeed, not only in the field of HIV/AIDS but in thinking about and organizing access to health care more broadly. This direct action group was primarily composed of various chapters in the United States, mostly in large metropolitan centers (New York, Los Angeles, Chicago, San Francisco). But ACT UP also had affiliate chapters outside the United States, such as in Montreal (established circa 1989 and preceded by the activist group Réaction SIDA) and Paris (established in 1999 and still active today).[28] In all these ways, it makes good intuitive sense for researchers and cultural workers to focus their attention on this particular group and its contributions.

That said, a focus of attention on ACT UP can obscure other forms of community organizing and mobilization that merit attention. To take one example, in April 1990 the US Food and Drug Administration announced a policy preventing all Haitians from donating blood. Haitians responded quickly to this announcement, which recalled earlier events in 1983 in which the American Red Cross had designated Haitians as a "risk group" and asked them to abstain from giving blood. Specific tactics to protest this policy included media interventions, petitions, and a massive demonstration in New York City. The latter was impressive in its scope and mandate: held on April 20, 1990, this demonstration brought together at least fifty thousand people, blocking the Brooklyn Bridge and paralyzing the downtown core.[29] The actions of the Haitian community were ultimately effective, as the policy was overturned after it was announced.[30]

I cite this example of community organizing for two reasons. First, the sheer size of the demonstration constitutes it as likely the largest public manifestation in relation to HIV/AIDS in US history, perhaps even in global history. Yet if one considers the scholarly attention paid to the history of community mobilizing and public demonstrations on HIV/AIDS, this event does not generally appear.[31] Rather, the focus is on activities organized by ACT UP, such as an intervention at Saint Patrick's Cathedral in New York City that brought together approximately five thousand people.[32] How and why, then, does community mobilizing by Haitians go unnoticed? What kinds of narratives and frameworks are privileged to understand AIDS activist history in the United States, and what might get left out of such accounts?

This event raises the important matter of sources for historians, and that is the second reason why I have chosen to include it here. The demonstration in question was not organized by or for ACT UP New York. It was located within Haitian communities themselves. This suggests that if we base our research primarily in the archives of self-designated AIDS activists, we may only access part of the story. To be sure, one could consult the archives of ACT UP New York and find much relevant information and documentation with regard to Haitians (see, for instance, the interview with Betty Williams in the ACT UP New York Oral History project[33]). Karma R. Chávez, in particular, delves into the ACT UP archives to examine questions of immigration, and finds ample documentation about Haitian migrants.[34] Such an approach is, of course, worthwhile and makes an important contribution by thinking through matters of migration and AIDS activism. But it would be greatly strengthened, I submit, by considering archival sources that are not primarily based in AIDS activist sites but are located in sites of migrant communities themselves. To offer one example from the New York context: an investigation of the history of Haitian AIDS activism would, I submit, necessarily need to base itself in the newspapers, community debates, and radio programs of the Haitian community (the latter are particularly important given the centrality of orality to Haitian culture).[35] Specifically with regard to AIDS in New York City, such an investigation might begin with a Haitian radio show, "L'Heure haïtienne," that aired on March 13, 1983.[36] Only days after the American Red Cross released its declaration, this radio show brought together several people: public health experts Dr. Friedman, Rebecca Reese, and James Monroe, as well as Lisa Watson of Union 1199 representing hospital workers. This radio show offers useful avenues for future research that might not be visible if one limits oneself to a more recognized AIDS archive. For example, in the exchange with Friedman, the interviewer maintains that public health ought to come out with a strong statement in favor of Haitians, given the lack of definitive information about transmission at the time.

> Mwen . . . te demande mesye, poukisa, *au fait*, depatman Lasante pa janm di anyen *sur le fait que la presse* isi ap blame refijye kòm kategori moun k ap pote maladi a. Msye di m ke li dakò pratikman ke pa gen ase enfòmasyon, ke, li pa pense ke *la presse* ta dwe ap blame ayisyen yo kòm kategori moun ki pote maladi a paske pa gen ase enfòmasyon.[37]

> [I asked . . . asked this man [Dr. Friedman] why, in fact, the department of public health has not said anything about the fact that the press blames refugees as a category of people with this disease. This man was more or less in agreement that there was not enough information, and he did not think that the press should blame Haitians as a category of people who carry the disease because there is not enough information.]

This radio show testifies to specific government policy that discriminated against Haitians, as well as to the negative presentation of Haitians in the media. But perhaps most significantly, the interview illustrates how Haitians challenged public health itself to intervene in the media and correct the misinformation that was circulating. Careful listening of this radio show thus illustrates a fundamental activist tactic: beyond dispelling myths in the media, or denouncing an institutional policy that is racist, this work challenges state institutions to provide accurate information about infectious disease in general, and specifically with regard to migrant populations. In consulting this radio archive, I submit, we can obtain a more complex analysis of Haitian activism than if we simply consult mainstream media representations and/ or the text of institutional policies.[38]

To take another example, the radio show included a representative from a union for hospital employees: this is especially relevant for Haitians given the large number of Haitians working as doctors or nurses.[39] This suggests that organizing occurred, from the get-go, with hospital workers within a Haitian context, a finding confirmed in my own research in the setting of Montreal, where the response to AIDS was organized first and foremost by Haitian nurses. A consideration of Creole-language community media, then, opens up sites of inquiry that may not be adequately explored if one simply consults the English-language archives of established AIDS groups.

My reflections on AIDS history and community mobilization seek to interrogate what we know about the history of the epidemic, and how we know it. Investigations of AIDS histories that base themselves in recognized sites of AIDS activism, notably ACT UP, can offer us many insights. But they might tell only some of the stories, and there is thus a danger that if we take these narratives to be the definitive history of AIDS activism per se, we tell a tautological story.[40] While the previous sections of this chapter considered the dangers of extrapolating US data and frameworks to those outside the United States, my work on community mobilizing suggests that the repetition of ACT UP as *the* site of AIDS activism flattens the complexity of AIDS organizing within the United States itself. In this process, Black and migrant bodies disappear from view, as do their collective actions and mobilizations.

Conclusion

This chapter takes up the thorny challenge of how we think about the history of AIDS, both within the United States as well as outside it. Initial knowledge of the epidemic was grounded in the epistemological frameworks of the United States, notably in disease surveillance and epidemiology. This way of understanding AIDS focused its attention on gay men in particular, as well as the opportunistic infections they presented, namely Karposi's sarcoma. This paradigm was taken up internationally, such that it is commonplace to claim that, at least in the context of North America, AIDS emerged in white gay male communities.[41] The data presented from the local context in Montreal offers a different story: AIDS was first observed primarily among Haitians, in addition to white gay men. Moreover, the clinical manifestations of the disease among Haitians was markedly different: while the US white gay men who were researched dealt in particular with Kaposi's sarcoma, Haitians in Montreal exhibited tuberculosis and toxoplasmosis. A mere application of a US knowledge framework to the local context in Montreal obscures both whom was affected by this epidemic as well as their bodily experiences. Aside from epidemiological and clinical health matters, my research demonstrates the ways in which certain versions of US AIDS history neglect the tremendous contributions of Haitian organizers in responding to this epidemic. A knowledge framework exclusively concerned with self-designated AIDS activists ignores the work that other organizers did in this field. Here, I caution against research that limits itself to ACT UP, since it obscures much of the complicated work done on the ground and as such is of limited value for understanding the complexities of dealing with AIDS *within* the United States.[42]

The objective of this chapter has been primarily to raise epistemological questions about how we know what we know. Scholarly inquiry in this vein needs to attend to matters of which paradigms are valued, and why. A double movement is here necessary: on the one hand, to think critically about the ways in which US narratives of AIDS history circulate outside the United States; and on the other hand, to generate local, grounded knowledge that might complicate such a vision (outside the United States, to be sure, but even within it). And in this light, epistemological reflection necessarily brings with it methodological innovation. Researchers, scholars, and cultural producers who wish to produce knowledge *otherwise* about the history of AIDS are faced with the challenge of consulting sources that can illuminate histories and realities heretofore unexplored.[43] In so doing, our understandings of AIDS will be deepened. Moreover, our knowledge production practices can offer something to displace the frameworks of empire. Therein lies the epistemological and methodological challenge for future AIDS histories.

Notes

This work has been supported by the Canadian Institutes of Health Research. The data was gathered in part by Elhadji Mbaye and Lilly Fanelli, whom I thank for their contributions. A preliminary version of some of these ideas was published in Namaste, *Oversight*; see especially chapter 1, pp. 15–17. A more developed exploration of these issues is available in Namaste, *Savoirs créoles*.

1 Hilderbrand, "Retroactivism"; Gould, *Moving Politics*.
2 See ACT UP Oral History Project, accessed May 17, 2017, www.actuporalhistory .org.
3 See AIDS Activist History Project, accessed May 17, 2017, https:// aidsactivisthistory.ca.
4 Projets hybris, "Propositions for the AIDS Museum"; Projets hybris, "More Propositions for the AIDS Museum."

5 Broqua, *Agir pour ne pas mourir!*; Lestrade, ACT UP.

6 "Pneunomcystis Pneumonia."

7 Auerbach et al., "Cluster of Cases."

8 Altman, "30 Years"; Harris, "Life after Death."

9 For an analysis of how epidemiological data on AIDS from San Francisco was extrapolated beyond that city, see Cochrane, *When AIDS Began*. For a medical history that debunks the myth of white gay male French Canadian flight attendant Gaëtan Dugas as Patient Zero, see McKay, *Patient Zero*.

10 Croix-Rouge canadienne, Communiqué de presse, March 10, 1983, archives, Bureau Communautaire des Haïtiens de Montréal (BCHM).

11 Flavien, "SIDA."

12 Mills, *Place in the Sun*; Massé, "L'émergence de l'ethnicité haïtienne."

13 Point 7b, Minutes of the meeting between the Red Cross and members of the Haitian community, April 13, 1983, archives, BCHM. Translations are mine unless otherwise noted.

14 See, for instance, the clinical definition of AIDS, in "Current Trends Update on Acquired Immune Deficiency Syndrome." For a critique of this definition, see LeBlanc et al., "Opportunistic Infections."

15 See Déjean, *Les Haïtiens au Québec*; Mills, *Place in the Sun*.

16 Fortin, "La transfusion sanguine."

17 See, for instance, "A.I.D.? Acquired Immune Deficiency," GMHC *Newsletter* 1 (1982). Specific epidemiological surveillance on Kaposi's sarcoma is especially noted in the section "A View from the Center for Disease Control."

18 See, for example, Hymes et al., "Kaposi's Sarcoma"; Friedman-Kien, "Disseminated Kaposi's Sarcoma Syndrome"; Durack, "Opportunistic Infections"; Jensen et al., "Kaposi's Sarcoma"; Marmer et al., "Risk Factors."

19 "KS: Latest Developments," *New York Native*, August 24, 1981; Citizens for Human Equality, *Kaposi's Sarcoma*.

20 Gorin, "Kaposi's Sarcoma."

21 For an overview of the history of this group, see the "Dossier SIDA" of the journal *Médica: Revue haïtienne de médecine*, no. 2 (June 1987).

22 For an analysis of this issue in the context of New York, see Carroll, *Mobilizing New York*.

23 Lamontagne, SIDA, 82.

24 Pape, "L'épidémiologie de l'infection," 2. See also Pape et al., "Acquired Immunodeficiency Syndrome (AIDS) in Haiti."

25 My argument here is grounded in the local specificity of Montreal. But a detailed, grounded analysis of AIDS in US cities with large Haitian populations (Miami, Boston, New York, and Chicago) would similarly complicate tremendously the official narratives of the US epidemic, locating it primarily among gay men. Similarly, a detailed ethnography of drug users and their communities would offer different ways to write and understand the history of this epidemic. On the latter subject, see, for instance, Rockwell, Joseph, and Friedman, "New York City." For a brief discussion on cases of Haitians living

in the United States, see McKay, *Patient Zero*. For a more developed overview of Haitians and AIDS in the context of Miami in the early 1980s, see Fournier, *Zombie Curse*.

26 Gould, *Moving Politics*; Hilderbrand, "Retroactivism"; Broqua, *Agir pour ne pas mourir!*; Hubbard and Schulman, *United in Anger*; France, *How to Survive a Plague*; Chávez, "ACT UP."

27 Epstein, *Impure Science*.

28 See ACT UP Paris, accessed May 17, 2017, http://www.actupparis.org.

29 For some video and news reportage of this demonstration, see "Haitian AIDS March," YouTube, 15:05, from the Haitians March on April 20, 1990, against FDA Blood Donor Rules Policy, posted by "cvolcy2006," January 10, 2011, https://www.youtube.com/watch?v=ot3MrHTVaHU.

30 Hilts, "F.D.A. Set"; Farmer, *AIDS and Accusation*.

31 A notable exception here is Farmer, *AIDS and Accusation*, 220.

32 See ACT UP, AIDS Coalition to Unleash Power, accessed May 17, 2017, http://www.actupny.org/YELL/stopchurch99.html.

33 My thanks to Sarah Schulman for this reference. See ACT UP New York interview #099, Betty Williams, August 23, 2008, http://www.actuporalhistory.org/interviews/index.html. While the ACT UP New York interviews include some work with Haitians, the index to the project does not contain any reference to Haitians or Haitian activism.

34 Chávez, "ACT UP."

35 See Tontongi, *Sèl pou dezonbifye Bouki*.

36 "L'Heure haïtienne," WKCR-FM, Columbia University, New York, March 13, 1983. A cassette copy of this program is available in the archives of BCHM.

37 "L'Heure haïtienne," WKCR-FM.

38 I cite this particular radio show, located in New York, as a point of entry to understand what kinds of stories may not make it into an Anglo-American public sphere. For a more developed analysis of the role of community radio in Haitian communities, specifically with regard to the HIV/AIDS crisis in Montreal, see Namaste, *Savoirs créoles*.

39 Massé, "L'émergence de l'ethnicité haïtienne."

40 Juhasz, "Forgetting ACT UP."

41 Altman, "30 Years"; Harris, "Life after Death."

42 See Román, *Acts of Intervention*; Brier, *Infectious Ideas*; Royles, "African American AIDS History"; Royles, *To Make the Wounded Whole*; Roque-Ramírez, *Queer Latino San Francisco*.

43 For excellent theoretical reflection in this regard, see Connell, *Southern Theory*.

Bibliography

Altman, Lawrence K. "30 Years In, We Are Still Learning from AIDS." *New York Times*, May 31, 2011.

Auerbach, David, William Darrow, Harold Jaffe, and James Curran. "Cluster of Cases of the Acquired Immune Deficiency Syndrome: Patients Linked by Sexual Contact." *American Journal of Medicine* 76, no. 3 (1984): 487–92.

Brier, Jennifer. *Infectious Ideas: U.S. Political Responses to the AIDS Crisis*. Chapel Hill: University of North Carolina Press, 2011.

Broqua, Christophe. *Agir pour ne pas mourir! ACT UP, les homosexuels et le sida*. Paris: Les Presses de Sciences Po, 2005.

Carroll, Tamar. *Mobilizing New York: AIDS, Antipoverty, and Feminist Activism*. Chapel Hill: University of North Carolina Press, 2015.

Chávez, Karma R. "ACT UP, Haitian Migrants, and Alternative Memories of HIV/AIDS." *Quarterly Journal of Speech* 98, no. 1 (2012): 63–68.

Citizens for Human Equality. *Kaposi's Sarcoma, Opportunistic Infections and the Urban Gay Lifestyle: Towards a Healthier Gay Lifestyle; What You Need to Know to Ensure Your Good Health*. Pamphlet prepared for the community by CHE (Citizens for Human Equality). Houston: Kaposi's Sarcoma Committee of Houston, 1982.

Cochrane, Michelle. *When AIDS Began: San Francisco and the Making of an Epidemic*. New York: Routledge, 2004.

Connell, Raewyn. *Southern Theory: The Global Dynamics of Knowledge in Social Science*. Crows Nest: Allen and Unwin, 2007.

"Current Trends Update on Acquired Immune Deficiency Syndrome (AIDS)—United States." *Morbidity and Mortality Weekly Report* 31, no. 37 (September 24, 1982): 507–14.

Déjean, Paul. *Les Haïtiens au Québec*. Montreal: Presses de l'Université du Québec à Montréal, 1978.

Durack, David. "Opportunistic Infections and Kaposi's Sarcoma in Homosexual Men." *New England Journal of Medicine* 305 (1981): 1465–467.

Epstein, Steven. *Impure Science: AIDS, Activism, and the Politics of Knowledge*. Los Angeles: University of California Press, 1996.

Farmer, Paul. *AIDS and Accusation: Haiti and the Geography of Blame*. Berkeley: University of California Press, 1992.

Flavien, Yves. "SIDA: Le courage de la vérité et de la rigueur." *Collectif paroles* 22 (1983): 2–6.

Fortin, Richard. "La transfusion sanguine et le SIDA: Une menace sournoise." *Le Courrier médical* 3, no. 7 (1983): 2.

Fournier, Arthur. *The Zombie Curse: A Doctor's 25-Year Journey into the Heart of the AIDS Epidemic in Haiti*. Washington, DC: Joseph Henry, 2006.

France, David, dir. *How to Survive a Plague*. Documentary film. New York: Public Square Films, 2012. 120 min.

Friedman-Kien, Alvin E. "Disseminated Kaposi's Sarcoma Syndrome in Young Homosexual Men." *Journal of the American Academy of Dermatology* 5, no. 4 (1981): 468–71.

Gorin, Isabelle. "Kaposi's Sarcoma without the U.S. or 'Popper' Connection." *The Lancet* 319, no. 8277 (1982): 908.

Gould, Deborah. *Moving Politics: Emotion and ACT UP's Fight against AIDS*. Chicago: University of Chicago Press, 2009.

Harris, Michael. "Life after Death." *The Walrus*, September 2011.

Hilderbrand, Lucas. "Retroactivism." *GLQ: A Journal of Lesbian and Gay Studies* 12, no. 2 (2006): 303–17.

Hilts, Philip. "F.D.A. Set to Reverse Blood Ban." *New York Times*, April 24, 1990.

Hubbard, Jim, and Sarah Schulman, dirs. *United in Anger: A History of ACT UP*. Documentary film. Los Angeles: The Film Collaborative, 2012. 93 min.

Hymes, Kenneth, Tony Cheung, Jeffrey Greene, Neils Prose, Aaron Marcus, Harold Ballard, Daniel William, and Linda Laubenstein. "Kaposi's Sarcoma in Homosexual Men—A Report of Eight Cases." *The Lancet* 318, no. 8247 (1981): 598–600.

Jensen, Olemøller, H. T. Mouridsen, Nielsstrandberg Petersen, Klaushou Jensen, Kristian Thomsen, and Kay Ulrich. "Kaposi's Sarcoma in Homosexual Men: Is It a New Disease?" *The Lancet* 319, no. 8279 (1982): 1027.

Juhasz, Alexandra. "Forgetting ACT UP." *Quarterly Journal of Speech* 98, no. 1 (2012): 69–74.

Lamontagne, Estelle. *SIDA*. Montreal: Leméac, 1986.

LeBlanc, R. P., M. Simard, K. M. Flegel, and N. J. Gilmore. "Opportunistic Infections and Acquired Cellular Immune Deficiency among Haitian Immigrants in Montreal." *Canadian Medical Association Journal* 129, no. 11 (1983): 1205–9.

Lestrade, Didier. *ACT UP: Une histoire*. Paris: De Noel, 2000.

Marmer, Michael, Alvine Friedman-Kien, Linda Laubenstein, R. David Bryum, Daniel William, Sam D'Onofrio, and Neil Dubin. "Risk Factors for Kaposi's Sarcoma in Homosexual Men." *The Lancet* 319, no. 8281 (1982):1083–87.

Massé, Raymond. "L'émergence de l'ethnicité haïtienne au Québec." PhD diss., Université Laval, 1983.

McKay, Richard A. *Patient Zero and the Making of the AIDS Epidemic*. Chicago: University of Chicago Press, 2017.

Mills, Sean. *A Place in the Sun: Haiti, Haitians, and the Remaking of Québec*. Montreal: McGill-Queen's University Press, 2016.

Namaste, Viviane. *Oversight: Critical Reflections on Feminist Research and Politics*. Toronto: Women's Press, 2015.

Namaste, Viviane. *Savoirs créoles: Leçons du sida pour l'histoire de Montréal*. Montreal: Mémoire d'encrier, 2019.

Pape, J. W. "L'épidémiologie de l'infection HIV en Haïti." *Médica: Revue haïtienne de médecine* (1987): 2.

Pape, J. W., B. Liautaud, F. Thomas, J. R. Mathurin, M. M. St. Amand, M. Boncy, V. Pean, M. Pamphile, A. C. Laroche, and W. D. Johnson Jr. "Characteristics of the Acquired Immunodeficiency Syndrome (AIDS) in Haiti." *New England Journal of Medicine* 309, no. 16 (1983): 945–50.

"Pneunomcystis Pneumonia—Los Angeles." *Morbidity and Mortality Weekly Report* 30, no. 21 (June 5, 1981): 1–3. https://www.cdc.gov/mmwr/preview/mmwrhtml/june_5.htm.

Projets hybris. "More Propositions for the AIDS Museum." Théâtre Lachapelle, Montreal, April 24–28, 2017. Accessed May 17, 2017. http://lachapelle.org/fr/morepropositionsforaidsmuseum.

Projets hybris. "Propositions for the AIDS Museum." Théâtre des Écuries, October 16–18, 2014. Accessed May 17, 2017. https://www.facebook.com/events/296925067158456/.

Rockwell, Russell, Herman Joseph, and Samuel Friedman. "New York City Injection Drug Users' Memories of Syringe-Sharing Patterns and Changes during the Peak of the HIV/AIDS Epidemic." AIDS and Behavior 10, no. 6 (2006): 691–98.

Román, David. Acts of Intervention: Performance, Gay Culture, and AIDS. Bloomington: Indiana University Press, 1998.

Roque-Ramírez, Horacio N. Queer Latino San Francisco: An Oral History, 1960s–1990s. Basingstoke: Palgrave Macmillan, 2013.

Royles, Dan. "African American AIDS History Project." Accessed September 2, 2019. afamaidshist.org.

Royles, Dan. To Make the Wounded Whole: African American Responses to HIV/AIDS. Chapel Hill: University of North Carolina Press, forthcoming.

Tontongi. Sèl pou dezonbifye Bouki: Esè politiko-literè sou ekrvien kontanporen ak sou trayizon demokrasi, mistifikasyon lengwistik ak lit istorik pou chanjman ann Ayiti. Cambridge, MA: Trilingual Press, 2014.

Weissman, David, dir. We Were Here. Documentary film. Weissman Projects. New York: New Yorker Films, 2011. 90 min.

SIX "A VOICE DEMONIC AND PROUD": SHIFTING THE GEOGRAPHIES OF BLAME IN ASSOTTO SAINT'S "SACRED LIFE: ART AND AIDS"

Darius Bost

Poet, playwright, dancer, musician, and performance artist Assotto Saint was born Yves François Lubin, in Las Cava, Haiti, in 1954. He moved to New York City in 1970 and became a prominent figure in US Black gay cultural arts movements of the 1980s and 1990s, until his death from AIDS complications in 1994. He began his exploration of the cultural arts as a dancer with the Martha Graham Dance Company. He self-published two collections of poetry, *Stations* (1989) and *Wishes for Wings* (1994), and his plays and poetry were published in numerous literary magazines and anthologies. He created a press, Galiens Press, and published two anthologies of black gay writing, *The Road before Us: 100 Black Gay Poets* (1991) and *Here to Dare: 10 Black Gay Poets* (1992). Saint founded the Metamorphosis Theater with his partner, Swedish American musician Jan Holmgren. Together they staged four multimedia performances: "Risin' to the Love We Need," "New Love Song," "Black Fag," and "Nuclear Lovers." Saint and Holmgren formed a band called Xotica, "which inflected the Brit techno-pop style of the 80s."[1] Saint was one of the founding members of the New York City–based, Black gay writers' groups Blackheart Collective and Other Countries Collective.

Despite Saint's important cultural and political contributions to US Black gay cultural arts movements in the early era of AIDS, he remains a marginal figure in historical and cultural analyses of this period. Saint's marginalization leaves intact questions regarding the damage that the AIDS crisis and subsequent state neglect had on the interior lives of Black gay men, and the methods used by Black gay men to resist psychological damage. This chapter explores how Saint drew upon sacred traditions to construct a sense of self in the context of AIDS discourses that converged to mark his being as a site of stigma and blame. Saint's nonnormative gender and sexual identity, white partner, and Haitian heritage marked him as multiply marginalized within the context of the AIDS epidemic in the United States. The Black gay cultural arts movements in which he participated grew out of Black nationalist ideologies of the previous decades, thereby categorizing Saint's interracial relationship as a betrayal of the sexual politics of Black gay nation-building. Saint's participation in the gay male sexual revolution of the 1970s, and his self-identification as a "snow queen" and "leather queen" who visited predominantly white gay spaces downtown, further stigmatized Saint's interracial desires, since Black gay men blamed the spread of HIV/AIDS in their communities on other Black gay men who maintained social and sexual relations with white men. Saint's gender deviance also relegated him to an outsider position within middle-class Black gay communities. This class-based exclusion rendered "drag queens" as more vulnerable to AIDS, as it deemed them illegible to state apparatuses and unworthy of community support. Assotto Saint's embodiment of multiple modes of marginality figured him as "the impossible Black homosexual," unable to fully belong within the Haitian nation or diaspora, the US nation-state, or even gay subcultural communities.[2]

Given Saint's embodiment of multiple modes of negation in the 1980s and 1990s, this chapter explores how Saint's writing both confronts and resists the violent global forces that figured him as multiply dispossessed. Through a close reading of Saint's essay "Sacred Life: Art and AIDS"—focusing in particular on his experimentation with the essay form—I examine how Saint drew upon notions of the sacred as a way of contesting the neoliberal ideologies that structured his political disenfranchisement and marked his ontological status as imperiled. Local, national, and global discourses of blame threatened Saint's sense of self, insofar as his (self-)negation was necessary for turning back to normality all the communities to which he belonged. In other words, Saint's social and corporeal death was necessary to bolster their claims to citizenship and subjective wholeness. Taking up E. Patrick Johnson's call to "expand notions of the sacred" and M. Jacqui Alexander's call for scholars to "examine how spiritual practitioners employ metaphysical systems to provide the moorings for their meanings and understandings of self," this chapter explores Saint's essay as a sacred text that draws on multiple spiritual traditions—Catholicism, Haitian Vodou, and ancestral presences—to construct a notion of self that is bound up with yet irreducible to these racialized, gendered, sexualized, and neo-imperial discourses of blame.[3]

Mapping the Geographies of Blame

In the 1980s and 1990s, dominant state and cultural discourses blamed gay men and Haitian immigrants for the spread of AIDS in the United States. Douglas Crimp demonstrates how state, media, and even discourses from within the gay community, especially the construction of "Patient Zero," labeled gay men's sexual irresponsibility as the "cause" of the epidemic.[4] Paul Farmer describes how US public health officials inferred that Haitian immigrants brought the AIDS epidemic to the United States. These researchers believed that unraveling the "Haiti connection" would lead them to discover the epidemiological origins of the disease. Because Haitians denied intravenous drug use, homosexual activity, and a medical history of blood transfusions, their contraction of the virus led US scientists to ascribe their illness to the deviance of Black culture, in particular to Vodou practices. Haitian immigrants in the United States and Canada were automatically deemed AIDS carriers, leading to anti-Haitian discrimination.[5] This double-bind meant that, as a gay Haitian American immigrant, Saint was doubly stigmatized.

In the context of the AIDS epidemic, interracial desire was also a site of blame within Black gay communities. Black gay writer and activist Joseph Beam wrote in the essay "Brother to Brother: Words from the Heart," published in his 1986 edited anthology, *In the Life: A Black Gay Anthology*, that "Black men loving Black men is the Revolutionary Act of the eighties."[6] For some this claim was understood, in the way Beam intended, as a declaration of the radical potential of love between Black men—in the form of creating networks of care and survival across difference. However, other Black gay cultural producers took up the quote to divided ends. Some Black gay men reduced the claim to the realm of the sexual and posited that the revolutionary act was in the disavowal of interracial relationships and sex, and that "prideful" Black gay identity could only be found in exclusive relationships with other Black men. The latter meant that queer interracial desire would be marked as "self-hatred" and detrimental to Black gay politics, in which "healthy" identity formation was expressed in acts of love between Black men. In the context of Black gay cultural movements that drew heavily on the cultural nationalist politics of the previous decades, Saint's long-term personal and professional relationship with Holmgren became a source of cultural shame.

Saint's interracial relationship amassed more import in the context of the AIDS epidemic's traumatic, yet largely unremarked, impact on Black gay men. In the context of the AIDS epidemic, "snow queens"—a pejorative term for Black men who exclusively date or have sex with white men—were constructed as exhibiting "self-destructive" desire, since the state apparatus and mass culture had constructed AIDS as a "white gay disease." Ideas about AIDS as a white gay disease were sustained within Black gay communities as well. In his ethnography of Black gay men in Harlem, William G. Hawkeswood notes how his research subjects were able to remain AIDS-free in the early years of the epidemic by relegating their social and sexual lives to other Black men in Harlem. Black gay men who were infected or died from AIDS-related complications were believed to have participated in the predominantly white sexual cultures taking place downtown in Greenwich Village.[7] Outing oneself as a "snow queen" not only signaled one's failure to fulfill his political role of loving and having sex with Black men, but it also meant that one was risking his own physical health and the health of the Black gay community. Thus, Saint embodied the contradictions of loving and lusting after white men in an era in which this practice was considered "bad" politics and "unhealthy" sexual behavior.

Saint's work also becomes significant in the context of the struggle over the meanings of masculinity within Black gay male communities. In 1980 Saint became a founding member of the Black gay writers' group Blackheart Collective, which reemerged as Other Countries Collective in 1986.[8] One of the reasons for Blackheart's formation was the conservative gender politics of other New York City–based, Black gay male organizations. Black gay historian Kevin McGruder notes that Blackheart formed, in part, because the Committee of Black Gay Men, a Black gay male support group that formed in New York City in the late 1970s, expressed an aversion to Black male performances of femininity.[9] While Saint found a home in Blackheart, and eventually became a leader in Other Countries, his gender deviant performances unsettled other members of the group. In an interview with Cary Alan Johnson, a founding member of both Blackheart and Other Countries, he describes Saint's flamboyance during a performance at the Harlem State Office Building. Because the group was performing above Seventy-Second Street, they tacitly agreed to perform according to normative conventions of middle-class Black masculinity, therefore making the group's sexual difference more palatable to the predominantly Black audience. However, Saint's gender fluidity and defiantly queer performance did not adhere to these standards, and Johnson admits that it made the group uncomfortable.[10]

Saint's embodiment of stigma was spatialized by New York City's municipal politics. In 1975 New York City experienced a fiscal crisis and state officials envisioned the city's economic recovery through tourism and building a more profitable service sector economy.[11] New York City officials blamed Blacks and Latinos for its economic woes, and the city sought to change its image as a crime-ridden city full of idle and unruly Black, Latino, and white ethnic populations.[12] Heightening this image of the city in "crisis," New York City also developed an image in the seventies as a "latter-day Sodom teetering on the verge of ruin."[13] Linking popular constructions of the city as "crime-ridden" and as a "latter-day Sodom" to the image of the city in (fiscal) "crisis" demonstrates how racial and sexual ideologies helped map New York City's economic and political landscape in the 1970s.

The racialization and sexualization of "urban crisis" also shaped Black leaders' responses to AIDS when it began to devastate the Black community in the early 1980s. Although AIDS hit in cities with Black elected officials, these officials were limited by the economic crisis already confronting urban Black communities. As Cathy J. Cohen argues, this complex political environment created cleavages in Black communities along class lines, creating distinctions between a good and moral middle class and those deemed unworthy or tainted by outside evils, such as "junkies, faggots, punks, and prostitutes." At the very least, Cohen argues, Black leaders could have used their bully pulpits to make AIDS a priority for their constituency, but instead they pursued a more aggressive campaign of denial and distance that marked Black people with AIDS as outside the community.[14] In this context, Saint's Black gay identity not only deemed him a threat to the economic recovery of the city, his seropositive status also marked him as an outsider within Black American communities. Given the matrix of stigma and blame that threatened to rob him of his personhood, Saint turned to the sacred to fashion a sense of self.

Expanding Notions of the Sacred

Assotto Saint's Haitian heritage and racialization as a Black man in the United States informed his cultural production and activism. Saint's migration from Haiti to New York City in the early 1970s was propelled by multiple dislocations—his sexual difference, an oppressive political regime, and the forces of global capitalism that structured Saint's mother's earlier migration to the United States to work as a nurse. Though Saint was seduced by gay liberation movements and the gay male sexual cultures of NYC, his queer Haitian diasporic subjectivity marked him as an outsider in gay communities and in New York's Haitian communities, even as these communities were publicly battling discrimination after being blamed for the spread of

AIDS in the United States. Saint refused to distance himself from any part of his identity, however. Erin Durban-Albrecht argues that Saint stood out among other prominent leaders of the Black gay cultural arts movement in the United States "for keeping Haiti, and by extension the larger 'geography' impacted by American imperialism, within the scope of the critique."[15] His ties to Haiti and his dispossession in the United States meant that he did not limit his political critique to the geopolitical boundaries of the United States. The widespread impact of the AIDS epidemic in Haiti meant that his political critique of the racial, class, gender, and sexual ideologies that structured state neglect necessarily extended to US imperial territories like Haiti.

Saint's diasporic cultural memories of Haiti also included its sacred traditions and its place in the Third World imaginary as a site of revolution against the forces of empire. That Yves François Lubin chose the name Assotto Saint after he began writing in 1980 demonstrates his identification with these sacred traditions. He describes why he chose the pseudonym Assotto Saint as follows:

> Assotto is the Creole pronunciation of a fascinating-sounding drum in the voodoo religion. At one point I had taken to spelling Assotto with one "t" but superstitiously added back the other "t" when my CD4 t-cell count dropped down to nine. Saint is derived from Toussaint L'Ouverture, one of my heroes. By using the nom de guerre of Saint, I also wanted to add a sacrilegious twist to my life by grandly sanctifying the loud low-life bitch that I am.[16]

Saint's nom de guerre brings together aspects of Haitian Vodou, superstition, the Haitian Revolution, and AIDS in a ceremonious attempt to reimagine himself as a sacred being despite the converging forces that inscribed his body as inherently deviant and pathological. But Saint refused to deny the pathologies that circumscribe blackness, queerness, gender nonnormativity, Haitianness, and AIDS. Rather than distance himself from anti-Black, heteropatriarchal, and xenophobic logics that marked him as a "loud low-life bitch," Saint embraced stigma and risked abjection. His embrace of both sainthood and the moniker "loud low-life bitch" brings together the sacred and profane, simultaneously perverting historical memories of the Haitian Revolution and sanctifying the perversities attached to Black gay social life.

Saint's embrace of two seemingly antithetical subject positions would not be possible without his embrace of non-Western forms of spirituality. While the surname "Saint" emerges from his Catholic upbringing, Saint expands notions of the sacred by shifting from the "prescribed place" of the

Catholic Church, and its predetermined meanings of how sainthood should be performed, to the "space" of the sacred, which allows for multiple interpretations and performances of selfhood.[17] M. Jacqui Alexander describes the sacred as being "both everywhere, as in the Wind, and at specific moments, as in dreams; they mediate a process of interdependence, of mutual beingness, in which one becomes oneself in the process of becoming one with the Sacred."[18] By renaming himself Assotto, after a fascinating drum used in Vodou ceremonies, Saint reveals that his notion of the sacred includes Vodou rituals and practices, the very same rituals and practices that US scientists demonized as the cultural origins of the AIDS epidemic. Jana Braziel argues that Saint's nom de guerre "is a performance or a possession of the lwa," ancestral African spirits of Haitian Vodou. Historically, practitioners of Vodou absorbed the Catholic saints into their spiritual traditions, as receptacles of the lwa.[19] Thus, it is only by expanding notions of the sacred to include Vodou that Saint can embrace his multiplicity and reimagine the geographies of blame that he inhabits as sacred spaces from which he might draw knowledge and energy to fight against the forces that promote his demise. As Alexander argues, "the Sacred is inconceivable without an aesthetic."[20] Thus, I now turn to analysis of the aesthetic and formal qualities of Saint's personal essay "Sacred Life: Art and AIDS."

Black/Queer/Diasporic Experimentation with the Essay Form

Marlon B. Ross argues that the personal essay has held an honored place in African American writing since at least the 1903 publication of W. E. B. Du Bois's *The Souls of Black Folk*, a legacy continued in the works of writers such as James Baldwin, Ralph Ellison, Audre Lorde, June Jordan, and Joseph Beam. Noting Du Bois's characterization of the Black race as stamped by the "red stain of bastardy," Ross demonstrates how "perverse sexuality as a touchstone of racial identity haunts the African American essay from the outset."[21] If we locate Du Bois's *Souls* as one origin story of the personal essay tradition in African American letters, then we might also note how central notions of the sacred have been to the tradition. Du Bois's first chapter, "Of Our Spiritual Strivings," and last chapter, "Of the Sorrow Songs," exemplify the importance of the sacred to the personal essay tradition. Saint's exploration of the intertwined relationship between blackness, perverse sexuality, and the sacred in his essay "Sacred Life: Art and AIDS" situates him within "the long essay tradition" in African American letters by "testifying to the texture and heft of cultural identity by fusing personal experience to polemics, philosophy, politics, and poetry."[22] Saint extends this tradition through his attention to ethnic, gender, and sexual difference and his reliance on non-Western forms of spirituality.

Saint also deviates from the long tradition of the personal essay in African American letters through the experimental form of the essay. Because the traditional essay form and its protocols of objectivity and rationality might reaffirm stigma and pathology, Saint experimented with this Western intellectual form to expand notions of the sacred. The essay consists of some complete sentences that might be said to reflect the normative conventions of an essay. But the majority of the essay oscillates between short declarative statements in all lower-case letters, sentence fragments without a subject or in some cases without a definite article, run-on sentences, and phrases that defy the logics of reason. "Sacred Life" also departs from the formal conventions of the essay form in its shifts from sentences punctuated with a period to free verse poetry separated by line breaks. Though the essay contains these breaks in form, it coheres through repetition with a difference of central themes of the essay. Explaining his experimentation with the essay form, Saint writes:

> Unlike a musician or a painter, a writer needs language. Obvious and not very interesting, until question which language. Our century is littered with examples of writers who have had to make a choice to stick to or abandon their mother tongue. Almost more poignant than these is the case of a writer whose language is all around him & who at the same time is driven away from his language by political rather than personal considerations.[23]

Saint's reference to the language all around him and to the writer being "driven away from his language by political rather than personal considerations" marks his experimentation as guided by his social dislocation as a gay, gender-deviant, HIV-positive Haitian living in the diaspora. France's and the United States' (neo-)imperial domination of Haiti structures Saint's "choice to stick to or abandon [his] mother tongue." The languages forced on Black people by New World slavery and global empire become necessary for their political work. Saint repetitively describes Black gay social life as a "relentless unreality" and proclaims that Black gay men must "create [their] own reality and invite [their] readers and audience to enter this reality."[24] In order for the audience to enter, in this case, "Western bourgeois Man," Saint must negotiate the languages of imperialism to articulate his being.[25]

But this reference to the "languages all around him" also suggests an engagement with the sacred, the spirit world that Alexander describes as "both everywhere . . . and at specific moments." Throughout the essay Saint discusses the "mystical forces" that inform his artistic work.

> I have access to the spirit world, to shadows, to animal understanding to guides & voices, visions, old ways of thinking, all the altered states of consciousness necessary for the core artistic creation/the main purpose of ritual as it developed in tribal life is the creation of shared images/ awareness far distant from the human/truth is beauty/something that lifts us above the everyday, meditate on the music/an artist being swept up by mystical forces he does not totally understand/artistic freedom & adventure embodies the concept of liberation/the song affirms mystical connection between primitive magic and modern technology, art & medicine, astrology and television, spiritual journey/terror of aloneness/ musical, spiritual, & political words transfigure one another.[26]

Here Saint describes the "spirit world" as his primary site of knowledge, which gives him "awareness far distant from the human." This knowledge is only possible if he allows himself to be "swept up by mystical forces he does not totally understand." And this knowledge is a decolonial knowledge insofar as it disrupts the disciplinary boundaries that would separate the "musical, spiritual, and political."

Saint turns to the sacred because the cultural, social, and political systems in his historical moment did not address the lived experiences of Black gay men.

> Contemporary culture, social, & political systems often countervail such fulfillment, whose spiritual institutions appear not to address the experience of living in the present age, & whose artistic milieu generally shuns the expression of that aspiration/our energies of the struggle ahead, idealist posture & utopian gesture/rebirth is basic need of revolutionary spirit/cataclysmic night of upheaval that precedes purification & freshness of dawn/trying to get whole perspective of myself, & work with it/a community celebrating and validating itself.[27]

The essayist implies that current cultural, social, and political systems— those governed by relations of capital and structured by the afterlife of slavery and ongoing forms of colonialism—do not nourish one's relationship to sacred forces because that relationship is one that might fuel revolution and give access to the sacred energies necessary for "the struggle ahead." Saint's embrace of the sacred, of knowledge derived from ancestral forces, enables his continuous "rebirth," which he defines as "the basic need of revolutionary spirit."

The languages readily available to Saint are insufficient because they deny him access to selfhood, which, according to Alexander, is only possible through the "process of becoming one with the Sacred." Saint's aesthetic and formal choices emerge from the limitations of existing literary forms for articulating the full range of his personhood. This struggle to write against the forces of negation, particularly in the context of HIV/AIDS, is evident in the works of other Haitian writers. In her analysis of representations of AIDS in contemporary Haitian cultural production, Regine Michelle Jean-Charles argues that "even as artists enter into their representation with overtly political intentions, they are unwittingly enmeshed in and implicated by the prevailing narratives of stigma."[28] Jean-Charles explicitly addresses how these artists, in their efforts to distance Haitian bodies from the pervasive narratives of stigma plaguing the country, often restigmatize the homosexual. The shifting form of the essay, and the repetition with a difference of various lines in the essay, reflect Saint's ever-shifting selfhood, an embodied mode of formal innovation in which "musical, spiritual, & political words transfigure one another."

Given the pervasive discourses of stigma and blame that afflict his being, Saint describes how difficult it is to "move into [him]self."

> Took me so long to move into myself/a vision of mythical consciousness/a voice demonic and proud/investigate other gods and cultures/today you begin the task of writing life as it is happening./everything is a thought first, triggered by some action somewhere, then registered on paper.[29]

Saint's move into himself can only come through "a vision of mythical consciousness/a voice demonic and proud." His embrace of mythical consciousness and the demonic aligns with the work of Black feminist scholars Katherine McKittrick and LaMonda Horton-Stallings, both of whom build on the work of Sylvia Wynter to interrogate how Western bourgeois Man has colonized Black women's geographies and sexualities. These scholars demonstrate how the demonic and the mythical—with their origins in the supernatural—offer an outside vantage point for viewing our current world-human organization, which "makes possible a different unfolding."[30] Horton-Stallings argues, "It is only in recognizing one's mythical status that the process of making inventive futures can begin. Black art, music, and culture, then, is not simply representation of a subject and object in the world for a celestial being. It is matter, energy, and forces to be codified into a method for creating new worlds and ways of being."[31] McKittrick argues that the demonic "re-presents the grounds from which we can imagine the world and more workable human geographies" and helps us "think about the ways that black women necessarily contribute to this geography."[32] Saint's claim that sacred forces create the possibility of "writing life as it is happening" anticipates McKittrick's conceptualization of the demonic as a "process that is hinged on uncertainty and nonlinearity."[33] Moreover, Saint's moving into himself conjures the forces of the demonic to counter "the historical spatial unrepresentability of Black femininity," even if that femininity is attached to a body sexed as male.[34]

Indeed, it is only through the mythical and the demonic that Saint can reimagine the "relentless unreality" of life as a gay, gender nonconforming, Haitian American "leather queen" and "snow queen," living with AIDS. Saint writes, "In the shadows of the empire state building, the world trade centers and myself/I begin this essay."[35] By situating the origins of the essay in the shadows of these symbols of neoliberal capitalism, figured as local and global, Saint signals that the essay is a critique of the ordinariness of crisis produced by life under capitalism. This critique is only possible when he is in the shadows of himself, when he is writing at the limits of being. The shadows form the supernatural vantage point for seeing a future that is not predetermined as life under capitalism, and one that might provide alternatives to our current world-human organization. Writing from the shadows also provides possibilities for reimagining the racial, class, gender, and sexual ideologies that undergird the neoliberal urban landscape. Saint writes, "This is where, one of us will have to come for solace / Jan: Sweden's pier island of Alno yves: Haiti, Cayes' piers / in search of solace and solitude / in search of sex . . . I hear a song within me: wind & waves / I hear the music all around me."[36] For Saint, the Christopher Street piers, a dense geographic site for multiple configurations of blame, becomes a site of Black queer diasporic memory, the "holy ground" for a sacred ritual celebrating all the parts of himself and those ancestors dwelling in the body, air, and sea. The wind, waves, and music, both within and without, evoke the sacred energies alive in humans and in nature. And it is here that he remembers the revolutionary spirit within, the song within himself that holds the power to resist the converging structural forces that usher him to premature death.

Saint's significance extends beyond his important role in US Black gay cultural movements in the 1980s and 1990s, and his political struggles against racism, heteropatriarchy, Western empire, and the global AIDS pandemic.

In his reliance on the sacred, Saint provides an alternative epistemological framework for thinking about how Western humanism and neoliberal capitalism structure the ongoing crisis of AIDS in Black communities across the globe. Becoming one with the sacred, as Alexander argues, "becomes a way of embodying the remembering of Self... a self that is neither habitually individuated nor unwittingly secularized."[37] This conception of self offers "otherwise possibilities" in its ability to disrupt modern categorical distinctions like race, gender, sexuality, ability, and nation, categories that structure one's relationship to the state and capital.[38] Furthermore, the sacred draws our attention to the memories of resistance and alternative modes of being that already exist, memories that must be extinguished so that capitalism and its crises seem inevitable.

Notes

1   Braziel, *Artists, Performers, and Black Masculinity*, 86.
2   See Saint's poem "The Impossible Black Homosexual (OR Fifty Ways to Become One)," in Saint, *Spells of a Voodoo Doll*, 169–72.
3   Johnson, "Feeling the Spirit," 400; Alexander, *Pedagogies of Crossing*, 295.
4   Crimp, "How to Have Promiscuity," 242.
5   Farmer, AIDS *and Accusation*, 1–4, 208–12.
6   Beam, "Brother to Brother: Words from the Heart," in *In the Life*, 240.
7   Hawkeswood, *One of the Children*, 169–70.
8   Bost, *Evidence of Being*, 67–68.
9   McGruder, "To Be Heard in Print."
10 Telephone interview with Cary Alan Johnson, November 14, 2014.
11 Greenberg, *Branding New York*, 7–17.
12 Preface to Finch, *Assassination of New York*, vii–xxi.
13 Braunstein, "'Adults Only,'" 130.
14 Cohen, *Boundaries of Blackness*, 89–91.
15 Durban-Albrecht, "Legacy of Assotto Saint," 245.
16 See Saint, *Spells of a Voodoo Doll*, 9.
17 Johnson, "Feeling the Spirit," 400.
18 Alexander, *Pedagogies of Crossing*, 301.
19 Dayan, "Querying the Spirit," 44–46.
20 Alexander, *Pedagogies of Crossing*, 323.
21 Ross, "Queering the African American Essay," 302.
22 Ross, "Queering the African American Essay," 302.
23 Saint, "Sacred Life," 264.
24 Saint, "Sacred Life," 256.
25 Wynter, "Unsettling the Coloniality," 260.
26 Saint, "Sacred Life," 258.

27 Saint, "Sacred Life," 258.
28 Jean-Charles, "Sway of Stigma," 65.
29 Saint, "Sacred Life," 260.
30 McKittrick, *Demonic Grounds*, xxv.
31 Horton-Stallings, *Funk the Erotic*, 211.
32 McKittrick, *Demonic Grounds*, xxv.
33 McKittrick, *Demonic Grounds*, xxiv.
34 McKittrick, *Demonic Grounds*, xxv.
35 Saint, "Sacred Life," 262.
36 Saint, "Sacred Life," 262.
37 Alexander, *Pedagogies of Crossing*, 298.
38 Ashon Crawley defines "otherwise possibilities" as "announc[ing] the fact of infinite alternatives to what is." See Crawley, *Blackpentecostal Breath*, 2.

Bibliography

Alexander, M. Jacqui. *Pedagogies of Crossing: Meditations on Feminism, Sexual Politics, Memory, and the Sacred*. Durham, NC: Duke University Press, 2005.

Beam, Joseph, ed. *In the Life: A Black Gay Anthology*. Boston: Alyson Books, 1986.

Bost, Darius. *Evidence of Being: The Black Gay Cultural Renaissance and the Politics of Violence*. Chicago: University of Chicago Press, 2019.

Braunstein, Peter. "'Adults Only': The Construction of the Erotic City in New York during the 1970s." In *America in the Seventies*, edited by Beth Bailey and David Farber, 129–56. Lawrence: University Press of Kansas, 2004.

Braziel, Jana. *Artists, Performers, and Black Masculinity in the Haitian Diaspora*. Bloomington: Indiana University Press, 2008.

Cohen, Cathy J. *The Boundaries of Blackness: AIDS and the Breakdown of Black Politics*. Chicago: University of Chicago Press, 1999.

Crawley, Ashon. *Blackpentecostal Breath: The Aesthetics of Possibility*. New York: Fordham University Press, 2016.

Crimp, Douglas. "How to Have Promiscuity in an Epidemic." *October* 43 (1987): 237–71.

Dayan, Joan. "Querying the Spirit: The Rules of Haitian *Lwa*." In *Colonial Saints: Discovering the Holy in the Americas, 1500–1800*, edited by Allen Greer and Jodi Blinkoff, 31–50. New York: Routledge, 2003.

Du Bois, W. E. B. *The Souls of Black Folk*. New York: Oxford University Press, 2007.

Durban-Albrecht, Erin. "The Legacy of Assotto Saint: Tracing Transnational History from the Gay Haitian Diaspora." *Journal of Haitian Studies* 19, no. 1 (2013): 235–56.

Farmer, Paul. *AIDS and Accusation: Haiti and the Geography of Blame*. Berkeley: University of California Press, 2006.

Finch, Robert. *Assassination of New York*. New York: Verso, 1996.

Greenberg, Miriam. *Branding New York: How a City in Crisis Was Sold to the World*. New York: Routledge, 2008.

Hawkeswood, William G. *One of the Children: Gay Black Men in Harlem.* Berkeley: University of California Press, 2007.

Horton-Stallings, LaMonda. *Funk the Erotic: Transaesthetics and Black Sexual Cultures.* Urbana: University of Illinois Press, 2015.

Jean-Charles, Régine Michelle. "The Sway of Stigma: The Politics and Poetics of AIDS Representation in *Le président a-t-il le SIDA?* and *Spirit of Haiti.*" *Small Axe* 15, no. 3 (2011): 62–79.

Johnson, E. Patrick. "Feeling the Spirit in the Dark: Expanding Notions of the Sacred in the African-American Gay Community." *Callaloo* 21, no. 2 (1998): 399–416.

McGruder, Kevin. "To Be Heard in Print: Black Gay Writers in 1980s New York." *Obsidian III* 6, no. 2 (2005): 49–66.

McKittrick, Katherine. *Demonic Grounds: Black Women and the Cartographies of Struggle.* Minneapolis: University of Minnesota Press, 2007.

Ross, Marlon B. "Queering the African American Essay." *GLQ: A Journal of Lesbian and Gay Studies* 11, no. 2 (2005): 301–7.

Saint, Assotto, ed. *Here to Dare: 10 Gay Black Poets.* New York: Galiens, 1992.

Saint, Assotto, ed. *The Road before Us: 100 Gay Black Poets.* New York: Galiens, 1991.

Saint, Assotto. "Sacred Life: Art and AIDS." In *Spells of a Voodoo Doll: The Poems, Fiction, Essays, and Plays of Assotto Saint,* 255–71. New York: Masquerade, 1996.

Saint, Assotto. *Spells of a Voodoo Doll: The Poems, Fiction, Essays, and Plays of Assotto Saint.* New York: Masquerade, 1996.

Saint, Assotto. *Stations.* New York: Galiens, 1989.

Saint, Assotto. *Wishes for Wings.* New York: Galiens, 1994.

Wynter, Sylvia. "Unsettling the Coloniality of Being/Power/Truth/Freedom." *New Centennial Review* 3, no. 3 (2003): 257–337.

SEVEN CRISIS INFRASTRUCTURES: AIDS ACTIVISM MEETS INTERNET REGULATION

Cait McKinney

In one of the most significant judicial cases in the history of US online content regulation, an AIDS activist explained the internet to a federal judge. Justice Stewart Dalzell asked Kiyoshi Kuromiya, director of Philadelphia's Critical Path AIDS Project, to help him understand: "I'm very curious to know, how exactly does the technology work? How do you build up this access to, as you say here, thousands of databases that go through your Web page?" The activist's patient response, as documented by the court reporter, begins with a simple sentence fragment: "Okay." The text is punctuated as a full stop, perhaps followed by a deep breath. The transcript suggests Kuromiya was gathering himself to explain a terribly complex and important idea to someone very different from himself.

Kuromiya, founder of the Critical Path AIDS Project, was testifying at Philadelphia's Federal District Court in the American Civil Liberties Union's (ACLU) challenge to the 1996 Communications Decency Act (CDA). This was the US government's first attempt at online content regulation. Within the terms of the act, *any* online information about sex—whether hard-core porn or explicit instructions on condom use—was potentially "indecent" and "patently offensive." The act required sites hosting or linking to these materials to verify that users were not minors, or face substantial penalties.

Kuromiya walked the judge through some internet basics (message boards, hyperlinks, webpages, and internet service provision), then repeated his objection to the CDA: the act would inhibit the work AIDS activists were doing online to circulate accurate, accessible information about HIV transmission and treatment—information that was not reliably available elsewhere. Online infrastructures linked by countless network connections could not impose technological safeguard against "indecent" and "patently offensive" content about sexuality without also limiting open communication about HIV.

The web was, by its very nature, indiscriminate in its network structures, and this was a good thing. As Kuromiya explained it, users seeking online information about HIV could connect to a wide range of sources through hypertext links. The ACLU drew on this assertion to argue that the web's linked data infrastructures exceeded existing definitions of individual liability that were grounded in discreet, one-to-many broadcast models for understanding media. Users who followed HTML links from one site to another often did so without knowing in advance that they were "leaving" one site for another. Analyzing Critical Path's website and Kuromiya's affidavit, Judge Dalzell asked the activist: "You seem to have entered into a number of arrangements, thousands of them, with institutions including research institutions. . . . Have you all changed anything in the way you communicate information to users [since the law was passed]?" Kuromiya replied, "No. We're constantly updating our site, but no, we haven't changed anything. . . . I'm not sure how to interpret that law. I do not know what indecent means. I don't know what patently offensive means in terms of providing lifesaving and life promoting information to persons with AIDS or persons at high risk for contracting AIDS, including teenagers."[1] The judge found the internet too promiscuous; for the AIDS activist, that was precisely the new medium's point.

Kuromiya's explanation to the court was simple and hard to dismiss: in order to teach young people about condom use, testing options, oral sex, and other low-risk sex practices, websites about HIV transmission needed to write about, and even depict, explicit sex acts. The internet was immediate, relatively cheap for marginalized content producers to access compared to broadcast or print, accessible to amateurs, and fundamentally collaborative; it was technology ideally suited to making and rapidly circulating information about HIV when access through traditional channels was precarious, uneven, and slow. Kuromiya's expert opinion was based on a decade of activism dedicated to building and sustaining what he called "Community-Based Infrastructure for AIDS Information Dissemination on the Internet."[2] This model offered nonprofit internet service provision and web hosting for AIDS service and activist organizations and individual users affected by HIV/AIDS. Critical Path also ran a website and Bulletin Board System (BBS), a twenty-four-hour telephone hotline, and a print newsletter aimed at rapid and accessible information distribution.[3]

This chapter mobilizes archival research in Critical Path's papers alongside court records related to the CDA, analyzing how Critical Path leveraged its community-based internet infrastructure model to challenge online content regulations about sex. The first section outlines how Critical Path used early computer network technologies to realize community-based responses to HIV. The second section situates this model in relation to Kuromiya's position as a formerly interned Japanese American, a gay man, and a prison abolitionist. I analyze how Kuromiya used Critical Path's infrastructure model in his instrumental testimony. AIDS provided a ready example for explaining to the court and the public that the formal and regulatory development of consumer internet infrastructure could fundamentally determine online communication's social utility.

The ACLU used Kuromiya and Critical Path to argue that online information about sex needed to be free and open, without any technologically enforced minimum age verification. This approach reflected outreach strategies activists and AIDS Service Organizations (ASOs) had developed over the previous fifteen years to reach young people. Targeting youth with information about sex was controversial because it acknowledged their sexual subjectivity, unthinkable within what Cindy Patton has named the "national pedagogy" of the AIDS crisis, which relied on stigma, the valorization of innocence, and binary thinking about "good" and "bad" sexuality.[4] Imagined as potential internet users, teenagers were simultaneously too young to *look at porn online* and old enough to *have actual sex offline* (and require information about doing so).

The CDA and AIDS internet activism were intertwined, sociotechnical phenomena, caught up in the rapidly unfolding, neoliberal information environments of the 1990s. Through this case, growing moral panics over sexual expression online were articulated to HIV and related perceptions of risk. I argue that during the 1990s, cultural understandings of HIV were inseparable from attempts to define the place of sexuality online and regulate "appropriate" internet use. The internet as we know it today has been imagined and recalibrated through AIDS. The "AIDS crisis," as it was understood during this period by US judicial and legislative systems and the wider public, continues to reverberate in the ways online infrastructures both provide and limit access to information about sex.

Community-Based AIDS Information Infrastructure

Critical Path's work building what they called information infrastructure is an opening to thinking about how precarious users perform sociotechnical work that matters to histories of networked computing. Critical Path's

"Community-Based Infrastructure for AIDS Information Dissemination on the Internet" offered alternatives to costly, telecom-controlled internet access, while the basic terms of information provision were being regulated and contested. Critical Path's model brought AIDS activists' resiliency and resourcefulness with media technologies to bear on computer network models. As a conceptual framework, this model explained why new information infrastructures mattered for people living with HIV. Practically speaking, it offered several unique approaches to service provision that allowed users with HIV to participate in new computer networks.

The model combined grassroots internet service provider (ISP) architecture with the development of accessible, shared communication tools and training for would-be users. The organization saw internet access as a basic communication need for people living with HIV during a period in which the web was considered either the domain of businesspeople and large institutions or an expensive and technologically sophisticated hobby. Critical Path began online work in the late 1980s, hosting an HIV-related Bulletin Board System. The organization also redistributed online information from BBS in a widely circulated print newsletter and via a twenty-four-hour telephone hotline.[5] This "analog" outreach focused especially on prisoners with HIV. Critical Path's multimedia activism extended online information to those less likely to become internet users because of poverty, disability, or carceral status. By the mid-1990s Critical Path's activism was bringing new users into online networks so that they could contribute to the larger "HIV/AIDS internet."[6] Critical Path offered instructions on how to dial up, participate in a listserv or BBS, host a website, or get and use an email address. In the CDA case, Kuromiya used Critical Path's model to put forward a working understanding of the internet as a networked infrastructure and, more precisely, as a shared technology for survival and making-do. This model challenged emerging, Clinton-era ideas about an "information superhighway" that promoted an efficient, globalized economy as the ideal outcome for internet use.

Studies of infrastructure examine developing information economies and networked publics to understand how people, systems, technologies, and standards of practice come together within specific lifeworlds under modernity.[7] Focused on infrastructure for addressing HIV, Critical Path's community model carved out ways for marginalized users to make do within technical systems that were not necessarily of their own making. This approach to infrastructure emphasizes the importance of friction and differential access and is exemplified by queer approaches in infrastructure studies that had begun to develop by the mid-1990s: for example, Susan Leigh Star's

"Misplaced Concretism and Concrete Situations," which queers understandings of how infrastructures and social worlds are co-constructed. Star was an information studies scholar and also a lesbian feminist who published on sexual politics and collaborated with the African American, lesbian-feminist poet Audre Lorde. This biography enriched Star's thinking about infrastructures beyond the academic science and technology studies orientations typical of the field.[8]

In "Misplaced Concretism," Star writes that "our collective experiences" working in and across queer, antiracist, and feminist publics are "one of the richest places for which to understand these core problems in information systems design: how to preserve the integrity of information without *a priori* standardization and its attendant violence." In the same paragraph, Star asks, "Why should computer scientists read African American poets?"[9] Star is not asking rhetorically—she is imploring us to do the work of thinking and theorizing across fields and communities of struggle to understand why, when, and for whom information infrastructures matter.

Star and Kuromiya were worlds apart, and yet they shared a fundamental commitment to exploring information infrastructures from the perspectives of those most vulnerable to their failures. For activists and users living with illness and disability, applying emergent internet infrastructures to HIV could offer radical support to those most vulnerable to information scarcity. Building on Star's work, Lauren Berlant, Steven Jackson, and Nicole Starosielski have each considered how infrastructures are maintained, repaired, or even purposefully broken by people and collectives trying to manage precarity within difficult conditions not of their own making.[10] Berlant, in particular, imagines infrastructures as forms for critical sociality, whether this looks like working in them, and on them, adjusting (to) them, or slowly transitioning them into something else, however provisionally or temporarily.[11]

AIDS activists and people living with HIV built and used community internet infrastructure as a resource, and a tool for adjusting to how stigma shaped both the distribution of information and the distribution of vulnerability to HIV. Activists during the 1980s and 1990s employed many media technologies to circulate information about HIV within these conditions. They used video and public-access television programs, posters, pamphlets and print ephemera, porn, and emergent online networks.[12] Critical Path's infrastructure model systematized an idea that was common across these practices—that media technologies could create alternative networks designed by and for those most vulnerable to HIV. The infrastructure concept allowed Critical Path to understand and address the AIDS crisis as being about state-sanctioned abandonment and the unequal distribution of vulnerabilities among people of color, queer people, and people who were poor, incarcerated, or did sex work, all of whom experienced limited access to new computing technologies that directly affected their life chances.[13]

Kuromiya explained the organization's turn to a community infrastructure model in the Critical Path newsletter. His words critiqued the inexorability of a corporate-controlled, economically rationalized internet.

> We decided that we must not only be content providers but provide free access to the Internet and do so by becoming Internet hosts ourselves. We understood that many of the persons we wanted to reach were on disability or lower incomes and would never be able to access the Internet if they needed to pay America On Line $20 a month. We also disagreed with those who felt that this new state-of-the-art technology was inappropriate for those without college educations and high incomes. After all, we knew that this whole generation had grown up learning from television and video games, not reading books and technical literature. We felt they deserved the best our technology could provide them.[14]

Kuromiya critiques Clinton-era approaches to communication infrastructure development, in which internet access was managed as a resource for economic advancement.[15] In other words, "Community-Based Infrastructure for AIDS Information Dissemination on the Internet" is a response to the ways in which access to communications infrastructures was deeply stratified by ability, income, and carceral status. By 1996 the "AIDS crisis" was just reaching a mature stage of biopolitical management, but only for those with privileged access, while the relatively undeveloped World Wide Web presented growing uncertainties about how online communication might fundamentally revolutionize social life.

The ease with which community-based AIDS information infrastructure could be articulated to larger concerns around the developing consumer internet revolution is indicative of infrastructure's broader sexual politics during this period. As Nancy Fraser argues, Clintonism imagined social welfare through "infrastructure development" as a new kind of public good, conceived within a neoliberal framework that pursued "investment" in "high-tech, fiberoptic communications systems" but not "public day care, public housing, or public health."[16] For the Clinton-Gore administration, designing an online regulatory framework presented an uncharted opportunity to demonstrate how government ought to treat infrastructure more broadly: regulate *content* minimally to ensure "decency" while staying out of the way of formal and technical development so that the private sector could manifest the medium's revolutionary trajectory.

There were, in a sense, two internets within Clinton-Gore infrastructure rhetoric: one focused on form, the other on content. The first emphasized the novelty of network technology itself, which would democratize access to information and revolutionize business and human communication. This version of the internet was fast-moving, inevitable, and would advance the economy while simultaneously reducing or eliminating inequalities among people.[17] The second version of the internet focused on problem content: pornography, hate speech, and gratuitous violence that could be eliminated through good regulation.[18] Children factored in both approaches, as either the beneficiaries of programs aimed at rebuilding a failed, inequitable public education system through internet access or as innocents threatened by unregulated online content.[19] The children Clinton-Gore invoked were not sexually active teenagers in need of honest, explicit information about HIV; rather they were younger, sweeter, more innocent future users who might dial up at their school library or virtually attend the first webcast White House Easter Egg Roll (1998).[20]

The desire to leave technical infrastructure unchecked combined with the drive to regulate sexual content led to cumbersome early regulatory frameworks, including the CDA and the 1996 Telecommunications Act.[21] The acts took a hands-off approach to regulating ownership structures and technical design, concentrating power and control over new communication technologies in the hands of corporations and government.[22] Wendy Hui Kyong Chun has shown that the CDA and the Telecommunications Act of 1996 promised to ensure open access to the internet for all citizens on the surface while deregulating technologies and their ownership structures at a deeper level. These regulations imposed surveillance and corporate content management by justifying digital certificates, age and identify verification measures, and other forms of data collection that ultimately aided online business development rather than community use.[23]

Chun argues that the CDA *appeared* to support access: "Congress decided that it must stop the free circulation of some obscene ideas in order to ensure the free flow of others, in order to make cyberspace truly public, where public means free from pornography."[24] This logic narrowed the terms for what access entails by sidestepping "the relationship between access and infrastructure/income/education."[25] Put simply, the CDA was a substantial step in the internet's ongoing neoliberalization, which Kuromiya directly critiqued. Through the CDA, Clintonism took a hands-off approach to the internet's technical development while imposing content restrictions that would limit speech about sex. Working against this framework, Kuromiya and Critical Path imagined alternative models for online access that would work around the gatekeeping measures presented by the CDA and corporate convergence. These frameworks threatened "Community-Based AIDS Internet Infrastructure's" potential as an accessible method for doing equitable, grassroots, and potentially anonymous communications among vulnerable user groups. Critical Path built community infrastructure that marginalized users could readily use, carving out ongoing enclaves for the internet as a public utility that needed to be actively built, maintained, and protected from private interests and conservative sexual values. This work marks infrastructure not as a background operation that keeps business operating as usual but as a field of struggle people living with HIV get by within, or build, in ways that materialize solutions to the shared vulnerabilities they care about.

Kuromiya Goes to Court: Community AIDS Infrastructure versus the CDA

Kuromiya's activist commitments emerged from his experiences as a gay, HIV-positive, formerly interned Japanese American. His biography contextualizes the political goals behind Critical Path's infrastructure model and the organization's critique of the CDA. Kuromiya (fig. 7.1) was born at the Heart Mountain Japanese internment camp in Wyoming, where his family was forcefully relocated from suburban Los Angeles. In a 1997 interview with historian Marc Stein, Kuromiya explained that while he could not remember the camp, "I'm sure it affected my own activism and my own attitudes toward our government, war, racial issues."[26] Kuromiya moved to Philadelphia in 1961 to start school at Penn State, and he came of age as an activist within civil rights–era Black freedom struggles and antiwar movements.[27] He spent 1964–71 under FBI surveillance for his antiwar activism, and information about his life, housed at Philadelphia's LGBTQ community archives, contains a redacted copy of these surveillance files, acquired by the archives through a Freedom of Information Act request after Kuromiya's death.[28]

When Kuromiya seroconverted in the late 1980s and became deeply involved in Philadelphia's AIDS activist communities, he brought commitments to antiracism, queer models for sexual expression, and anticarceral consciousness drawn from his family's history of incarceration. As I argue in detail elsewhere, Kuromiya discovered that information systems could be an outlet for addressing these intertwined issues through his relationship

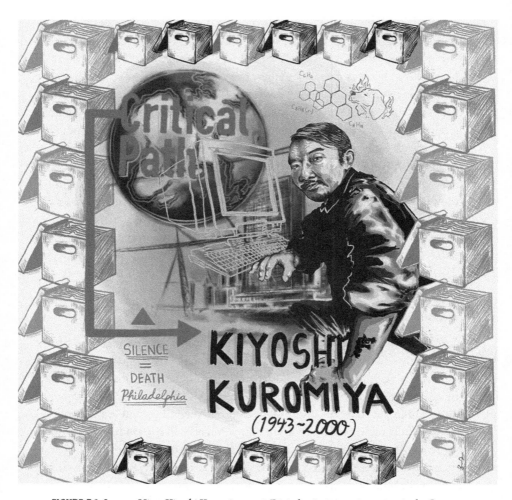

FIGURE 7.1. Lauren Higa, *Kiyoshi Kuromiya*, 2018. Digital painting, 1920 x 1080 pixels. Courtesy of the artist.

with the technological philosopher and architect Buckminster Fuller, most noted for designing the geodesic dome.[29] Kuromiya was Fuller's assistant in the early 1980s and helped him write the book *Critical Path* (1981), which argues that social problems could be addressed through thoughtful information systems.

Thinking through Fuller's systems theories, Kuromiya understood social problems and their solutions as intertwined within sociotechnical networks. For example, his anticarceral internet activism imagined the prison as a space not just of confinement but also one walled off from internet access. Bringing prisons into existing AIDS information networks could address the unique health needs of incarcerated people. Such integration also enables those who were incarcerated to share their own activism and strategies of survival with the wider HIV/AIDS community. To do this, Critical Path's newsletter featured regular articles by incarcerated writers, also published online through the organization's ISP. The newsletter was also free for subscribers in prisons (and all subscribers living with HIV/AIDS).[30]

Kuromiya's identity as an Asian American committed to antiracist organizing also shaped Critical Path's infrastructure model. As Che Gossett argues, to understand Kuromiya as solely an AIDS activist would "invisibilize the contributions and theorizations of queer of color activists."[31] Gossett argues that Kuromiya's multiple, entwined positions in social justice movements manifested a capaciousness for thinking across communities of struggle and imagining otherwise, characteristic of queer of color theory and activism.[32] In a way, Kuromiya *was* the computer scientist (or "skilled amateur," as he put it) reading African American poets who Susan Leigh Star had imagined.[33] Critical Path's infrastructure model, designed from within and also across these political orientations, developed out of enmeshment in multiple social justice worlds and an attendant understanding of HIV as a larger resource-distribution problem. In other words, Kuromiya could manifest his particular vision of the internet because he was able to imagine, through AIDS, other ways of being in collaborative relations of difference with people, systems, and problems.

The CDA put forward a vision of the internet that threatened this community infrastructure model. Specifically, the act would impose technological limitations on Critical Path's goals of networking across various sites, reducing barriers to access, and building online spaces where diverse sexualities could proliferate. The act's implications were unthinkable within Kuromiya's vision of what online communication ought to be doing for people living with HIV, hence his frustrated incredulity to the judge: "I'm not sure how to interpret that law. I do not know what indecent means."

Hobbyist, tinkerers, and internet activists like Kuromiya worked away at building and maintaining their own online infrastructures while large institutions fought publicly about what the internet would become. The mid-1990s was a period of regulatory scrambling in which government, telecom and tech companies, and lobby groups like the ACLU and Electronic Frontier Foundation vied to put in place policies and protocols to support their visions for online communication. Focused on free-speech concerns, the ACLU announced that it would seek a temporary restraining order (TRO) against the CDA's "indecent" and "patently offensive" clauses even before the law was passed. This TRO was granted by a Philadelphia federal judge one week after the CDA passed, and the case was heard by the three-judge Federal District Court just two months later. On June 12, 1996, this court ruled in favor of the ACLU.

When the government appealed this decision, the United States Supreme Court agreed to review the case, ultimately striking down these clauses in June 1997. As the earliest attempt at online content regulation, the CDA was part of a larger public education campaign about the internet as a public utility and a form of basic infrastructure; journalists covering the ACLU's challenge to the act were tasked with explaining to readers the ins-and-outs of how online communication worked, and why this technology warranted a political debate that ought to matter to the public. Ultimately, this case set a precedent for content regulation online and informed how a developing user base thought about the web as inseparable from communication about, and through, sexuality.

The Supreme Court's opinion, striking down the CDA's indecency clauses, understood online communication as personal telecommunications rather than broadcasting or publishing. Restricting access to sexually explicit materials was found unconstitutional under the First Amendment: as Justice John Paul Stevens, author of the majority opinion put it, "In order to deny minors access to potentially harmful speech, the CDA effectively suppresses a large amount of speech that adults have a constitutional right to receive and to address to one another."[34] These sexually explicit forms of speech might include porn but also "serious discussion" about "birth control practices," "safe sexual practices," "homosexuality," "artistic images that include nude subjects," "the consequences of prison rape," "and arguably the card catalog of the Carnegie Library" (if it were to be transmitted online).[35] Materials that might be "obscene" or "patently offensive" to some had clear public utility that justified deregulating sexual expression online.[36]

The court agreed with the ACLU's argument that the internet presented a unique community-based form of communications infrastructure because it could be used easily and inexpensively by regular people. Internet users, even amateurs, could circulate information on a wide scale, including information about all kinds of sex practices, not limited to sharing porn. Demonstrating the court's understanding of the niche social worlds that could thrive online through technologies like Critical Path's website and bulletin board, Justice Stevens wrote, "There are thousands of such groups, each serving to foster an exchange of information or opinion on a particular topic running the gamut from, say, the music of Wagner to Balkan politics to AIDS prevention to the Chicago Bulls."[37] This odd, flippant sandwiching of HIV-related information between German opera and a 1990s sports dynasty perfectly demonstrates how AIDS activism came to matter in *ACLU v. Reno*: as a limit case for why online infrastructures needed to remain open to sex as just another everyday topic of vital interest to many different kinds of users. Kuromiya's affidavit and testimony listed a range of potentially "indecent" topics that were at risk for censorship. These acts and subjects were critical to doing meaningfully sex-positive HIV education aimed at a wide range of people, and included sex work, needle exchanges, massage parlors, "rimming," "blow-jobs," anal sex, sex toys, gags, and dildos, to name just a few.[38]

Kuromiya was the first of forty-six ACLU plaintiffs to address the Philadelphia district court, including Planned Parenthood and the Electronic Frontier Foundation. Journalists' accounts of the court proceedings highlight how Kuromiya's position resonated most clearly with judges. The *New York Times Cybertimes* blog cited Kuromiya's testimony as the most significant in informing the court's decision.

> While it is difficult to say which of the witnesses most influenced the judges in their trail-blazing decision, the first major opinion about free speech and the Internet, lawyers agree that Kuromiya played a pivotal role. Time after time while hearing the case, judges cited Kuromiya's testimony when questioning government lawyers. Several times during the decision, they mentioned the problems the law would create for him. "I think he was the perfect symbol of speech that is about sex and has strong social value," said Christopher A. Hansen, an American Civil Liberties Union lawyer and one of the lead attorneys in the case. "He also symbolized that speech is of value to minors as well as to adults. Somehow, Kiyoshi came to symbolize the essence of what this case is all about."[39]

The details behind this ACLU lawyer's "somehow" are key to understanding AIDS activism's role in online infrastructure development. Reading across court transcripts, news coverage, and Justice Stevens's majority opinion, AIDS-related community internet infrastructure successfully shored up the ACLU's case in a few distinct ways. First, the model demonstrated in concrete terms what marginalized users could do with access to computer networks, within the very timely rhetoric of a mature "AIDS crisis." Kuromiya succeeded at showing the court that AIDS activist work online was both vital and too large in scale and dispersed in its network structure to reasonably monitor within the act's terms; as one activist stretched for time and money,

Kuromiya could not possibly vet content on thousands of databases Critical Path amalgamated for its users or censor the message boards built collaboratively by these users. A grassroots organization like Critical Path would collapse under this manual content moderation workload. While intended to protect small organizations from this burden, this argument has had lasting repercussions for the CDA. Section 230 has shielded corporate platforms from liability for users' speech and more recently has encouraged platforms to ban sex workers from communicating with clients under 2018's SESTA/FOSTA amendments to the act.[40]

Second, Kuromiya used Critical Path's model to systematically dismantle the CDA's vague definition of what was "indecent" or "patently offensive." He critiqued the idea that tagging or filtering technologies, or even well-meaning people, could make good judgments about the value of sexually explicit information. As Kuromiya, out to the court as a gay man, warned in his affidavit, discussion of sex acts and diverse sexual orientations necessary for doing HIV outreach "may be considered by some to be 'offensive' or 'indecent'" under the act's terms.[41] Internet users living with HIV/AIDS were creating useful, explicit, and community-specific information about how to have and enjoy sex within a broader public-health climate that singularly preached monogamy, abstinence, or condom use, despite the unpalatability of these measures to many.[42] As Kuromiya explained it, reaching these users with information that made sense to them might require "colloquial street terms that would be widely recognized in particular communities" or visual and written material at "a range of levels to be understood by various groups in our community, either people with low literacy levels, (or) people for whom English is a second language."[43]

Teenagers represented the most significant and controversial of these community groups within the CDA's terms, which did not ban "indecent" or "patently offensive" materials outright but rather criminalized their circulation to minors. Kuromiya was unequivocal in asserting that young people needed explicit information about sex, precisely because they were *having explicit sex*. When questioned by Department of Justice lawyers, Kuromiya gave what transcripts suggest was an impassioned response.

I can only repeat what I said. I know the difficulties of living with this disease. I've been infected for something like 15 years, and have had full-blown AIDS by the CDC definition since 1993. And yes, I would want to protect people who are potentially going to contract HIV and we know that from current Government statistics that two-thirds of all high school students are sexually active. And so yes, we're providing the information for people who are sexually active and are potentially exposing themselves, maybe because of lack of information or the lack of a source where they can get anonymously information that they need to protect themselves.[44]

Within Patton's "national pedagogy," youth of color and queer youth are figured as sexually active and in need of information about HIV "in order to inscribe the heterosexual [white] teen as safe from AIDS."[45] Critical Path's community infrastructure model implicitly challenged this division between "good" and "bad" sexuality by promising anonymous access to sex-positive information, without judgment. Technologies that restrict young people's access to online spaces through age verification or other forms of identity management threatened to dismantle this community health model. The idea that sexual-health information for youth ought to be explicit in order to be meaningful challenged the logic behind designing technological systems that could sort "bad" porn from "good" sexual health materials.[46] Critical Path's model showed that building conservative sexual values into developing internet technologies would diminish HIV prevention for young people. Here, AIDS activism hoped to ensure a "free and open" internet, and ultimately, the proliferation of diverse sexualities online, including through internet porn.

While the Supreme Court's decision did ensure AIDS activist approaches to sexuality online could continue unfettered by age verification, the terms through which the case was argued may have ultimately paved the way for future technological regulations in this vein. The CDA required sites hosting "indecent" or "patently offensive" materials to place them behind some kind of age-verification interface, the technological details of which were vague, in part because legislators writing the act did not understand how the web worked. Many of the submissions put forward by both the ACLU and the government at both levels of court involved explaining "hyperlinks," "websites," and "email" to the court. To do this work, both sides grilled expert witnesses on the technical details of potential tagging schemes, widespread "parental" controls, and credit-card verification systems.

The ACLU argued, relying on Critical Path's affidavit, that "barring older minors from access to explicit safer sex information or other communications that may help them deal with the onset of sexuality" was unethical. But their case laid out a secondary, technological critique of the act that was perhaps equally convincing to the court.[47] Through an argument titled "Future

Technology Cannot Save a Statute That Criminalizes Speech Today," the ACLU built in a fail-safe to their case: the government's proposal is moot because it is not technically possible . . . yet.[48] In their brief to the court, the ACLU wrote, "Industry continues to invent new ways to empower parents— from the user end—to control Internet content, illustrating that less restrictive alternatives to the CDA's draconian burdens are clearly available."[49] Filtering technologies that could sort porn from G-rated sexual health materials would become widely available in the decade to follow. Case in point: in 2003 the Supreme Court upheld the Children's Internet Protection Act (CIPA), which requires all K–12 schools and public libraries to install internet filters for materials that are "obscene" or "harmful to minors." This act prevents any young person without the means to obtain private internet access from finding the kinds of meaningful, potentially "indecent" information about sexuality, including HIV, that Critical Path's model worked to protect and circulate.

Conclusion

The CDA brought together two of the great "crises" of the 1990s: the AIDS crisis and the infrastructure crisis, which justified many transformations in public spending and utility (de)regulation. This approach strategically disarticulated public investment in new internet infrastructure from the material, gendered needs of women, people of color, and people living with HIV. Kuromiya made explicit that the internet's utility for these users depended on access to information that the CDA would prohibit. He understood the internet as an infrastructural resource that reconfigured existing communication paradigms. Conversely, the CDA's authors understood the internet through previous media systems: the highly regulated and controlled broadcasting and publishing industries.

Since the CDA decision, the internet has become a utility that AIDS service organizations use regularly for outreach, particularly within men who have sex with men (MSM) communities. At its best, this work translates community health-care models to networked digital environments, taking what Sharif Mowlabocus, Craig Haslop, and Rohit Dasgupta call "contextually relevant harm reduction work" online.[50] But as these authors argue, this work is constrained by the corporate-driven sexual politics of apps and platforms—the mature online infrastructures enabled by the commercialization Chun traces back to the CDA.[51] Other online tools for HIV outreach, such as viral-load trackers, leverage personal risk-management models that are far from the community-based resource and information sharing Kuromiya imagined. Alexander McClelland argues that these apps support surveillance, exert biopolitical control over data, facilitate HIV criminalization, and are ultimately only useful to those with the capacity to actively and routinely measure and manage their health.[52] The 2017 end to net neutrality regulations further threatens those living with HIV who rely on accessible and affordable broadband to learn about and access public services, especially nonjudgmental, queer and/or antiracist health information.[53] Net neutrality protects the affordability of broadband access and ensures the content agnostic treatment of online information by ISPs.

In the shadow of this context, Critical Path continues to help marginalized internet users get online. The organization has transitioned into a publicly funded community service that provides basic training and free internet access to low-income people at computer centers across Philadelphia.[54] The contrast between smartphone-based apps within already networked MSM communities and the basic community infrastructures Critical Path continues to maintain for poor or street-involved users shows that within a mature internet era, communities vulnerable to HIV use the internet in many different ways. The technological inequities of access Kuromiya worked against persist, as do community infrastructure models for interrupting them.

Critical Path's model placed vulnerable users at infrastructure development's center. People living with HIV/AIDS not only *needed* a particular kind of community-oriented internet; they had already built this for themselves, within crisis conditions, and through movement-based labor that exceeded the CDA's narrow sexual politics. AIDS activists' work to adjust to, adapt, and even transform new computer networks placed sexuality, social justice, and crisis conditions at the center of how online communications developed.

Notes

1 Kuromiya, *Testimony of Kiyoshi Kuromiya*.
2 Kuromiya and Bauer, "AIDS Information Dissemination."
3 Broader in scope today, Critical Path continues to operate as a digital literacy center and free computer lab for traditionally marginalized user groups. See http://criticalpath.org.
4 Patton, *Fatal Advice*, 38.
5 McKinney, "Printing the Network."
6 TheBody is perhaps the best-known online information source about HIV/AIDS during the 1990s; however, more participatory listservs and BBS use by

AIDS activists and PWAs was also substantial. See Brown, "Norman Brown's List."

7   Star, "Misplaced Concretism and Concrete Situations"; Star and Ruhleder, "Steps toward an Ecology of Infrastructure"; Edwards, "Infrastructure and Modernity."

8   Star and Lorde, "Sadomasochism."

9   Star, "Misplaced Concretism and Concrete Situations," 152.

10 Berlant, "The Commons"; Jackson, "Rethinking Repair"; Starosielski, *Undersea Network*.

11 Wakeford, "Don't Go All the Way," 70. Wakeford suggests the "prefiguring" of Berlant's work on intimacy and affect in Star's "Misplaced Concretism."

12 Chávez, "ACT UP"; Juhasz, *AIDS TV*; Whitbread and McClelland, "Claiming Sexual Autonomy"; Patton, *Fatal Advice*.

13 Geary, *Antiblack Racism and the AIDS Epidemic*. Geary's recent work on anti-Black racism, HIV, and the prison industrial complex provides a strong model for thinking about HIV and infrastructure and includes some attention to questions of information.

14 Critical Path AIDS Project, "AIDS Information on the Internet," 7.

15 Chun, *Control and Freedom*.

16 Fraser, "Clintonism, Welfare, and the Antisocial Wage," 16.

17 McOmber, "Technological Autonomy," 145–46.

18 McOmber, "Technological Autonomy," 147–48.

19 "Statement by Vice President Al Gore," July 16, 1997, https://clintonwhitehouse5.archives.gov/WH/new/Ratings/19970716–6884.html.

20 The administration's annual NetDay event encouraged tech companies to wire public schools for internet access (1996–2004). Clinton and Gore rolled up their sleeves and ran ethernet cable through the ceiling of a California high school to celebrate the first NetDay. See also "The White House 1998 Easter Egg Roll," April 13, 1998, https://clintonwhitehouse2.archives.gov/WH/glimpse/Easter/1998/index.html.

21 The CDA was a distinct section of the updated 1996 Telecommunications Act.

22 Chun, *Control and Freedom*. Chun also argued that these laws need not stand up to constitutional scrutiny in order to have lasting effects on internet infrastructures because of how they inspire forms of corporate self-regulation aimed at compliance (120). She gives the example of digital certificates, produced in reaction to the CDA to establish user authenticity but also support e-business.

23 Chun, *Control and Freedom*, 77–120.

24 Chun, *Control and Freedom*, 112.

25 Chun, *Control and Freedom*, 113.

26 Stein, "Philadelphia LGBT History Project."

27 Stein, "Philadelphia LGBT History Project."

28 "Federal Bureau of Investigation File on Kuromiya," box 44, Kiyoshi Kuromiya papers on HIV/AIDS research and organizations, John J. Wilcox Jr. GLBT Archives of Philadelphia.

29 See McKinney, "Printing the Network." Kuromiya remained a devotee after Fuller's death in 1983. He co-administrated a BBS board dedicated to Fuller's work, and Critical Path's newsletter included many attempts to think about the problem of HIV through Fullerian systems thinking.

30 Smith, "Tales from behind the Wall." This column was written by Gregory Smith, prisoner #22043 at Trenton State Prison. Smith authored a webpage on Critical Path's server, which the newsletter described as "the nation's first Internet website operated by an incarcerated PWA."

31 Gossett, "We Will Not Rest in Peace," 36.

32 Gossett, "We Will Not Rest in Peace," 46.

33 Kuromiya, *Deposition of Kiyoshi Kuromiya*, 25.

34 Stevens, "Opinion of the Court," 874.

35 Stevens, "Opinion of the Court," 871–78. "The consequences of prison rape" is not a random addition but reflects the affidavit of another expert who ran an activist site called Stop Prison Rape.

36 The CDA vaguely defined the terms of indecency according to "contemporary community standards." Communications Decency Act, 47 U.S.C. § 502 2B (1996).

37 Stevens, "Opinion of the Court," 851.

38 Kuromiya, *Deposition of Kiyoshi Kuromiya*, 83–105.

39 Mendels, "AIDS Activist's Dilemma."

40 Gillespie, "Governance of and by Platforms." See, in particular, controversy over section 230 of the act.

41 Kuromiya, "Critical Path Affidavit," item 16.

42 On these community sex education techniques outside the context of the internet, see Brier, *Infectious Ideas*.

43 Kuromiya, *Deposition of Kiyoshi Kuromiya*, 76–89.

44 Kuromiya, *Testimony of Kiyoshi Kuromiya*.

45 Patton, *Fatal Advice*, 54.

46 For a literature review on the pedagogical potential of porn, see Albury, "Porn and Sex Education." Patton's "Visualizing Safe Sex" in *Fatal Advice* gives an excellent overview of the relationship between HIV education and porn aesthetics.

47 American Civil Liberties Union, *Brief of Appellees*, 41.

48 American Civil Liberties Union, *Brief of Appellees*, 33.

49 American Civil Liberties Union, *Brief of Appellees*, 34.

50 Mowlabocus, Haslop, and Dasgupta, "From Scene to Screen," 4.

51 Chun, *Control and Freedom*, 86.

52 McClelland, "Big Data, Bodies and Health Risk."

53 For a selection of takes on how the end of net neutrality might harm Americans living with HIV, see Scurato, "Who Will Be Hit"; Vanderlee, "Net Neutrality Is a Queer Issue"; and Planned Parenthood, "Planned Parenthood Opposes FCC Efforts."

54 Critical Path Learning Center, "About Us."

Bibliography

Albury, Kath. "Porn and Sex Education, Porn as Sex Education." *Porn Studies* 1, nos. 1–2 (2014): 172–81. doi:10.1080/23268743.2013.863654.

American Civil Liberties Union. *Brief of Appellees: ACLU v. Reno*, Pub. L. No. 96–511 (1996).

Berlant, Lauren. "The Commons: Infrastructures for Troubling Times." *Environment and Planning D: Society and Space* 34, no. 3 (2016): 393–419. doi:10.1177/0263775816645989.

Brier, Jennifer. *Infectious Ideas: U.S. Political Responses to the AIDS Crisis*. Chapel Hill: University of North Carolina Press, 2009.

Brown, Norman. "Norman Brown's Consolidated List of AIDS/HIV Bulletin Boards." February 1, 1993. http://textfiles.com/sex/abbs9302.txt.

Chávez, Karma R. "ACT UP, Haitian Migrants, and Alternative Memories of HIV/AIDS." *Quarterly Journal of Speech* 98, no. 1 (2012): 63–68. doi:10.1080/00335630.2011.638659.

Chun, Wendy Hui Kyong. *Control and Freedom: Power and Paranoia in the Age of Fiber Optics*. Cambridge, MA: MIT Press, 2006.

Critical Path AIDS Project. "AIDS Information on the Internet: Critical Path Internet Services—An Update." *Critical Path AIDS Project Newsletter*, 1998. John J. Wilcox Jr. GLBT Archives of Philadelphia.

Critical Path Learning Center. "About Us." Accessed August 23, 2017. https://www.critpath.org/about-us/.

Edwards, Paul N. "Infrastructure and Modernity: Force, Time, and Social Organization in the History of Sociotechnical Systems." In *Modernity and Technology*, edited by Thomas J. Misa, Philip Brey, and Andrew Feenberg, 185–225. Cambridge, MA: MIT Press, 2003.

Fraser, Nancy. "Clintonism, Welfare, and the Antisocial Wage: The Emergence of a Neoliberal Political Imaginary." *Rethinking Marxism* 6, no. 1 (1993): 9–23.

Fuller, Buckminster. *Critical Path*. New York: St. Martin's Press, 1981.

Geary, Adam. *Antiblack Racism and the AIDS Epidemic: State Intimacies*. New York: Palgrave Macmillan, 2014.

Gillespie, Tarleton. "Governance of and by Platforms." In *SAGE Handbook of Social Media*, edited by Jean Burgess, Alice Marwick, and Thomas Poell, 254–78. London: SAGE, 2017.

Gossett, Che. "We Will Not Rest in Peace: AIDS Activism, Black Radicalism, Queer and/or Trans Resistance." In *Queer Necropolitics*, edited by Adi Kuntsman, Jin Haritaworn, and Silvia Posocoo, 31–50. New Brunswick, NJ: Routledge, 2014.

Jackson, Steven J. "Rethinking Repair." In *Media Technologies*, edited by Kirsten A. Foot, Pablo J. Boczkowski, and Tarleton Gillespie, 221–40. Cambridge, MA: MIT Press, 2014.

Juhasz, Alexandra. *AIDS TV: Identity, Community, and Alternative Video*. Durham, NC: Duke University Press, 1995.

Kuromiya, Kiyoshi. "Critical Path Affidavit in ACLU, et al v. Reno." American Civil Liberties Union (ACLU), February 1996. https://www.aclu.org/legal-document /critical-path-affidavit-aclu-et-al-v-reno.

Kuromiya, Kiyoshi. *Deposition of Kiyoshi Kuromiya in the Matter of ACLU v. Reno.* Pub. L. No. 755229922, 191 (1996).

Kuromiya, Kiyoshi. *Testimony of Kiyoshi Kuromiya.* Director of Critical AIDS Path Project (1996). https://w2.eff.org/legal/cases/EFF_ACLU_v_DoJ/960321 _kuromiya.testimony.

Kuromiya, Kiyoshi, and Richard Bauer. "Building a Community-Based Infrastructure for AIDS Information Dissemination on the Internet: Three Years Later." Critical Path AIDS Project, n.d. Box 35, folder "Internet Funding." Kiyoshi Kuromiya papers on HIV/AIDS research and organizations, John J. Wilcox Jr. GLBT Archives of Philadelphia.

McClelland, Alexander. "'Lock This Whore Up': Public Health Legislation and Other 'Risks' to Public Safety." Paper presentation, Big Data and Risk Conference, Concordia University, Montreal, November 6–7, 2015. https:// bigdatariskconference.wordpress.com/program/abstracts/.

McKinney, Cait. "Printing the Network: AIDS Activism and Online Access in the 1980s." *Continuum: Journal of Media and Cultural Studies* 32, no. 1 (2018): 7–17. https://doi.org/10.1080/10304312.2018.1404670.

McOmber, James B. "Technological Autonomy and Three Definitions of Technology." *Journal of Communication* 49, no. 1 (1999): 137–53.

Mendels, Pamela. "AIDS Activist's Dilemma Proved Decisive in Decency Act Case." *New York Times Cybertimes Blog*, June 18, 1996. Box 40, folder "ACLU Class Action." Kiyoshi Kuromiya papers on HIV/AIDS research and organizations, John J. Wilcox Jr. GLBT Archives of Philadelphia.

Mowlabocus, Sharif, Craig Haslop, and Rohit Dasgupta. "From Scene to Screen: The Challenges and Opportunities of Commercial Digital Platforms for HIV Community Outreach." *Social Media and Society* 2, no. 4 (2016): 1–8. doi:10.1177/2056305116672886.

Patton, Cindy. *Fatal Advice: How Safe-Sex Education Went Wrong.* Durham, NC: Duke University Press, 1996.

Planned Parenthood. "Planned Parenthood Opposes FCC Efforts to Repeal Net Neutrality Rules." December 14, 2017. https://www.plannedparenthood.org /about-us/newsroom/press-releases/planned-parenthood-opposes-fcc-efforts -to-repeal-net-neutrality-rules.

Scurato, Carmen. "Who Will Be Hit Hardest by Net Neutrality? Marginalised America." *The Guardian*, December 18, 2017.

Smith, Gregory. "Tales From behind the Wall." *Critical Path AIDS Project Newsletter*, Summer 1997. Kiyoshi Kuromiya papers on HIV/AIDS research and organizations, John J. Wilcox Jr. GLBT Archives of Philadelphia.

Star, Susan Leigh. "Misplaced Concretism and Concrete Situations: Feminism, Method, and Information Technology." In *Boundary Objects and Beyond: Working with Leigh Star*, edited by Geoffrey C. Bowker, Stefan

Timmermans, Adele E. Clarke, and Ellen Balka, 143–70. Cambridge, MA: MIT Press, 2016.

Star, Susan Leigh, and Audre Lorde. "Sadomasochism: Not about Condemnation; An Interview with Audre Lorde by Susan Leigh Star." In *A Burst of Light: Essays*, by Audre Lorde, 11–18. Ithaca, NY: Firebrand Books, 1988.

Star, Susan Leigh, and Karen Ruhleder. "Steps toward an Ecology of Infrastructure: Design and Access for Large Information Spaces." *Information Systems Research* 7, no. 1 (1996): 111–34.

Starosielski, Nicole. *The Undersea Network*. Durham, NC: Duke University Press, 2015.

Stein, Marc. "Philadelphia LGBT History Project: Kiyoshi Kuromiya, June 17, 1997." Oral History Interview, 2009. http://outhistory.org/exhibits/show /philadelphia-lgbt-interviews/interviews/kiyoshi-kuromiya.

Stevens, John Paul. 521 U.S. 844. "Opinion of the Court, Reno v. American Civil Liberties Union." June 26, 1997.

Vanderlee, Juliana. "Net Neutrality Is a Queer Issue." *Lambda Legal*, December 7, 2017.

Wakeford, Nina. "Don't Go All the Way: Revisiting 'Misplaced Concretism.'" In *Boundary Objects and Beyond: Working with Leigh Star*, edited by Geoffrey C. Bowker, Stefan Timmermans, Adele E. Clarke, and Ellen Balka, 69–84. Cambridge, MA: MIT Press, 2016.

Whitbread, Jessica, and Alexander McClelland. "Claiming Sexual Autonomy for People with HIV through Collective Action." In *Mobilizing Metaphor: Art, Culture, and Disability Activism in Canada*, edited by Christine Kelly and Michael Orsini, 76–97. Vancouver: University of British Columbia Press, 2016.

EIGHT DISPATCHES FROM
THE PASTS/MEMORIES OF AIDS

A Dialogue between Cecilia Aldarondo, Roger Hallas,
Pablo Alvarez, Jim Hubbard, and Dredge Byung'chu Kang-Nguyễn,
with an Introduction by Jih-Fei Cheng

If I were not "queer," I would not know AIDS. Without knowing AIDS, I could not be "queer." I would also not be "queer" if it were not for the Cold War. If it were not for the Cold War, AIDS could not exist. The past lives in memories like a narrative missing transitions.

As Marita Sturken writes, "Both the Vietnam War and the AIDS epidemic have profoundly affected the experience of nationality. America is inconceivable without them."[1] Sturken explains that the traumas borne of the Vietnam War and AIDS interrupted once commonly held "truths" as well as progress narratives: "those of American imperialism, technology, science, and masculinity."[2] In turn, there has been widespread cultural productions to revisit these memories and traumas in order to seek a modicum of healing, even where healing must first draw anger, and even when healing—nevertheless a cure—has remained impossible.

Both of my parents were born in Nanjing, China, during World War II. At the end of World War II, followed by the Civil War and the ascendancy of the People's Republic of China under Mao, they evacuated to Taiwan as children of the politically privileged Nationalist Party of China (Kuomintang, or KMT). Although they grew up under what they would describe as modest means, they did not experience the most devastating effects of more than thirty-eight years of martial law—the second-longest period of military rule in modern history after Syria and Israel—installed by the KMT to violently suppress Native resistance, leftists, Taiwanese independence, and/or pro-Japanese agitators.

As adults, my parents immigrated individually and met in the United States, where my mother pursued the field of nonprofit finance and my father public health. Despite their own careers, they never predicted that their eldest son would not only be "queer" but also work at the intersections of nonprofit and public health in AIDS social services and research.

My first intimate encounter took place in 1995 and was with an older HIV-positive white gay man and graduate student of anthropology who emphasized his fetish for, and research interests in, Asians. For our first date, he rented on VHS director Lino Brocka's *Macho Dancer* (1988), a pivotal and controversial film about the queer and trans sex industry in the Philippines made possible by the exploitations of ethnic, regional, and class differences; tourism; and the long arms of Spanish and US empires and military occupation. In the context of my first sexual experience, and prior to the advent of highly active antiretroviral therapy (HAART) to effectively treat HIV infection, viewing the film through this white man's anthropological gaze organized much of my psychic, emotional, and intimate world into the seemingly inextricably tied categories of "queer," "Asian," "HIV/AIDS," "tragedy," and enduring "loneliness." Tom stopped returning my phone calls after our second encounter. However, he had also taught me how to use condoms.

In 1996, during my second year in college, gynecologist Dr. Gao Yaojie discovered that her patient had become infected with HIV from a blood transfusion supplied by my paternal grandfather's home province of Henan, China. Pervasive poverty led many in Henan to sell blood that was left unscreened or contaminated during the collection process, which transformed my grandfather's province into an epicenter for the People's Republic of China's AIDS epidemic, if not an epicenter for the global pandemic.

As an undergraduate student, I led multiple queer and trans student organizations and volunteered as a peer counselor facilitating weekly support groups for gay/bi/questioning men. I also took courses in ethnic studies, feminism, and queer theory and became involved in AIDS initiatives as a community advisory board member for Kyung-Hee Choi's early research on HIV prevention among men who have sex with men (MSM). I continued my involvement and research on HIV/AIDS literary productions as an MA student in Asian American studies at the University of California, Los Angeles. Meanwhile, I worked in HIV-prevention outreach and education, and then emotional support services for people living with HIV/AIDS, at the Asian Pacific AIDS Intervention Team in Los Angeles. That was followed by several years of work at the Asian & Pacific Islander Coalition on HIV/AIDS in New York City, where I was also involved in the Fabulous Independent Educated

Radicals for Community Empowerment (FIERCE!) and the Gay Asian & Pacific Islander Men of New York (GAPIMNY).

It would take me two more decades to realize that coming out in the mid-1990s as a teenager meant that I was walking into a war zone where the bombs are still going off and everyone is scattering. I did not realize that arriving in the midst of the precocktail AIDS epidemic would so closely mirror what it was like growing up in an immigrant family that still seemed focused on how to survive war. You hear about family, neighbors, and community members who live afar, some who have disappeared, and those whose remains may never resurface except through the occasional memories told late at night across the kitchen table or when the DJ plays an old song. Do not ask questions. No one will answer them. Just feel lucky that you are here. Meanwhile, be ready, again, for war.

I was trained and politicized vis-à-vis AIDS, women of color feminist, queer of color, and trans of color politics. I have lost lovers, friends, colleagues, mentors, comrades, and leaders to HIV/AIDS—all women, queer, and trans people of color—during a period when HIV/AIDS was no longer supposed to be a death sentence because of HAART. I have also lost *potential* lovers, friends, colleagues, mentors, comrades, and leaders to the systematization of HIV stigma and criminalization; compulsory serosorting; biomedical interventions that simultaneously save some lives while also embedding toxins deep within our bodies, psyches, and communities; as well as the violences of racism, misogyny, transphobia, classism, ableism, and more that imbue the pandemic with its force. There are many times where I have felt that I lost my immediate blood kin, who see me as selfish and even turn their anger and violence upon me because they cannot understand what I have endured and why I have spent so much time away from them while failing to fulfill their expectations. Ethnic studies, feminism, and queer theory, alongside films, poetry, novels, and short stories produced by those women, queer, and trans people of color who came before me, have served as my teachers, my guides to help me navigate loss, and my connections to communities of the past. These pasts, and their memories, matter to the present because they reveal the interruptions into imperial, capitalist, nationalist, military, patrilineal, and technoscientific narratives of progress.

"Dispatches from the Pasts/Memories of AIDS" figures between individual and collective experiences with HIV/AIDS. As you will see, the section title itself ignited pain, fury, resentment, fear, determination, and more. The first prompt for this asynchronous set of "dispatches" commenced in September 2016. The second prompt was initiated in December 2017 and registers the anxiety and impassioned responses to what was then the new election of US president Donald Trump. For reasons delineated in some responses, there is also anger expressed toward me and toward others who were not a part of this recorded discussion. There were times during the process of soliciting responses where I quietly fumed at a participant for misunderstanding, mischaracterizing, and even belittling the prompts while seemingly dismissing my experiences and work with HIV/AIDS. Meanwhile, I became further disturbed by a furious email from a somewhat well-known white gay cis-male documentary filmmaker (not featured here), berating me for including his latest AIDS film in my essay critiquing the recent mainstreaming of AIDS activist historiography.[3] He accused me of being an irresponsible and opportunistic academic. Furthermore, he called me "racist" for pointing out that he featured only one person of color in his film and in very limited fashion. I offered to have a phone conversation, which he refused and continued angrily demand from me an apology. To critique white men is to face their vehemence, stark entitlement, and the institutional violence they can wield as self-entitled gatekeepers.

During my years in HIV/AIDS social services, behavioral research, cultural productions, and activism, I felt lost, isolated, and extremely frustrated at the corporatization of AIDS and the waning public interest in the pandemic. People of color were still becoming infected at high rates and dying, but in the age of HAART there was a rush to abandon the AIDS crisis in communities of color and the Global South in order to embrace military service and marriage. As a doctoral student in American studies and ethnicity at the University of Southern California, and now assistant professor, I have been treated with some disdain for having left the AIDS industry for academia. Suddenly, I have been constituted as an "outsider" to AIDS by some who remain within AIDS social services, science research, and/or cultural productions precisely because my choice to pursue a humanities approach to the pandemic is read as abstract and idealistic, if not out of touch with AIDS itself.

However, it is precisely the obfuscation of the overlapping pasts of AIDS, queerness, and the Cold War that I continue to pursue in the historicization of cultural memory. Cultural memory, Sturken submits, is distinct from both personal memory and history: "It is a field of contested meanings in which Americans interact with cultural elements to produce concepts of the nation, particularly in events of trauma, where both the structures and the fractures of a culture are exposed. Examining cultural memory thus provides insight into how American culture functions, how oppositional politics engages with nationalism, and how cultural arenas such as art, popular culture, activism, and consumer culture intersect."[4] Here, you will see these contestations emerge and even sharpen as shards of memory meant to pierce the present. Sometimes, these memories end up cutting even further into already deepened wounds.

I met Cecilia Aldarondo through Facebook, after activist and writer Sarah Schulman posted my article "How to Survive: AIDS and Its Afterlives in Popular Media." Pablo Alvarez and I became acquainted after my coeditor and mentor Alexandra Juhasz introduced us at one of her talks. I have had the honor of serving as a faculty committee member reviewing his brilliant dissertation proposal. I met Alexandra Juhasz and Nishant Shahani at the 2014 Society for Cinema and Media Studies Conference in Seattle, Washington, where I presented a paper that led to the above article, on a panel formed by Lucas Hilderbrand. I was introduced to Lucas by my friend and peer in graduate school Patty Ahn. Roger Hallas and I have never met, but while in graduate school, I became intimately familiar with his book *Reframing Bodies: AIDS, Bearing Witness, and the Queer Moving Image*. Jim Hubbard and I met upon introduction by Sarah, but, prior to these dispatches, only ever exchanged emails and talked on the phone. In the fall of 2015, I spoke with and interviewed Jim at length as I prepared the research and writing for the article. Dredge Byung'chu Kang-Nguyễn and I have known each other since about 2002 when we both attended a men of color institute in Washington, DC, that commenced prior to the annual National Conference on AIDS. We were assigned as roommates.

Each of these memories invokes the pasts of AIDS. Whether their edges are left coarse or worn soft, these memories refuse to be resembled—to look exactly like one another or simply reflect one another. They also refuse assembly into a singular or coherent past. We trace these memories of shattered pasts with our fingertips. We struggle to love and hold each other with barriers; we struggle to love and hold each other without barriers.

Without the Cold War, there would be no AIDS. If it were not for the Cold War, I would not be queer. If AIDS did not exist, I would not be queer. If I were not queer, I would not know AIDS.

—*Jih-Fei Cheng*

Prompt 1

Jih-Fei Cheng: The increased visibility of AIDS cultural productions in recent art shows, such as the traveling exhibition *Art AIDS America*, and in widely distributed feature-length films, including *We Were Here* (David Weissman,

2011), *Vito* (Jeffrey Schwarz, 2011), *United in Anger* (Jim Hubbard and Sarah Schulman, 2012), *How to Survive a Plague* (David France, 2012), and *The Normal Heart* (Ryan Murphy, 2014), has prompted inquiries into the AIDS past. Theodore (Ted) Kerr and Alexandra Juhasz, among others, have described this in various ways as "AIDS crisis revisitation." Is this framing apt? If not, why? If so, what is being revisited and in what forms? Who is prompting this revisitation and who is the audience?

Cecilia Aldarondo: My instinct is to respond to this question in personal terms, because I feel as though I've been up to my neck in AIDS revisitation for the last eight years. Since 2008 I've been making a film about my uncle Miguel, who died at thirty-one of AIDS when I was only six years old. *Memories of a Penitent Heart* (2016) is a documentary that reexamines Miguel's death in 1987, specifically the rumor—perpetuated by my ultra-Catholic grandmother—that Miguel "repented" of his homosexuality on his deathbed, thereby securing a righteous place in heaven. Propelled by the sense that there was something amiss in my family's collective memory of Miguel, I decided to make a film in order to reexamine the conflict around Miguel's sexuality with a generation's worth of hindsight.

It's as though this period—in which I spent years chasing down the remains of my uncle's life—has cracked open a gateway to the past, enabling my adult self to observe a history I did not directly live. It's an unruly sort of revisitation, for I was barely old enough to meet Miguel before he died, and at the time I had no idea that his death had anything to do with AIDS. Because of my family's euphemistic ways of speaking about Miguel's death—he died of "cancer," et cetera—I first learned about AIDS through the distorted lens of my parents' *Newsweek* magazine, and through the public hysteria and moralizing that characterized the 1980s and 1990s in the US. Before making this film, I had only the most superficial understanding of AIDS and its impact. And I was completely unprepared for what I'd encounter when I started asking questions.

By going back to 1987, I've been brutally confronted with what I have come to call a "memorial black hole": not merely the tragedy of Miguel's death but the added injustice of my family's obliteration of his life as a gay man. I see it in the euphemisms of Miguel's death certificate—"natural causes," "never married"—in the wholesale exclusion of Miguel's partner from his obituary, and in Miguel's burial in the family plot in Puerto Rico, while Miguel's chosen family was left with no public memorials to speak of. It's as though I have come to sketch the outline of a terrible nothingness, a negative space where Miguel and his rightful memory should have been. And along with that nothingness, I've come up against a feeling that my family has not simply forgotten Miguel or selectively remembered him—my family has helped to create a mountain of unresolved grief for those friends and lovers who lacked the legitimacy to properly mourn him.

I see an undeniable parallel between my family's very personal forgetting and the national forgetting of AIDS that currently afflicts the United States. I did a great deal of research in preparation for making *Memories of a Penitent Heart*—I read every book on AIDS I could find; I interviewed veteran AIDS activists; I watched and rewatched films such as Derek Jarman's *Blue* (1993) and Gregg Bordowitz's *Fast Trip, Long Drop* (1994). I went to see *How to Survive a Plague* during its New York premiere; I rented *We Were Here* and *Dallas Buyers Club* (Jean-Marc Vallée, 2013) on Netflix. I consumed every primary and secondary text on the AIDS crisis that I could get my hands on.

This research has taught me three things: (1) the space occupied by the AIDS crisis in our national memory is disproportionately tiny relative to its horrors; (2) this national ignorance of AIDS serves to reperpetuate the notion that AIDS was never everyone's problem, a fact that helped to create the genocide in the first place; (3) we are at a particularly sensitive cultural moment, with an aging population of survivors actively working to countermand this cultural ignorance before it's too late.

While we seem to need revisitation badly, I'm very concerned that all this focus on AIDS as a historical phenomenon is simultaneously producing a false and dangerous dichotomy between past and present—that the very act of remembering AIDS serves to embalm it, to produce AIDS as a thing of the past when the opposite could not be farther from the truth. While they do undeniably important work, most of the recent cultural texts on AIDS are overwhelmingly white, overwhelmingly male, and overwhelmingly bourgeois. If we allow these representations to dominate this moment of revisitation, then we risk many things. We risk implying that AIDS never touched people of color and non-Americans, those very communities for whom stigma, disclosure, HIV criminalization, access to medical care, and family dynamics are ever present.

I'm reminded of a young Puerto Rican man, maybe twenty years old, who came to see *Memories of a Penitent Heart* when it screened in New York. He'd left the island three months before and was profoundly homesick. After the screening was over he came to talk to me, shaking and crying. Pointing excitedly at the screen, he said, "This is my life!" I think of this kid often—for him, what happened to Miguel is *not* a historical phenomenon. It is not then. It is now.

So how do we "revisit" AIDS without fossilizing it? When, how, and why should we revisit our losses? Is it about vengeance, redemption, closure, or all of the above? What could we gain from this kind of return, and whom do we put at risk?

Roger Hallas: I think this notion of "AIDS crisis revisitation," which Alex Juhasz and Ted Kerr have elaborated, is a profoundly useful one, but we should also be mindful of what it might potentially obscure or reify. Stripped of its theological baggage, the dual meaning of the term *visitation*, as either official visit or disaster, is strangely apt for the kind of cultural production that has emerged in the last decade.

On the one hand, many of these films and exhibitions work to gain wider recognition of the historical significance of AIDS activism and cultural production not just to the 1980s and 1990s but also to the present. It is about claiming a place of agency and achievement in the national narrative of the epidemic. Here I recall Sarah Schulman's anecdote about the origins of the ACT UP Oral History Project: in 2001, on the twentieth anniversary of the epidemic, she heard a respected radio program in Los Angeles that completely whitewashed the history of AIDS in the US. It has also been about placing AIDS at the center of American culture, as exemplified in Jonathan Katz and Rock Hushka's exhibition *Art AIDS America*, which claimed to be "the first exhibition to examine the deep and ongoing influence of the AIDS crisis on American art and culture."[5]

On the other hand, some of these works articulate how the individual and collective trauma of that time remains open, unresolved. For example, Cecilia's incredible documentary *Memories of a Penitent Heart* delves into her painful family history around her uncle's death from AIDS in 1987, which has remained an agonizing trauma, laden with secrets, guilt, and recrimination, for both her family and her uncle's lover, whom she tracks down at the beginning of the film. The film culminates in Cecilia's attempt to bring about reconciliation between her mother and her uncle's lover. But rather than generate the anticipated scene of redemptive bonding between the two, the encounter seems disappointing and anticlimactic. We are left with the poignant image of the mother and the lover sitting separately on a pleasure boat as it meanders through the suburban backwaters of Florida.

Trauma theory also provides a way to understand AIDS crisis revisitation. One of the core arguments I made in my book *Reframing Bodies* was to challenge the idea that the act of bearing witness to historical trauma was intrinsically belated. Unlike the Holocaust, which served as the historical case upon which trauma studies were founded, the AIDS epidemic generated prolific acts of bearing witness in the immediate midst of the crisis. Now, if we look back, maybe the decade following the arrival of antiretroviral (ARV) combination therapy in the late 1990s, what Ted has dubbed the "second silence," facilitated the conditions for AIDS crisis revisitation to emerge as a kind of belatedness that followed traumatic silence, numbness, and oblivion.

My experience teaching queer AIDS media in documentary film and queer studies courses has certainly changed over the last decade. In the early 2000s, my undergraduate students were resistant to films like *Zero Patience* (John Greyson, 1993) as "too gay" and AIDS activist videos like *Stop the Church* (Robert Hilferty, 1990) as "too angry." Their difficulty in recognizing the historical nature of the very recent past caused them to often dismiss the work as "outdated." In the past few years, student responses have been quite different. Screening *United in Anger* generates in my students a palpable and indignant sense of betrayal by an education and a culture that has denied them access to such a significant social movement for not just queer but also US history. They clearly see the relevance for and continuity with more recent movements like Occupy and Black Lives Matter.

The recent films about AIDS activism, whether documentary or narrative, have all explored—with varying degrees of success—the relationship between individual and collectivity regardless of whether they were focused on a single person (*Vito* and *Larry Kramer in Love and Anger* [Jean Carlomusto, 2015]), a small group of activists (*We Were Here* and *How to Survive a Plague*) or a whole activist group (*United in Anger* [Hubbard and Schulman]). With the exception of Jim and Sarah's documentary, these films about activists and artists in the AIDS crisis are overwhelmingly white and male. Where are the films about Essex Hemphill, Rotimi Fani-Kayode, Félix González-Torres, or Zoe Leonard? In that sense, AIDS crisis revisitation is just as much subject to the dynamics of white male privilege as are most contemporary cultural phenomena, queer or otherwise.

As useful as AIDS crisis revisitation is as a mode of historical periodization, it also has its limitations. It is premised on a prior period in which AIDS cultural production was largely absent, the "second silence" that Ted dates from 1996 to 2008. Yet that framework seems rather US-centric if we look at the proliferation of media production around global AIDS activism during this period, especially in relation to Southern Africa: for example, John Greyson's video installation *Fig Trees* (2003); Anne-Christine D'Adesky, Shanti Avirgan, and Ann T. Rossetti's *Pills, Profits, Protest: Chronicle of the Global AIDS Movement* (2005); and *Steps for the Future* (2002), the thirty-three-film series focused on southern Africa produced by Don Edkins. In its stark dialectical montage between his increasingly normalized life on ARVs and the urgency of global activism at the 2000 AIDS conference in Durban, Gregg Bordowitz's video *Habit* (2001) eloquently articulated the geopolitical discontinuities of the global AIDS pandemic at that historical moment. Arguably, one of the most valuable aspects of the recent resurgence in looking back at the AIDS past is precisely the work that rethinks the established historicity of the pandemic, such as Ted's recent piece, "AIDS 1969: HIV, History, and Race," about Robert Rayford, the Black teenager from St. Louis who died from HIV-related causes in 1969.[6]

Pablo Alvarez: As a Brown queer Chicanx growing up on the ancestral land of the Indigenous people, the sacred land later named Pico Rivera after the last Mexican governor of California, located thirteen miles southeast of downtown Los Angeles against the backdrop of the San Gabriel Mountains, I ask: What are the stories of AIDS that have yet to be unearthed in this city? What documentations of AIDS reveal the history of the crisis in my neighborhood? How do stories of Chicanx AIDS ancestry emerge? Who will visit Latinx histories of AIDS?

As I reflect upon the current cultural production of AIDS and the "AIDS crisis revisitation," my thoughts merge collectively with other activists, artists, writers, and scholars who have critiqued the current moment of AIDS revisitation as a moment all too limiting. I too see these forms of revisitation as moments of reentering dominant representations of the gay white experience or as a return to ACT UP as the standard representation of AIDS activism, and in this regard I revisit Alexandra Juhasz's article "Forgetting ACT UP." Juhasz indicates that "when ACT UP is remembered—again and again and again—other places, people, and forms of AIDS activism are disremembered. . . . When ACT UP is remembered as the pinnacle of postmodern activism, other forms and forums of activism that were taking place during that time—practices that were linked, related, just modern, in dialogue or even opposition to ACT UP's 'confrontational activism'—are forgotten."[7] Because it is quite obvious who is being revisited and who is doing most of the visiting in the current cultural production of AIDS, except for those brief moments offered to women, gender-fluid, trans people, and people of color activists who continue to be denied full visitation rights, I would like to explore the possibilities of expanding visiting hours.

The late Los Angeles writer Gil Cuadros left us with a collection of short stories and poetry that documents a history of AIDS in Los Angeles through a Chicanx and queer experience. In a poem titled "There Are Places You Don't Walk at Night, Alone," published in *City of God* by City Lights in 1994, Cuadros documents the reality of AIDS signification, homophobic violence, love, and Chicanx desire on the streets of Los Angeles. Written in three parts, each part locates main intersections of Los Angeles that are located near my home. These are the streets that I have traveled throughout my life. Part 1 of the poem starts: "Whittier Blvd., Beverly, Atlantic, / over by Johnson's Market, / or the Projects on Brooklyn. (112)" Part 2 begins with "Manzanita, Hoover, Del Mar, / The Detour's After Hours. (113)" Part 3 begins with "Marengo, Arroyo, Colorado. / I walk like a police man / to the bus bench / and some homeboys are waiting." Cuadros became one of the very few Chicanx to document, through the creative act of writing, a historical time in Los Angeles during the AIDS epidemic of the 1980s and 1990s. His collection of short stories and poetry reflects how the creative act of writing promotes social and cultural survival in a time of great loss. How do we revisit Cuadros's narratives? Who revisits the street intersection of Los Angeles and AIDS? Or the intersection of Chicanx and AIDS?

Los Angeles performance artist Luis Alfaro asks, "Where are my heroes? Where are my saints?" in the literary documentation of "Downtown," published in 1998 in *O Solo Homo*. The vignette "Heroes and Saints" in "Downtown" begins in a populated dance floor of Circus Disco, the famous Latinx queer club of Los Angeles that was established in 1975. (Not too long ago I revisited Circus Disco only to find that it had been demolished, furthering the mechanisms of gentrification and capital investment.) By the closing of "Heroes and Saints," Alfaro finds the once crowded dance floor virtually empty. Alfaro moves from dancing at the club among other queer Brown bodies to working at an AIDS center in South Central Los Angeles. The shift from dancing among other queer Latinx to returning to an empty Circus Disco honors an early history of AIDS among Latinx in Los Angeles.

Started working at an
AIDS center in South Central.
But I gotta,
I gotta,
I gotta
get out of here.
'Cause all of my boys
All of my dark-skinned boys

All of my cha-cha boys
are dying on me.
And sometimes I wish
it was like the Circus Disco
of my coming out.

Two thousand square feet
of my men.
Boys like me.
Who speak the languages,
who speak the languages
of the border
and of the other.
The last time I drove
down Santa Monica Boulevard
and I passed by Circus Disco,
hardly anybody was there.
And I ask you,

Where are my heroes?
Where are my saints?[8]

In revisiting Alfaro's and Cuadros's work, I ask: Where are *my* heroes? Where are *my* saints, in the current AIDS crisis revisitation? By revisiting the creative work of Cuadros and Alfaro, I come to understand the ways in which these writers have disrupted the homogenous representation and activist geography of AIDS.

How do we revisit a history that is not visibly present in the current cultural production of AIDS? How do we visit the stories untold? Who will offer ancestral medicine upon visiting? I call upon the ancestry of AIDS, the activist forces, and I seek their guidance; ask for their permission to visit with great gratitude. I am brought to reflect upon Johanna Hedva's "Sick Woman Theory" and recall her memory of the day she lifted her fist. While the rest of her body remained on the bed, she lifted her fist in solidarity to the Black Lives Matter protest happening on the streets below her apartment in MacArthur Park, Los Angeles. Through the complexities of Sick Woman Theory, Hedva asks, "How do you throw a brick through the window of a bank if you can't get out of bed?" According to Hedva, Sick Woman Theory is a political identity. In sickwomantheory.tumblr.com, the transcript of Hedva's talk (which includes the memory mentioned) on Sick Woman Theory indicates that "The Sick Women are all of the dysfunctional, dangerous and in danger, badly behaved, crazy, incurable, traumatized, disordered, diseased, chronic, uninsurable, wretched, undesirable, and altogether dysfunctional bodies belonging to women, people of color, poor, ill, neuroatypical, differently-abled, queer, trans, and gender-fluid people, who have been historically pathologized, hospitalized, institutionalized, brutalized, rendered unmanageable, and therefore made culturally illegitimate and politically invisible."[9] I refer to Hedva's theory in order to prompt other forms of AIDS revisitation and to illuminate the stories of AIDS that have been left outside visiting hours.

When I show the documentary *United in Anger* (a documentary that does not erase the experiences of sick women, of poor people, of people of color) in my Introduction to Gender Studies course, the majority of the students (whose age range is approximately between eighteen and twenty-five) visit the history of AIDS for the first time. During our discussion of the film, a number of students express outrage at the fact that the history of AIDS remained hidden from their previous education. Students express a tremendous sadness and an urgency to organize. Students express anger upon learning that AIDS had been excluded by the state as a critical component to women's reproductive health and as a result, women were misdiagnosed if diagnosed at all. Every semester for the past two years, I revisit the history of AIDS through *United in Anger*; the students in the classroom bear witness through AIDS activist video.

The framing of "AIDS crisis revisitation" offers an opportunity to unpack the forms that visiting AIDS takes shape. The framing offers an opportunity to revisit a historical moment of AIDS activism while simultaneously seeking out the stories that have yet to be remembered.

Jim Hubbard: First, I think the premise of the prompt has it completely turned around. These exhibitions and the films have not prompted inquiries into the AIDS past; they are the result of examinations of the past.

When I first started putting together the AIDS Activist Video Collection of the New York Public Library in 1995, it was because Patrick Moore, the head of the Estate Project for Artists with AIDS, who originated the idea and project, feared that the videos had been forgotten, were being neglected and in grave danger of being lost. In retrospect, this is remarkable because the tapes at that point were only a few years old. The collection and the subsequent interest in other videotapes shot during the period made those films mentioned in the prompt possible by providing an enormous resource of actuality footage.

In 2001, when Sarah Schulman and I first conceived the ACT UP Oral History Project, we did so because so little accurate information about ACT UP and AIDS activism in general was available. The AIDS activism that saved thousands of lives and changed the world was in danger of being forgotten.

To be generous, one can say that these works have prompted a more general inquiry into the AIDS crisis, but none of the more recent productions would have been possible without this preexisting examination of the past.

Furthermore, you can't just group these works together without an analysis of how they position the past and how they fit into the larger cultural structure. Clearly, the works that adhere most closely to the power structure's accepted narrative are the works that will gain the most support from that power structure, and consequently, the most media attention. Hence, works that focus exclusively on cis white men and present the story as a triumphalist narrative will garner the most positive attention and support.

To take an example that is not on the list, *Dallas Buyers Club*, a film that is a tissue of lies from countdown leader to copyright notice, won three Oscars and was nominated for three others. The buyers' club movement was a direct result of the collective nature of the AIDS movement and a heroic community effort to save the lives of friends and lovers, but the dominant straight white culture would not have been comfortable with—indeed, would not have understood—a story about queers and people of color banding together to help one another in the face of an uncaring government. It was necessary to twist it into some preposterous version of cowboy capitalism embodied by a fabricated bisexual drug addict and an inauthentic portrayal of a trans person in order for it to be lauded by the larger culture.

The tortuous thirty-year route of *The Normal Heart* from Off-Broadway phenomenon to mass media cable TV extravaganza is also illustrative. It offers a fascinating example of how a work transforms so that it is no longer threatening to the power structure. The TV version of *The Normal Heart*, directed by Ryan Murphy, invites an interpretation where the depredations of the government are firmly in the past and not an ongoing pattern of neglect. It allows viewers to think that it was those awful people back then who prevented a better response to AIDS and leaves the audience feeling that we're not like that anymore.

At first I thought "AIDS crisis revisitation" wasn't a frame; it's just a phrase. But the more I thought about it, the more I was upset by it. First, the phrase is inaccurate. The current efforts to look at the AIDS crises of the 1980s and 1990s are actually a first attempt to understand it historically. To me, the word *revisitation* has a certain nostalgic tinge that I find condescending and an attempt to belittle the efforts of traumatized people to reexamine their past, try to understand what happened, and historicize it. The way Americans perceive the past has a kind of spiral structure, returning periodically to revise and reuse. At its best, a reexamination of the past would correct prior errors and include those who were left out the first time. This effort usually begins twenty or thirty years after the events, so the reexamination of the AIDS crisis is, if anything, a bit overdue.

There is also a tendency for current AIDS activists to feel that this historicization is somehow stealing all the oxygen from the current AIDS movement. The lack of attention to the current social and political problems around AIDS is not the result of trying to understand and make peace with the past but rather a somewhat different manifestation of the same problems that we had to deal with in the 1980s—unequal access to health care, extreme inequality of wealth, pharmaceutical company greed, government indifference, and racism.

Finally, if you are dissatisfied with the media being made now about the AIDS crisis, there is a solution—make your own. That's what AIDS activists did in the 1980s and 1990s and with the ubiquity of cell phones and computerized editing systems, it's even more possible today.

Dredge Byung'chu Kang-Nguyễn: In conversing with my partner, film scholar Nguyen Tan Hoang, if we base the "AIDS crisis revisitation" on the examples cited in the prompt (the art exhibition and the cycle of films), it would seem to be a very limited project. Nevertheless, we suggest that this has happened due to several factors: the idea that AIDS is over; AIDS was a long time ago; and the assimilation of LGBT communities into majoritarian culture, most clearly demonstrated by the recent legalization of same-sex marriage. Especially in the films mentioned in the prompt, we see an impulse to present testimony, a witnessing, to put forth a reminder in an era of AIDS amnesia, of active forgetting. In that way, these documentaries' revisitation serves an important pedagogical function. We were also struck by the nostalgia in the tone of the films, in the texture of degenerated archival footage (in the case of the docs), not to mention the passionate reminiscences of the interview subjects. We don't think this nostalgia is a bad thing, for the historical actors and for the contemporary viewers, especially those who did not live through the events narrated. This nostalgia can inspire action; it can be productive—

especially since too often these kinds of sentiments and affects get dismissed as unproductive, idealizing sentimentality.

Going back to the films, it's clear that there is one dominant narrative that is being revisited (not all of them follow this storyline exactly, and some do so more than others): the narrow cast of characters are well-educated, well-heeled white men based in the United States (specifically cities like NYC or San Francisco); they were at the front lines of direct-action activist struggles (ACT UP), who heroically battled the medical establishments, challenged government inaction, and debunked societal stigmatization, who against all odds survived to the present day (David France's *How to Survive a Plague* is exemplary here). For those who are supposed to identify with this narrative arc, AIDS as a crisis is indeed over. We think the histories and stories of these courageous activists are important and necessary, but the danger here is to privilege them as the only narratives worth telling. Where are the other stories, about those who were not so lucky, who did not survive; whose battles with HIV/AIDS were mundane, took place outside urban gay ghettos, and did not have a happy Hollywood ending? What about those folks disenfranchised by race, ethnicity, class, gender, region, whose struggles were not documented and archived; those without institutional connections; those who did not leave anything behind? Perhaps art museums and galleries, international film festivals, arthouse theaters, cable TV, Netflix are not the most appropriate places to find, produce, exhibit, and distribute these missing stories? For instance, we might point to the work of many community-based organizations across the US in the late 1980s and 1990s targeting people of color, sex workers, queer youth in efforts around HIV/AIDS education, prevention, and direct care—that is, a significant part of AIDS responses without clear villains, victims, and heroes; no sexy sound bites or slogans; no spectacular archival footage.

The framing of the prompt as "AIDS crisis revisitation" suggests that there was a specific time and place that certain folks are now returning to, to revisit someone or something that happened at a place in the past. It assumes that there had been an interruption or a cleaving between the AIDS past and the post-AIDS present. For those folks for whom AIDS has never gone away, never ended, the framing of the renewed attention to AIDS as a revisitation would be inaccurate. To be sure, I am aware the phrase is meant to denote that there is now renewed attention to the history of AIDS (whether it be cultural, political, activist, artistic), and this development is welcomed. At the same time, it's important to point out that inequities around HIV/AIDS continue to exist; so it's necessary to resist the knee-jerk embrace of medical developments as an unquestioned good, as progress.

I am not ignoring the medical advances that have rebranded AIDS as a "manageable disease" for some fortunate people. However, it's the case that HIV/AIDS remains central to gay male communities in the US, in spite of grandiose pronouncements about the "post-AIDS era." AIDS is not making a comeback, since it has never gone away. The hotness and transgression of barebacking in gay porn video and fucking "bare" or "natural" in real life do not make any sense without the danger and stigma that is still attached to HIV/AIDS. Some people of our generation become very alarmed when they see eighteen-year-old guys on Grindr announce that they refuse to use condoms because they are "clean," or they want to fuck "bare" because they are on PrEP—as if these were foolproof protection. It's alarming for me, because we're not sure whether these are self-determined, informed choices, or they are made without access to information about HIV/AIDS and other sexually transmitted infections (STIs). One might say the project of HIV/AIDS education and prevention is not finished.

To return to my uneasiness about the word *revisitation* and the linear timeline that it implies, it might be more useful to talk about multiple epidemics, with different casts of characters and narratives, within various temporalities (linear or cyclical). Such a consideration allows us to account for epidemics that occur alongside one another, some declining while others are on the rise—thus troubling discourses about progress and development that inevitably center the Global North and marginalize the Global South.

Prompt 2

Cheng: In distinct and powerful ways, each of your responses refuses AIDS memory, and the structural violence in which its crises remain lodged as temporally past. The very act of forgetting and remembering—"AIDS revisitation"—centers white, cisgender male, and North American heroic narratives of survival that obfuscate the ongoing pandemic. AIDS revisitation, then, is a condition of the constellation of globalized crises that *is* AIDS and which most adversely impacts women, queer, and trans people of color and those living in the Global South. Yet each of you recalls the necessary cultural, political, and scholarly work undertaken to collectively sustain perception of the uneven and devastating presence of AIDS. In turn, you offer questions and examples that challenge the enduring racial, gender, and structural violence of AIDS revisitation. This includes intervening narratives, fragments of memory, invocations of those invisibilized in the pandemic, critical embodied practices, and more. Can you elaborate further upon your specific strategies for resisting totalizing narratives of AIDS? What work needs to be done to underlie the constellation of these crises to prevent their expressions from being consumed as discrete units of culture, politics, or scholarship?

Aldarondo: Something has happened since I first received everyone's comments. Two days ago Donald Trump was elected president of the United States. And I find that I cannot respond to these thought-provoking comments in any other light. In the same way that politics is always already part of intellectual work—a truism that AIDS makes plain—this news about our new world order is necessarily coloring everything I do. And somehow, it makes our conversation all the more urgent.

There are uncanny yet not accidental parallels between Reagan—a two-bit actor to whom no amount of scandal could stick—and our new president, a second-rate attention whore who frames hate speech as free speech, commits flagrantly illegal acts, and yet has managed to become the most powerful person in our country. And in considering the relationship between HIV/AIDS "then" and HIV/AIDS "now," it occurs to me that there are now glaringly parallel issues of presidential power determining who lives and who dies, who survives and who thrives. Suddenly we are in a situation where HIV-positive people are at risk of losing their health care, their disability benefits, of being deported or thrown in jail, and, indeed, of dying. These were risks before—but in a Trump world, they are all the more acute.

Last night I was on a national conference call that was brainstorming ways to react to a Trump presidency. Although the people on the call represented a variety of constituencies and issues, the call was initiated by HIV/AIDS activists. On the call I heard voices of activists old and young, movement "veterans" and people who weren't even alive when the epidemic first began. This told me several meaningful things: First, AIDS activists have an institutional memory, a wealth of organizational discipline and political knowledge that we will be able to draw on in the coming months and years. Second, I realized that the only way of looking at AIDS, in my mind, is by categorically refusing a divide between past and present. We have to pay attention to time's ability to fold, to repeat, to return. We have to constantly interrogate the way that remembrance relies on forgetting—that when we remember some, we risk obliterating others in material ways. It seems to me more important now than ever to recognize the dangerous correlation between the "AIDS is over" narrative and the constituencies that will be disproportionally vulnerable under a Trump presidency—people of color, the poor, immigrants, drug users, sex workers, women, trans people.

I also want to say something about pedagogy. This semester I have been teaching a course on HIV/AIDS for the first time. I am doing so at the suggestion of a fellow academic who presented at a symposium on AIDS activism earlier this year. He exhorted any of us in the room who'd ever considered teaching HIV/AIDS to do so. I thought to myself, what do I know about HIV/AIDS? I just made a film about my uncle. But I chose to do it anyway. Now, midsemester, I realize I know a lot more than I thought. And I can honestly say that teaching HIV/AIDS is the most challenging and enlivening thing I've ever done as an educator. Every week my students come to class increasingly dismayed by their ignorance about AIDS. They feel cheated and duped by their education. They come angry. But they also come hungry. They say things like "Why don't I learn these kinds of things more often?" "What are we supposed to do with this knowledge?" These questions are openings—cracks in time that allow for transformation.

The night before the election, I asked my students how they felt. No one was excited. They waxed nostalgic about Obama, wished they had more inspiring choices. But no one, including me, was expecting the outcome we got. Now, my students are at a loss. And now I have to guide them.

It occurs to me that the classroom will be one of the most important spaces we have moving forward. The classroom is a space of oral history. It is a space of mis/remembering, of communal, corporeal witnessing. Of relying on the archive and resisting its sepulchral effects at the same time. I see my classroom as the hinge between past and present, the space where then and now commingle. And while I may not necessarily feel hope, I feel a sense of purpose in this space. Because a whole generation of young people is coming of age. And in the dark days to come, it will be our responsibility to give them tools, the space to reckon, to remember people and events they never knew in the first place, and, perhaps most importantly, to provide a bulwark against ignorance. Knowledge may just be what saves us.

Hallas: To understand how "AIDS crisis revisitation" could be framed as the commemoration of a past safely anterior to the present, we also need to consider the complementary discourses of futurity pervading the institutions of biomedicine and public health at the same time. The rhetorical temporality of scientific and policy discourses has clear bearings on how the cultural politics of memory play out. When I attended the 2012 International AIDS Conference in Washington, DC, the official conference theme was "Turning the Tide Together," and there was much talk of finally envisioning the possibility of the "end of AIDS" through the combination of biomedical advances in treatment, scientific momentum toward a cure, and upscaling treatment access globally. While some global institutions, such as the Joint United Nations Programme on HIV/AIDS (UNAIDS), have continued to promote this future-oriented discourse, others have returned to emphasizing the exigency of the present historical moment. In June 2016, the United Nations (UN) General Assembly adopted a "Political Declaration on Ending AIDS" based on UNAIDS's "Fast-Track" initiative, which included highly ambitious targets to be reached by 2020, in order to facilitate the possible end of the AIDS epidemic by 2030. However, a month later in Durban, the 2016 International AIDS Conference convened under the theme of "Access Equity Rights Now," marking a return to an explicit discursive emphasis on the present, which had marked the 2008 and 2010 conferences (respectively "Universal Action Now" and "Right Here, Right Now"). Reports from the conference expressed growing concerns over infection rates, rising drug resistance, and austerity-driven cuts in global funding. Declaring the 2020 target "unrealistic" and potentially "counterproductive," former UNAIDS director Peter Piot stressed that biomedicine alone could not end the epidemic and that the social and cultural transformations needed to combat stigma, discrimination, and exclusion would take much longer.[10] With all its racism, homophobia, misogyny, and isolationism, the nativist ascension to power in the United States and elsewhere in the Global North will undoubtedly savage the international cooperation necessary to make any real progress in the global struggle against the pandemic.

To offer examples of recent visual works generating complex yet non-totalizing pictures of the epidemic and its history, I want to highlight two very different projects: queer Portuguese filmmaker Joaquim Pinto's almost three-hour essay film *E Agora? Lembra-me* (What Now? Remind Me, 2013) and *Through Positive Eyes* (2007–16), a participatory photography project by South African photographer and activist Gideon Mendel and David Gere of the UCLA Art and Global Health Center. In *What Now?* Pinto records and reflects upon his yearlong experimental drug treatment for Hepatitis C, which has been complicated by two decades of living with HIV. The film clearly draws from the legacy of queer AIDS cinema from the 1990s: like Tom Joslin and Peter Friedman's *Silverlake Life: The View from Here* (1993), this autobiographical documentary is constructed around the intimate intersubjective relay of the camera between Pinto and his lover Nuno Leonel (also a filmmaker); like Jarman's *Blue*, Pinto's essay film shares his friend's expansive vision of sensuous experience, philosophical reflection, and political perception. What I find most impressive about *What Now?* is its sheer ambition not only to articulate the day-to-day challenges of living long-term with HIV but also to try to comprehend such human precarity in relation to a bewildering range of contexts, past and present—from Pinto's personal history in the queer cultural world to the dire impact of European austerity on healthcare provision to the biological recency of the human species.[11] Although one would hardly consider the film an activist work, it nevertheless faces seropositive precarity with an undoubtedly political expression of queer intimacy, eroticism, and solidarity. Pinto's philosophical and historical reflections are always in the service of sharpening the stakes of the present rather than diffusing them. *What Now?* never devolves HIV/AIDS into a universal allegory of the human condition; human thought and history are complexly brought to bear on HIV/AIDS through Pinto's philosophical engagement with his immediate lived experience of the virus.

Through Positive Eyes also focuses on the everyday lived experience of living with HIV, but its authorship is decentered and collaborative, its scope both local and global. In ten cities across the globe over the period of a decade (including Mumbai, Johannesburg, Rio, London, and Los Angeles), Gideon Mendel and Crispin Hughes ran photography workshops for a small group of people living with HIV/AIDS. Selected by local AIDS service organizations for their willingness to share their seropositive status publicly to fight stigma, more than one hundred participants learned to explore their own worlds and express themselves through photography. Mendel also visited them at work or home to film them and make a moving-image portrait of them. On an aesthetic level, the often uncanny combination of still and moving images in the participants' short videos provides a subtle but powerful means to sensuously convey seropositive experiences with instability, precarity, and alienation. Indebted to the diversified forms and synergies of earlier AIDS cultural activism that were designed to intervene simultaneously into multiple publics and institutions, this multiplatform project has generated a range of forms, including gallery exhibitions with live tours by the local participants, a database-structured website, photo-essays in major print publications, and a forthcoming book publication. Over the course of almost three decades documenting the AIDS pandemic, Mendel has developed a set of practices that can adapt flexibly to local and global frameworks. The specificity of the local is never sacrificed in the service of putting a universal or global "face" to HIV/AIDS. In fact, when organized together in a nonlinear, searchable interface, the specificities of these local micronarratives provide powerful, comparative testimony to the global inequities of access to health care as well as the variation in the experience of living with HIV/AIDS.

Alvarez: When I read that I would be included in this roundtable, I initially felt that the editors had made a mistake. To be included among remarkable filmmakers, longtime activists, academics, and writers of AIDS is humbling and I enter with great gratitude. I came into AIDS awareness at a young age, and it was limited to registering people to walk and raise funds for AIDS research. As a sophomore in high school, I did a presentation on AIDS in my social history class. The presentation highlighted the racist ideologies embedded within the US's tropical narratives of AIDS. I began my academic research on queer Chicanx sexuality and AIDS as a first-generation college student in the McNair Scholars program, a program designed to increase graduate degree admissions among underrepresented students in higher education by providing research opportunities and mentorship. In this research, I mostly came across work from the social sciences that depicted queer Chicanx sexuality as a binary of sexual positioning (assertive/passive or top/bottom). These academic writings reinforced patriarchal examinations of Latinx sexuality through white lenses. Yet these writings remain insensitive of language, class, citizenship status, culture, and faith. What could I do to resist these representations and to challenge them through my own writing and with the writings of other Brown queer people? In my search for Brown queer storytellers, I came across Gil Cuadros's collection of short stories and poems in *City of God*. I came across the scholarship of Lionel Cantú, who challenged the eroticism of Brown queer men by focusing on the multiple complexities of Latinx identity. Like many queer Chicanx, I read Francisco X. Alarcón and Gloria Anzaldúa. I found in their writing incredible acts of resistance, a cosmic spiritual invocation of ancestry, a return and departure from home. I found death and an urgency to document our histories of survival as Brown and queer people. What I discovered in this search for other Brown queer storytellers was the sacredness of sexuality. These writings revealed an ancient technology: the sacred act of creating as a tool for survival. I began to understand my own survival, as a queer Chicanx, linked to the legacies of queer and AIDS activism. Because of these legacies, I believe that part of my responsibility is to continue the work of resistance. And part of that work is to unearth the stories that remain hidden from larger narratives of survival. Gil Cuadros's writing solidified my commitment.

In one way or another we have all responded to AIDS revisitation in a manner that critiques the white gay representations that dominate the narratives or current cultural production of AIDS. Following this critique we are asked to elaborate on specific strategies for resisting a totalizing narrative of AIDS. We are asked: What work needs to be done to underlie the constellation of these crises to prevent their expressions from being consumed as discrete units of culture, politics, or scholarship? To this I reference Jim Hubbard and his response to our initial prompt, "Make your own!" We make our own. We create our own. We offer space for people to contribute and create in the same way I was offered space in this roundtable discussion.

I recently had a conversation with a friend regarding both our efforts to produce work that honors queer Chicanx and Latinx ancestry. Though our projects are different, our projects entail revisiting a past. Our methodologies consist of archival investigations, collecting and documenting stories through the tradition of oral histories, and visiting sites connected to our projects. Equally important to our methodologies is the act of ceremony. These ceremonies regard the burning of *copal*, the lighting of a candle, raising an altar, and days of ritual practices. In our conversation we had asked each other: Why are we doing this research at this particular moment in time? Why are we revisiting these past legacies of survival and struggle? We realized that the concerns of that past are the ones that are most important today. We agreed that we are visiting a historical past because it is calling us in the present. It is the present moment of neoliberal capitalist white supremacy in which new technologies of mass deportations, incarcerations, as well as new modes of racism, gendered, and sexual violence are refueling the act of forgetting. It is the present moment that is at stake of eradication. So, then, how do we survive this current time? How do we resist? We do what our ancestors did: we create and we document. We create acts of resistance through writing, filmmaking, storytelling, painting, photography, digital art making, protesting, and through radical acts of self-care, by loving.

I want to end by referencing a recent documentary film that was completed by Dr. Osa Hidalgo de la Riva. Hidalgo de la Riva's film *Me and Mr. Mauri: Turning Poison into Medicine* (2015) unearths and illuminates legacies of Brown queer resistance to illness, shame, homophobia, and colonization. Her work is a sacred act of ceremony and storytelling created through a personal video archive and political consciousness. *Me and Mr. Mauri* is accomplished entirely using raw personal video footage of Hidalgo de la Riva's friends and their experiences impacted by the early AIDS pandemic while living in the Bay Area, California, during the early 1990s. The documentary is not male-centered and revisitation of the past extends further to recall Mayan and Zapotec knowledge of sacred sexualities. The documentary begins with the ceremonious act of body healing through massage and the burning of sage shared between Hidalgo de la Riva and Mauricio Delgado. Throughout the documentary I came to understand the significance of ancestral medicine; Indigenous and Native American knowledge of nonheteronormative sexualities and healing; ritual, dance, and commitment as the critical manifestations of AIDS political consciousness; and activism that emerges from an intimate place called home. One of the most powerful moments for me in Hubbard and Sarah Schulman's *United in Anger* was the footage of the Ashes Action at the White House lawn staged by ACT UP activists in 1992. Just as powerful was the footage of Hidalgo de la Riva and Veronica Delgado placing the ashes of Mauricio into a pre-Columbian clay sculpture in *Me and Mr. Mauri*. For ACT UP activists, the Ashes Action is significant on multiple levels, ones that place the responsibilities for AIDS-related deaths at the hands of government. I interpret Hidalgo de la Riva and Delgado's action in *Me and Mr. Mauri* as a ceremonious return to ancestry, linking Mauricio to the legacies of his Nicaraguan ancestry, an ancestry that experienced a history of colonization and yet survives through acts of creation, including this film.

At the end of the film, Hidalgo de la Riva offers words to her friend Mauricio and states,

> Hey, *flaco* dude, you know for those of us left behind remaining on the plane of the physical, existing on this planet Earth, we need to continue daily to be creative, to act in nonviolent ways, healing eternally ourselves, each other, one another, show love for our planet. We are so far from perfect. I watch the political and economic disasters made by men reflect on the ecological ones as well. We are in a hurricane, in the depths of crevices left by meteors and earthquakes. I live in the memory of your laughter and dancing self, sweet little brother. I'm sitting here writing a script portraying you, Mr. Mauri, one of my contemporary heroes. In this role we simultaneously live and die and live again as brother and sister and friend.

These final words in the documentary, and my recollection of the documentary reiterated in this roundtable discussion, perform the multiple ways we can resist a totalizing narrative of AIDS. When I asked Hidalgo de la Riva why she had decided to complete the documentary in 2015, she said, "Because it is not over."

Hubbard: I wish we were having this interchange in person instead of asynchronously. I feel as if I've been thrown in the deep end and ordered to swim. Perhaps it's because I'm not an academic that I find this all so mystifying.

Perhaps it's because I'm an experimental filmmaker who has never respected the limitations of enforced notions of narrative or documentary filmmaking, nor allowed the extreme limitations on access to larger audiences prevent the work from getting done. Perhaps it's because when I came out it was into the world of 1960s/1970s gay liberation, which sought to transform the way *everyone* felt about sexuality and gender instead of aspiring to assimilate into some humdrum version of pseudo-heterosexuality. Perhaps it's just that I'm old and my ears can no longer hear the dog whistles.

First, I do not refuse AIDS memory. That is all I have left of my dead friends and the extraordinary effort of thousands of AIDS activists of all genders, all colors, and many nations to force the governments of the world to live up to their responsibilities to provide services and health care and to do the research that has, in turn, utterly changed the face of the epidemic. None of this is to say that AIDS is over or that allowing millions of people around the world to struggle with HIV without medicines or proper health care is not a crime. Furthermore, we can't ignore that certain individuals and communities have far greater access to the means of media production than others. I can't help thinking that to an observer anywhere in Africa or Asia, this discussion would seem awfully US-centric. I am also sensitive to the fact that every work mentioned by name in the first prompt was made by a cis white male. Nevertheless, to feel that people remembering their own history and trying to make sense of it steals all the oxygen from present-day efforts to deal with the disease is to surrender too easily to despair and inaction. Nor is that to say that there aren't real political critiques to be made of certain efforts to obscure the true nature of the epidemic and the struggle against it. Nevertheless, it is absolutely crucial to remember that when AIDS was first recognized, it was killing people who had no rights and no power and those people fought back and changed the world.

Further, to refuse AIDS memory is to forget the important lessons of the AIDS crisis of the 1980s and 1990s. It is to forget the triumphs and the losses and to forgo the analysis necessary to understand which strategies and tactics worked and which would not work today and to use that knowledge to further the vital work being done today.

However, I find the assertion that "the very act of forgetting and remembering . . . centers white, cisgender male, and North American heroic narratives of survival that obfuscate the ongoing pandemic" utterly stupefying. Every word in the responses to Prompt #1 belies this. As someone who has spent a lifetime rejecting "North American heroic narratives," I understand the political and social power of those narratives. The accolades and rewards that accrue from adhering to heroic narratives are powerfully seductive, but it is our responsibility as artists to reject those and tell the stories that reflect our unique understanding of the world and paint the pictures that we truly see.

In making *United in Anger*, I worked extremely diligently to counter heroic and totalizing narratives. In order to reflect accurately the ever-changing membership and leadership of ACT UP, many people had to speak in the film. It was crucial to show how the activism was done, to highlight the nuts and bolts of grassroots political organizing and to emphasize that effective direct action is hard work. When I first began making the film, I was told that I had to choose five or six "characters" to represent ACT UP and through them to tell the story of the AIDS activist movement. However, to do so would have been to reject the reality of ACT UP and the film would have perpetrated a lie. The implied threat, however, was that if I did not present history in the prescribed manner, I would not receive funding and the film would not be shown in the major festivals or on television. In fact, the funding for the film came almost exclusively from social justice organizations, not from film grants, and the film has only shown on one local, independent station.

Furthermore, if there are inaccuracies and lacunae in the recent historicizing of the AIDS crisis, then it is our responsibility to fix them. However, I think it is a terrible strategic error to believe that the HIV epidemic of 2017 is the same as the AIDS crisis of the late 1980s and early 1990s. To think that is to ignore two massive changes since then—the introduction of HAART in 1996 and the bureaucratization of HIV/AIDS. Other aspects of the world's relationship to HIV/AIDS, such as stigma and lack of access, have been disturbingly persistent. The continuing power of racism, classism, homophobia, and transphobia allows some people to benefit from medical advances but prevents millions of others from having access. I don't know how to address the lack of access to medication and services outside the larger issue of health-care provision either in the United States or in developing nations. Prevention, in order to be effective, must be culturally specific. Efforts to thwart the creation and dissemination of culturally specific prevention techniques have been a consciously homophobic and erotophobic part of US AIDS policy since the very beginning. I find it astonishing that the stigma of having HIV in your body has persisted and even worsened in some places such as in Canada, with its epidemic of HIV criminalization, but I don't have any solutions to the problem. What seems to be forgotten is the very foundation of the AIDS activist movement, which fought against the dominant homophobic, racist, sexist power structure and transformed the nature of the epidemic.

Let me speak as a filmmaker. The period when attention is paid to most films is actually very short. If you're doing well on the festival circuit, where most films garner public attention, the life of a film is a year and a half or perhaps two years. Probably, YouTube has extended that somewhat, but it's easy to get lost in the fractiousness and cornucopia of the online world. Of course, a film that's made for television will have a much larger initial audience. Because they are made for that larger audience, they will reflect the politics of the ruling class, but even those films fade away rather quickly. When was the last time anyone seriously considered *An Early Frost* (John Erman, 1985) or even *Philadelphia* (Jonathan Demme, 1993)? It's interesting that the lazy analysis and internalized homophobia of Randy Shilts's 1987 book, *And the Band Played On*, and the 1993 movie of the same name directed by Roger Spottiswoode are finally being exposed for what they were—a glorification of the power of straight white men rather than a useful or insightful exploration of the first years of AIDS.

But where films and books and posters do have an extended life is in academia. Academics have the power to decide what's important and which films get shown, which books are read, and to shape the worldview of the next generation and the next. Academics have the power to resist this totalizing narrative of AIDS by presenting works that tell a more complex, subtle, and diverse set of stories. Of course, it increases your students' media literacy to critique work that obscures the complexity of life in favor of a socially acceptable comforting narrative, but it is far more important and ultimately more inspiring to show and write about work that stands in opposition to that narrative. Show films about people of color and people outside the United States in your classes. If you feel they are not being made now, dig up the ones from the past. The AIDS activist movement generated an extraordinary flowering of angry, smart, creative video making that refused the dominant narrative and told the story of AIDS from the grassroots multiethnic point of view. I know it's difficult to obtain copies, but the demand will create accessibility.

And perhaps, most importantly, encourage your students to make films about AIDS today or about an alternative view of the past. To add to Roger's list of missing work, I would include films about the Asian and Pacific Islander Coalition on HIV/AIDS (APICHA), Brooklyn AIDS Task Force, Treatment Action Campaign, AIDS in Asia, et cetera. Considering the tenor of this discussion, I think it's crucial to make films about the inspiring work of the People with AIDS self-empowerment movement, starting with the Denver Principles and the founding of the People with AIDS Coalition (PWAC) and continuing to the present moment.

There is a current problem in terms of media and that is we live in an era when raw footage instantaneously uploaded to the internet grabs people's attention most of all. I don't know what that means for AIDS media. Unless there are demonstrations that lend themselves to uploading raw footage, I don't know what can be done. I still believe, however, that thoughtful, well-edited documentaries, whether about the current epidemic or the past of the AIDS crisis, can be useful educational tools to garner attention for the movement.

Finally, for me, politics is not simply the way we vote but the way we view and live in the social world. It is not possible to separate culture or scholarship from politics. If you don't continuously, consciously, specifically assert the political nature of your art or your scholarship, you are reinforcing and accepting the dominant worldview and the power of the ruling class. It is to abjure your moral responsibilities as a human being, as a scholar, and as an artist.

Kang-Nguyễn: These responses emphasize the tensions between global/local perspectives and their associated temporalities. There have always been multiple HIV epidemics, each with their own contours, stakeholders, and interests. Each of these is, in turn, made visible or invisible in different ways. In particular, I'm thinking of Cecilia's summary of what she learned in researching her film. Who are the "them" of the "thens" and the "theys" of the "now"? Whose stories get told and pictured? Following Pablo, ACT UP is very special, but how is it also representative of broader social justice activism? Roger reminds us of the "second silence" and Jim's rejoinder to point out that the inequitable conditions that structure the AIDS epidemic persist are also important reminders to be vocal and remain angry. Ryan Conrad's analysis of shifting AIDS metaphors, from genocide to plague, state to moral responsibility, and testimony to witnessing, seems very appropriate at this time.[12]

When I remember and imagine AIDS activism during the early crisis years, what comes to mind most readily is the excitement of ACT UP from its New York center: Gran Fury, actions there, as well as at the National Institutes of Health (NIH), the White House, and at the Centers for Disease Control (CDC). I came out in 1990 in Washington, DC, started working for the "AIDS Industrial Complex" the year after, and participated in DC protests toward the end of ACT UP's heyday. Queer Nation had also emerged. There were many kiss-ins, die-ins, and other actions that built up to the 1993 March on Washington for Lesbian, Gay and Bi Equal Rights and Liberation. AIDS activism was already waning when I moved to Los Angeles. A few years later, one of the ACT UP activists I admired in DC threatened many of my San Francisco colleagues and actively advocated with conservative congresspeople to defund HIV prevention in the city. He also supported South African president Thabo Mbeki's AIDS denialism. The latter is estimated to have cost hundreds of thousands of lives. That is when ACT UP was over for me. Two decades later, I've used video from the CDC protests when teaching public health courses at Emory University in a building across the street from the CDC building that no longer exists and has been replaced by a much larger, more modern, more secure facility that no one could get into or climb up any more. I'm reminded of having taught Vito Russo's famous 1988 "Why We Fight" speech. Now, I mourn the irony of the last line: "And then, after we kick the shit out of this disease, we're all going to be alive to kick the shit out of this system, so that this never happens again."[13] I'm reminded of the postprotease Los Angeles context in which the demand became for "drugs and jobs." I teach what ACT UP and AIDS activism did: produced a system in which patients knew more about the disease than their doctors; reframed patient-doctor interactions, and then moved this to the clinical trials process and beyond; but, most importantly, linked disease status with ideas of social inequality and deservedness. AIDS activism has fundamentally changed how Americans conceive of themselves as diseased/disabled, their health care, and human rights. The changes are fundamental and groundbreaking, though they have also enabled new biocapitalist modes of therapeutic citizenship, ways of being in the world based on disease status and reliance on expensive pharmaceuticals.

I spent most of my years working in HIV/AIDS social services in Los Angeles and San Francisco. Each city had its own way of engaging activism and developed local models for prevention and care. In San Francisco, the epidemic was heavily concentrated among white gay men more so than other cities in the United States. Combined with the existing gay political clout and medical research and service infrastructure, the city fostered a more compassionate and evidence-based system for HIV care. The "San Francisco model" was based on collaboration. There was tremendously concentrated suffering but without the same level of anger seen elsewhere. Great efforts at inclusive access, however, did not always lead to equitable outcomes. There has always been a conflict in HIV work among those who want to stop the epidemic and those who want to alleviate the inequalities in the world that shape the epidemic. This is an oversimplified dichotomy that pits disease intervention against social justice work. Neither strategy, in and of itself, will end the epidemic. But the positions are, for some, intractable. Social justice work by itself doesn't stop epidemics, but epidemics like HIV take advantage of social vulnerabilities. We've always needed to do both kinds of work simultaneously, but activists have fought over the proportions as the strategies get rationalized into divisible pie charts and Venn diagrams. There has been a move to incorporate sexual health into broader programs, to shift HIV prevention to sexual wellness, but the resources for such work are shrinking all over the world. Funding in the United States and through our international development programs is now under existential threat.

I think that we can identify broad patterns in the HIV pandemic (e.g., the role of structural violence, the attachment of stigma) and also see the specificities of the many local epidemics that we experience. In many ways, HIV has been the exemplary story of the oppressed (I don't like the term *affected* to describe communities) taking control over representations, practices, and policies about ourselves. I'm thinking about the situation for Asian American (or men of color) and Asian (or Global South) gay men more broadly. I think Cecilia's comment about an "aging population of survivors" is apropos in the US context and this is put in tension with her statement about producing "AIDS as a thing of the past when the opposite could not be farther from the truth," both from a minority perspective in the United States and from a Global South perspective. I sit uneasily in this position, living through and being part of multiple localized epidemics among gay men: among Asian and Pacific Islander gay men in the United States and, now, among gay men in Thailand, where I am reliving the epidemic as a crisis. These two epidemics have always been linked, but they also point to how the epidemics are extremely localized and differentiated.

Thailand is one of the global models for HIV prevention, especially in regard to its 100 percent condom use policy among brothel-based sex workers. But the program's success was only attainable because it operationalized under a military dictatorship. That is, strict enforcement was made possible because human rights were not considered. But now the situation has shifted dramatically. Military rule may have reasserted itself, but the "heterosexual" epidemic (injection drug users have never benefited from this progress narrative) has shifted to one that has reemerged among gay men and trans women. During my fieldwork engagements from 2004 to 2011, the prevalence of HIV among gay men in Bangkok rose from less than 5 percent to more than 30 percent. HIV prevention programs sponsored by the US government redirected funds toward the *most* "at risk" populations (MARP) to differentiate the wide array of needs between various populations but concentrated efforts on those who were actually becoming infected: that is, males who have sex with males (gay/bi men and heterosexual men who work as sex workers with them) and trans women (MSM and TG).

One of my best friends in Thailand is suffering from schizophrenic dementia. She is a trans woman, sex worker, and HIV positive. She has been a migrant sex worker in Singapore and Hong Kong over the years, remitting money to her mother in Thailand. This has prevented her from being able to regularly access anti-HIV drugs through the national Thai scheme. People generally think that she is going crazy. During a visit last year, I brought up the issue with some of her closest friends. I told them that I believe her dementia is caused by HIV. Her Thai friends replied that they think it is methamphetamine-induced dementia. I told them that she is not using drugs frequently anymore but the symptoms are getting worse and that I suspect it is HIV-related as she has not been on medication. In fact, it is probably a synergy of both effects. Her other friends' response was that she is not open about her HIV status, so they can't broach the topic with her. They cannot help her in this situation. Inside, I wanted to scream, but I kept my composure. What I wanted to say was that their inability to even broach the subject could cause her to die faster. I wanted them to stage an intervention on her, to get her on medication and support adherence, and what I got was the perpetuation of the culture of silence on HIV. I've had friends die this way before and now I am seeing this pattern repeating in another context. An ethics of engagement is not negated by cultural respect.

There is increasing recognition that HIV is not just about what you do but who you are, something that was buried in earlier campaigns, which operated under generalized assumptions about the risks suffered by everyone. This partially explains why Black gay men in the United States are still experiencing the epidemic much more brutally, as they are less likely to have regular access to health care, are less likely to be undetectable, and are thus more likely to experience negative health consequences and pass on the virus to their partners, who are more likely to be other Black men. MARP sounds weird, but in essence, the term reminds us that groups like "faggots, junkies, and whores" continue to "out-die" others, even where the epidemics currently affect the greater population. The epidemic among MSM and TG is resurging in developed countries and exploding in the developing world. In many parts of the developing world, the HIV-prevalence rates for MSM and TG are fifty times that of other "high-risk" groups.

AIDS activism recast HIV prevention from a biological model to a social model in the United States. This was replicated in much of the developing world. But there is a sense that the social model has failed, been exhausted, or is too difficult to pursue because it requires too many social changes. With increasing information on the success of treatment as prevention (treating HIV-infected individuals to suppress their viral load so that they do not infect their partners)—postexposure prophylaxis (PEP), preexposure prophylaxis (PrEP), microbicides, and ongoing discoveries in vaccine research—more and more people are promoting biological interventions as prevention (e.g., mobilize all gay men, trans women, sex workers, and other MARPs to take a preventative pill every day rather than use condoms). I think context is really important. In some places, access to medical services is pretty easy, even for relatively disenfranchised groups (not to say it is great or that it can't be improved). Though PrEP advocates often forget that adherence is a behavioral issue, realistically, it is often easier to get people to pop a pill daily than do other things like use a condom for every penetrative sexual act. The danger is we further medicalize society (if you do think that is a bad thing) and create challenges to ongoing access, including costs for the meds (especially where patents and insurance make them relatively inaccessible), provider reluctance to prescribe, and sex stigma. More than two decades ago, I presented a talk: "Let the Semen Flow." In it, I advocated advances in barrier-free semen exchanges (without condoms), modeled at that time on anal microbicides. This was before I ever imagined that PrEP, which is currently only approved using Truvada, might be priced at $1,000 per month in developed nations.[14] We need to successfully use drugs without letting pharmaceutical companies control the terms. Use of these medications can integrate with or bypass the wellness model of sexual health, which takes a more holistic approach than the prevention of specific diseases like HIV. However, the latter seems more likely.

Back to the issue of representation, I think part of the issue lies in narratives of heroes and villains (the cowboy capitalist embodied in *Dallas Buyers Club* or Patient Zero, Gaëtan Dugas, in *And the Band Played On*). These stories rely on narrative tropes in general: the hero is a person who individually accomplishes amazing things against all odds and should be praised for it. America's focus on individualism naturalizes these stories. These narratives, however, fail to register the power of social institutions and their historical contexts. We don't need another hero, but we do need a lot of action.

Notes

1 Sturken, *Tangled Memories*, 14.
2 Sturken, *Tangled Memories*, 15.
3 Cheng, "How to Survive."

4   Sturken, *Tangled Memories*, 2–3.
5   Bronx Museum of Arts, "Press Release."
6   Kerr, "AIDS 1969."
7   Juhasz, "Forgetting ACT UP," 7.
8   Alfaro, "Heroes and Saints," 331.
9   Hedva, "My Body Is a Prison."
10 Boseley, "Hope for 'End of Aids' Is Disappearing."
11 I am using the term *precarity* in Judith Butler's sense: "'Precarity' designates that politically induced condition in which certain populations suffer from failing social and economic networks of support and become differentially exposed to injury, violence, and death." Butler, "Performativity, Precarity and Sexual Politics," ii.
12 Conrad, "Reviving the Queer Political Imagination," chapter 2, "Revisiting AIDS and Its Metaphors."
13 Russo, "Why We Fight."
14 In the United States, private health insurance will cover the cost with a copayment of around fifty dollars per month. Some public and community clinics will provide it for free, depending on income and local availability. Activists have been fighting the National Health Service in the United Kingdom to cover the prescription. A generic is available in Thailand for approximately thirty dollars per month through public and private clinics. Gay men in places such as Singapore and Hong Kong can purchase the generic in Thailand and illegally export it for use at home.

Bibliography

Aldarondo, Cecilia, dir. *Memories of a Penitent Heart*. POV, 2016

Alfaro, Luis. "Downtown." In *O Solo Homo: The New Queer Performance*, edited by Holly Hughes and David Román, 313–48. New York: Grove, 1998.

Alfaro, Luis. "Heroes and Saints." In *O Solo Homo: The New Queer Performance*, edited by Holly Hughes and David Román, 331. New York: Grove, 1998.

Bordowitz, Gregg, dir. *Fast Trip, Long Drop*. 1994.

Bordowitz, Gregg, dir. *Habit*. 2001.

Boseley, Sarah. "Hope for 'End of Aids' Is Disappearing, Experts Warn." *The Guardian*, July 31, 2016.

Brocka, Lino, dir. *Macho Dancer*. Culver City, CA: Strand Releasing, 1988..

Bronx Museum of Arts. "Press Release: Art AIDS America: July 13 to October 23, 2016." Accessed November 20, 2018. http://www.bronxmuseum.org/exhibitions/art-aids-america.

Butler, Judith. "Performativity, Precarity and Sexual Politics." *Antropólogos Iberoamericanos en Red* 4, no. 3 (2009): i–xiii.

Carlomusto, Jean, dir. *Larry Kramer in Love and Anger*. HBO, 2015.

Cheng, Jih-Fei. "How to Survive: AIDS and Its Afterlives in Popular Media." *Women's Studies Quarterly* 44, nos. 1/2 (2016): 73–92.

Conrad, Ryan. "Reviving the Queer Political Imagination: Affect, Archives, and Anti-normativity." PhD diss., Concordia University, 2017.

Cuadros, Gil. "There Are Places You Don't Walk at Night, Alone." In *City of God*, 112–14. San Francisco: City Lights, 1994.

D'Adesky, Anne-Christine, Shanti Avirgan, and Ann T. Rossetti, dirs. *Pills, Profits, Protest: A Chronicle of the Global AIDS Movement*. Outcast Films, 2005.

Demme, Jonathan. *Philadelphia*. TriStar Pictures, 1993.

Edkins, Don, dir. *Steps for the Future*. Jacana Media, 2002.

Erman, John. *An Early Frost*. NBC Productions, 1985.

France, David, dir. *How to Survive a Plague*. Sundance Selects, 2012.

Greyson, John, dir. *Zero Patience*. Strand Releasing, 1993.

Greyson, John, dir. *Fig Trees*. Berlinale, 2003.

Hallas, Roger. *Reframing Bodies: AIDS, Bearing Witness, and the Queer Moving Image*. Durham, NC: Duke University Press, 2009.

Hedva, Johanna. "My Body Is a Prison of Pain so I Want to Leave It Like a Mystic but I Also Love It & Want It to Matter Politically." February 1, 2016. https://sickwomantheory.tumblr.com/.

Hidalgo de la Riva, Osa, dir. *Me and Mr. Mauri: Turning Poison into Medicine*. Royal Eagle Bear Productions, 2015.

Hilferty, Robert, dir. *Stop the Church*. Frameline, 1990.

Hubbard, Jim, and Sarah Schulman. *United in Anger: A History of ACT UP*. United in Anger, 2012.

Hughes, Holly, and David Román, eds. *O Solo Homo: The New Queer Performance*. New York: Grove, 1998.

Jarman, Derek, dir. *Blue*. Zeitgeist Films, 1993.

Joslin, Tom, and Peter Friedman, dirs. *Silverlake Life: The View from Here*. 1993.

Juhasz, Alexandra. "Forgetting ACT UP." *Quarterly Journal of Speech* 98, no. 1 (2012): 69–74.

Kerr, Theodore. "AIDS 1969: HIV, History, and Race." In "AIDS and Memory," edited by Ricky Varghese, special issue, *Drain* 13, no. 2 (2016). http://drainmag.com/aids-1969-hiv-history-and-race/.

Mendel, Gideon, and David Gere. *Through Positive Eyes*. 2007–16.

Murphy, Ryan, dir. *The Normal Heart*. HBO, 2014.

Pinto, Joaquim, dir. *E Agora? Lembra-me* [What Now? Remind Me]. CRIM Produções, 2013.

Russo, Vito. "Why We Fight." 1988. https://actupny.org/documents/whfight.html.

Schwartz, Jeffrey, dir. *Vito*. First Run Features, 2011.

Shilts, Randy. *And the Band Played On: Politics, People, and the AIDS Epidemic*. New York: St. Martin's, 1987.

Spottiswoode, Roger. *And the Band Played On*. HBO Pictures, 1993.

Sturken, Marita. *Tangled Memories: The Vietnam War, the AIDS Epidemic, and the Politics of Remembering*. Berkeley: University of California Press, 1997.

Vallée, Jean-Marc, dir. *Dallas Buyers Club*. Focus Features, 2013.

Weissman, David, dir. *We Were Here*. Netflix, 2011.

NINE BLACK GAY MEN'S SEXUAL HEALTH AND THE MEANS OF PLEASURE IN THE AGE OF AIDS

Marlon M. Bailey

The Anything Goes Party

Raheim, a Black gay man who lives in Detroit, demonstrated for me the "secret knock" that he used to gain access to the "Anything Goes" sex party to which he had been invited. [1] He received the instructions for attending the sex party the previous night through a text message from the organizer. Unlike other sex parties Raheim has attended, this Anything Goes party was not advertised through any of the usual websites that gay men use, such as Adam4Adam, Black Gay Chat, or Jack'd. This party is "double underground." The only way Raheim learns about it is because he knows the organizer and has fucked at his parties before. Other Black gay men find out through word of mouth since it is a get-together that happens regularly, albeit in secret.

Raheim arrives at the hotel located in a nearby suburb of Detroit, right off Highway 10, also called the John C. Lodge Expressway. He does the secret knock once he arrives at the door of the hotel room. There are a variety of measures taken to keep Anything Goes parties private and thus outside various forms of surveillance, such as the attention of the hotel staff or police. Parties like these are typically illegal in a Midwestern state like Michigan or at the very least they are against hotel regulations, if exposed. The term *anything goes* also signifies "raw sex." So, given the stigma associated with condomless sex and busting nuts inside one another, these parties also remain secret to avoid a potential "outing" from those who Raheim refers to as "condom Nazis."

Immediately after he knocks, Raheim sees a guy look through the peep-hole and then open the door of the hotel room. Upon entering, Raheim is asked to show the text message he received before he is allowed to proceed into a suite. Only then is he allowed to approach a makeshift reception area in the sitting room of the suite. He immediately sees a bucket of some alcoholic concoction and a bowl full of condoms and lube.

Raheim is entering a sex space in which, as he describes it, *nothing really matters*. Perhaps this is a way for him to experience those ephemeral moments of sexual bliss, a temporary escape from a world in which *everything matters*, but the standards of what matters are defined by others, even for his own body. The Anything Goes sex party is a *situation* and *space* in which Black gay men "have the right to fuck" and fuck raw if they want, because, as writer Herukhuti rhetorically asks in his provocative essay on raw sex, "Whose booty is this?"[2] Herukhuti gets to the heart of what is at stake for Black gay men in this particular HIV/AIDS moment, sexual autonomy, which is the focus and the central question of this chapter.

Elsewhere, I explore the extant literature on raw sex (and barebacking) and propose a theoretical edifice to examine the possibilities for conceptualizing sexual health that emphasizes sexual pleasure, as opposed to mandatory—one-size-fits-all—safe sex for Black gay men.[3] In this chapter, I think through, *aloud* (and with others like me), the messy, complicated, and complex relationship between risky sex, HIV, and sexual health for Black gay men. I query what sexual health actually means to Black gay men on their own terms and what it looks like in their quotidian lives from their own perspectives. I bring into focus Black gay men's sexual participation in and experiences of "high-risk" sex and the spaces and situations in which it occurs. But rather than doing so with judgment and from a distance, to then advocate for a continuation of decades of failed interventions into this community, I do so from among communities of Black gay men, drawing from perspectives grounded in their experiences. Perhaps, most importantly, I emphasize Black gay men's views on their own sex practices. My ethnographic study forces us to rethink sexual health where risk and pleasure are not placed in binary opposition. Instead, for the Black gay men in my study, sexual health consists of risk and pleasure as co-constitutive. Ultimately, I argue that sexual practices, spaces, and situations in which Black gay men are engaged allow them to claim and enact sexual autonomy during this HIV crisis that disproportionately impacts them.

Much of this chapter is drawn from a pilot study that my colleagues and I conducted on raw sex and semen exchange practices among Black gay men and men who have sex with men (MSM) communities in the Midwest.[4] In this study, we used both semistructured interviews and ethnographic methods. Our sample consisted of a total of twenty-four Black gay men or MSM participants, between the ages of eighteen and forty-five, twenty of whom we referred to as *key informants* and four as *interlocutors*. We held two hour-long interviews with twenty key informants who self-disclosed as participating in raw sex and semen exchange. We asked the participants to discuss their sexual practices in detail. For example, we asked the participants to describe the kind of sex they have and what brings them pleasure. Many of the participants were taken aback by our questions because they had never been asked by service providers or researchers to discuss what they like to do sexually. The ethnographic dimension of this study also included four interlocutors, Black gay or MSM, who engage in raw sex and semen exchange in public/private sex venues (i.e., sex clubs, bathhouses, and parties like Anything Goes). Using an observation guide, each interlocutor undertook two visits to sex venues and audio-recorded a detailed description of experiences, observations, and the space in a private location after leaving the event. My research assistants and I debriefed with the participants after each of their two visits to a sex club or sex party. Our overall aim was to explore the meaning of sex and sexual health for Black gay men to engender more knowledge about and strategies for HIV prevention that embrace and enhance their sexual health and wellness while still emphasizing pleasure.

HIV/AIDS, Black Gay Men, and Social Inequalities

Social inequality and health disparities due to convergent racism and homophobia contribute to Black gay men's structural vulnerability to HIV. It is well documented that Black gay men disproportionately experience the consequences of institutional racism, such as poverty, under/unemployment, incarceration, health disparities, and violence perpetrated by law enforcement and civilians. While Black gay men live and navigate the realities of structural racism that, in part, underpin their health outcomes, they also simultaneously experience structural homophobia that includes gay- and HIV-related stigma, linked to violence, abuse, and exclusion. In her intersectional study of Black gay and bisexual men, Lisa Bowleg captures the ways in which many Black men's experiences are shaped by the race, gender, and sexual oppression that challenge their mental health and overall social well-being.[5] Since many Black gay men experience convergent racism and homophobia in society at large, they rely upon their families and communities of origin for support, acceptance, and affirmation. Yet in these settings many Black gay men experience sexuality as an aspect of their lives that they should hide or be ashamed of, and as a potential source of their social exclusion and ostracization. The simultaneity of structural anti-Black racism and homophobia, grounded in the intersections of race, gender, and sexuality, undermines the health and well-being of Black gay men.[6]

HIV/AIDS prevention and sexual health paradigms developed by public health have neither worked to reduce HIV nor improved the sexual health and well-being of Black communities, let alone Black gay men. While public health has ostensibly led the charge against HIV/AIDS, according to Chandra L. Ford and Collins O. Airhihenbuwa, the field of public health has and continues to use theories and methodologies that inadequately address the complexity with which structural racism influences health and health disparities experienced by communities of color, as well as the knowledge produced about these communities.[7] Research and interventions in public health overemphasize individual and interpersonal behavioral modification, without seriously accounting for the ways in which structural racism impacts social inequities and health disparities experienced by entire communities, particularly those who are simultaneously marginalized by race, socioeconomic status, gender, sexuality, and HIV status.[8]

Black gay men's disproportionate representation in the HIV/AIDS epidemic in the United States is the most vivid example of the severity of health disparities that Black gay men and MSM continue to experience after nearly four decades of the epidemic. For instance, in 2005 the CDC conducted a five-city study and released a startling report concluding that 46 percent of Black gay men were infected with HIV and 67 percent of those infected were unaware of their HIV infection.[9] In 2006 Black gay men and MSM accounted for 63 percent of new infections among all Black men and 35 percent among all MSM.[10] Nearly two decades later, the CDC concluded that "if current HIV diagnosis rates persist, about 1 in 2 black gay men and MSM in the U.S. will be diagnosed with HIV during their lifetime."[11] Black gay and bisexual men remain more affected by HIV than any other group in the United States, accounting for 37 percent of all new HIV diagnoses in 2017.[12] What does such a staggering and tragic projection from public health say about the sexual health of Black gay men? Ford and Airhihenbuwa suggest that critical race theory would help public health research investigate the root causes of social inequality and health disparities so as to alter the conditions under which Black gay men engage and express their sexuality, and instead advance an approach that is underpinned by social justice principles.

Indeed, many Black gay men engage in high-risk sex, but there are many factors that make them more vulnerable to HIV beyond their sexual practices. These forms of high-risk sex include infrequent to no condom use with multiple sexual partners, the mixing of sex and drugs, and group sexual situations in which raw sex is practiced. The many social and structural factors that make Black gay men vulnerable to HIV and other sexually transmitted diseases/infections (STDs/STIs) include the small social/sexual networks in which Black gay men socialize and have sex (with higher HIV and STD prevalence), barriers to prevention and treatment services, and the social stigma experienced within and beyond their families and communities of origin. Hence, social inequalities make Black gay men more vulnerable to HIV and other STDs, not their sexual behavior, necessarily. This is why strategies designed to change and reduce these men's "risky" sexual behavior, such as promoting consistent condom use, the main focus of prevention strategies, have not proven effective in reducing HIV prevalence among these gay men. For some Black gay men at least, the aforementioned sexual practices, sites, and situations are designed to heighten sexual pleasure and satisfaction, even as they also bring heightened risk for HIV and STD infections. But for other Black gay men, all sex makes them vulnerable to HIV and STDs due, in part, to the conditions under which they live.

When Black gay men struggle to find connection, meaning, and intimacy, sex becomes the means through which many seek and find these essential and healthy experiences. Black gay men face discursive and material obstacles to sexual satisfaction in their quotidian lives. Daily barriers go unexamined due to an overemphasis on sexual behavioral change, largely shaped by the promotion of sex practices that run counter to the actuality of these men's sexual aims and experiences. Given these contradictions and the ongoing rates of high seroprevalence within this community, I am interested in the structural and systemic conditions that constrain and limit Black gay men's sexual pleasure and possibilities. Overall, we must attend to the role that structural and social factors play, as they align or do not with desire, pleasure, and risk, in how Black gay men ascribe meaning to sex, and how this influences the sexual choices they make and the options and experiences they have.

Sexual Health and Homosex Normativity

What constitutes sexual health for Black gay men? What discourses define it and how does this definition impact HIV-prevention policy? As national HIV-prevention efforts move toward strategies such as "find (HIV positives), test, and treat" to lower viral loads so as to reduce infections, there is also concurrently an international discussion around the meaning of *sexual health*. According to the World Health Organization (WHO), sexual health is the state of physical, emotional, mental, and social well-being in relation to sexuality.[13] The WHO also suggests that sexual health promotion requires an understanding of the complex factors that shape human sexuality, which include both risk and pleasure and simultaneous barriers and facilitators of sexual satisfaction.[14] Furthermore, the WHO emphasizes that fundamental to sexual health is the right to information and pleasure.[15] Yet the WHO definition does not seem to apply to Black gay men. In their everyday lives and encounters, many Black gay men receive messages from their peers and service providers that if having pleasurable and satisfying sex means unprotected sex and sexual situations that involve multiple partners and drug and alcohol use, they should not be having it, especially if they are HIV positive. As writer Abdul-Aliy A. Muhammad suggests in his essay "Moralism, Plentiful in HIV Prevention, Is the Fuel of Stigma," people are sometimes shocked to learn that someone who is HIV positive is still having sex. Yet understanding how Black gay men think about, negotiate, and make decisions around risk and pleasure can help public health devise prevention strategies that better promote these men's sexual health, satisfaction, and well-being, whether they are HIV negative or positive. Clearly a definition of sexual health has to consist of more than reducing risk of STDs/STIs, particularly HIV, while not losing sight of it entirely.

In addition to convergent forms of anti-Black racism and homophobia that structure Black gay men's experiences with public health and other social institutions, dominant discourse and related approaches to HIV/AIDS prevention draw from and advance what I refer to as a homosex-normative discourse. Public health paradigms for HIV prevention and overall sexual health promote/require repressing sexual urges and focusing on fear of contracting not only HIV but other STDs as well. It is worth mentioning that although most STDs are common and are not life-threatening, if/when Black gay men get an STD they are often demeaned and shamed not only by their peers but by some service providers as well.[16] Instead of a primary emphasis on sexual desire, urges, and pleasure as healthy sexuality, emphasis is placed on reducing or eliminating STD/STI risk at the expense of pleasure.[17] As Brandon Andrew Robinson observes, for public health in the United States, sexual health discourse is centered on subordinating sexual urges to rational thinking and behavior. Too often white heterosexual health officials function as the paternalistic authorities on and managers of the behaviors of Black gay men.[18] These encounters with public health authorities cause these gay men to internalize repressive and disciplinary discourses about their sexuality. By using the term *homosex normativity*, I bring into focus the management of gay sex practices as part of the neoliberalization of gay life, marriage, and kinship, undergirded by an anti-Black racism.

In her canonical 1984 essay, "Thinking Sex: Notes for a Radical Theory of the Politics of Sexuality," Gayle Rubin deftly theorizes heteronormativity (the primary target of critique of many queer theorists) by constructing a "charm circle" to map the ways in which regimes of sexual regulation and management distinguish between "charmed" sexual practices and those "uncharmed." Although HIV/AIDS appeared in the United States in the early 1980s, and Rubin focuses on the epidemic's impact on mostly white gay men's lives, she does not include HIV/AIDS as a part of her theoretical framework of sexual stratification.[19] Rubin also occludes race, particularly racial blackness, as constitutive of sexual stratification. However, as they intersect with other categories of sexual identities and acts that are charmed and uncharmed (i.e., approved or disapproved), race and HIV status also function to determine good sexual subjects versus bad ones. Thus, one can extend Rubin's fecund theory to understand where Black gay men line up on the hierarchy of sex acts and sexual subjecthood then and now. For my purposes here, I use a homosex-normativity charm circle that my students developed in a Gay Histories, Queer Cultures course that I taught at Indiana University to apply and extend Rubin's framework for these current times (see figure 9.1).

Our homosex-normativity charm circle consists of categories that break down into good sexual subjects and practices versus bad sexual subjects and practices. The inner "charmed" of the circle includes HIV-negative status, protected sex, and linear life progression. The outer dimension of the circle consists of bad sexual subjects and practices, such as HIV-positive status, unprotected sex (raw sex), and nonlinear life progression. We could imagine that other bad sex or uncharmed sex includes all condomless sex, serodiscordant sex (negative with positive), group sex, and those people who like to "catch nut" in their ass or in their throat, or "swallow the kids," as we say in Black gay sexual vernacular.

Black gay men who engage in raw sex are viewed and treated as bad sexual subjects in public health HIV-prevention discourse. Various forms of unprotected or what is now called "condomless sex" hover in the outer limit, the uncharmed realm, primarily for Black gay men and trans women. Public health interventions in the United States that target Black gay men and MSM operate from a premise that condomless anal intercourse is problematic and

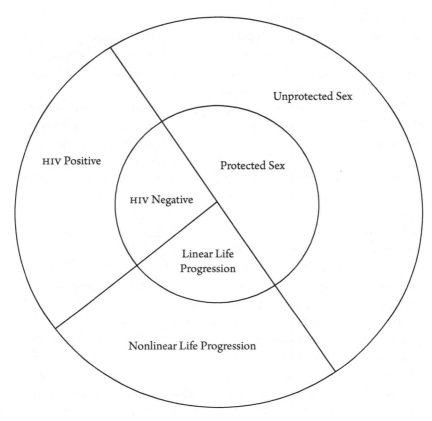

FIGURE 9.1. Homosex-normativity charm circle.

dangerous, regardless of other risk reductive strategies such as strategic positioning, withdrawal, and sex partner reduction that many Black gay men already deploy. In larger society, those Black gay men who engage in raw sex are viewed as reckless, dangerous, and uncivilized and in need of punitive social ridicule and management. According to some Black gay men—who see themselves as the respectable and moral stewards of Black gay life and representation—those who have raw sex are deeply retrograde and demonstrative of Black gay men's self-hatred and self-destruction. As Drew-Shane Daniels argues in his July 2013 article in *Mused*, because of the disproportionate impact of the HIV/AIDS epidemic on Black gay men, "barebacking [assuming he means raw sex too] is never a safe bet for black gay men."[20] However, for the Black gay men in my study, condoms undermine and prevent sexual pleasure and physical and social connection and intimacy.

For public health and other service providers, HIV-positive Black gay men who have any kind of sex are viewed and treated as bad, dangerous, sexual subjects, and in some states also as criminal, if they do not compulsorily disclose their status to their partners. But for HIV-positive Black gay men like Vibe Issues from Indianapolis, condoms are intolerable and counter to the pleasurable feeling and meaning of Black gay sex. For instance, Vibe Issues said, "I don't like nothing about condoms; I don't like the way they feel; I don't like the way they smell; I don't like anything about them." Vibe Issues added, "When I let a nigga bust in me, I can feel the nut in me and it feels good as fuck. Like sometimes I can feel his dick pulsating in my ass and I can feel the nut." According to the homosex-normativity charm circle, Vibe Issues is a bad sexual subject, a sexual outlaw, who should be contained, disciplined, and managed, not so much because he is a threat to himself but because he may be a threat to others, including general populations read as white and/or heterosexual. Even with the advancements and development of antiretroviral (viral suppression) therapy that, if taken effectively, can suppress the HIV virus to an undetectable and noninfectious level, the stigmatization ascribed to HIV-positive people, particularly Black gay men, remains extremely high.

Those Black gay men who neither place a premium on the longevity of life nor pursue a linear life trajectory are also considered to be bad sexual subjects, in HIV-prevention discourse. The basic assumption that underpins a homosex-normative logic to sexual health, the one promoted by public health and larger society, is one that assumes that for all rational, self-loving gay men, avoiding seroconversion or discontinuing sex if one seroconverts is more important than satisfying and pleasurable sex. For instance, when asked about the role that HIV and awareness play in his sexual decision-making, Tyrone, who is HIV positive and from Indianapolis, said, "I just don't see it as, I guess, that big of a deal because I got so much knowledge about HIV I feel like it's not the end of the world. It's a lot more worse stuff out there. I'd rather have HIV than diabetes or some other stuff, you know." In addition, for many of the interlocutors in my study, including those who were HIV negative at the time, the fear of or concern about contracting HIV was not always a primary factor in their sexual decision-making. Johnthon from Indianapolis, who is HIV negative, made this point:

There's a risk with sex either way it go. You know what I'm saying? So it's a choice I had to make. If I'm gonna have no sex or if I'm gonna have sex that I want to have and enjoy it. And if I'm gonna do it, if I'm gonna take the risk, I wanna enjoy it. I don't wanna take a risk and be like, damn, I took this risk for nothing and now I'm like, what the fuck did I do it for. So I'm gonna take the risk, I'm gonna make it mean somethin'.

I do not suggest that Black gay men do not think about or fear seroconversion and that HIV never plays a role in their sexual decision-making; instead, I suggest that other needs and priorities such as sexual pleasure, intimacy, connection, and satisfaction are also key factors, and in some cases, more important ones. Ultimately, the assumption that as a Black gay man one's goal is to remain HIV negative at any cost and adhere to an anti-Black homosex-normative regulatory regime that requires unsatisfying sex to make others feel comfortable and safe at their own expense should not be the logic that underpins all HIV-prevention and sexual health models.

Black Gay Sexual Autonomy

The vast majority of the research on Black gay men and HIV pathologizes their sexual behavior.[21] Rarely does the HIV-prevention discourse in public health treat Black gay men as active informed sexual agents who, with very limited resources, navigate through obstacles, negotiate risk, and pursue erotic and sexual pleasure on their own terms. Elsewhere, I theorize that some Black gay men engage in raw sex as an act of sexual autonomy that is based on the meaning and function of sex in their lives (or what Black gay men want). I extend that argument here by placing at the center of analysis an articulation and deep description of Black gay men's experiences of sexual pleasure and risk. Given the ways in which homosex normativity underpins public health's definition of sexual health as consisting of the reduction or elimination of risk of HIV seroconversion, as well as how many Black gay men police (stigmatize) their own behavior, I highlight how some Black gay men resist these logics to forge sexual lives on their terms for their own purposes. Black gay men create a counterdiscourse that critiques the public health dominant logic of sexual health (and HIV prevention) through their profiles on popular sex, hookup, and dating websites for gay men. I demonstrate how others create and participate in spaces and situations wherein heightened sexual risk and pleasure are co-constitutive.

In her groundbreaking essay "Erotic Autonomy as a Politics of Decolonization: An Anatomy of Feminist and State Practice in the Bahamas Tourist Economy," M. Jacqui Alexander mostly focuses on regimes of sexual normativity that impact Black women's sexuality in the Caribbean. Here, Alexander offers her theory of *erotic autonomy* and sexual agency to explain what marginalized and stigmatized Black women do to engage in erotic and sexual pleasure on their own terms despite the often institutional, communal, and familial influences against it. For Alexander, Black lesbian women in the Bahamas reject and resist the ideological anchor for the state that positions the heteropatriarchal nuclear family as the cornerstone of society.[22] Alexander calls for a "feminist emancipatory project" that creates discursive and material spaces where "women can love themselves, love women, and transform the nation simultaneously.[23] Drawing from Alexander's theory of erotic autonomy and sexual agency, I argue that in part through sex, Black gay men create opportunities through which to not only experience sexual pleasure in the midst of an anti-erotic/antipleasurable sex HIV arena but to also create ways to experience deep intimacy with other Black gay men. This is what I theorize as Black gay sexual autonomy.

One way to imagine and forge an antihegemonic epistemology of Black gay sex and sexual health is to create a discourse that exposes and critiques the homosex-normative basis of dominant HIV-prevention discourse. In this sense, Black gay men undertake this task, sometimes unwittingly, through gay profiles on gay sex websites. Similar to the Anything Goes sex party in which Raheim participates, a raw sex profile on sex websites not only tells a would-be suitor basic information about a person, such as his race/ethnicity, age, height, weight, and endowment and so on, but also his HIV status and whether or not he uses substances and engages in group sex situations, among other information that someone may find pertinent. Furthermore, the profile reveals a lot, both explicit and implicit, about his sexual desires, practices, and identity. Consider this profile from a Black gay man:

> i jus wanna fuck raw . . .
>
> 33, 6'0", 190lb, 34w, Athletic, Black Hair, Some Body Hair, Black, Looking for 1-on-1 Sex, 3some/Group Sex, Misc. Fetishes, Cam2Cam.
>
> I like to fuck raw only . . . get at me . . .
>
> Conservative, Out No, Smoke Yes, Drink Occasionally, Drugs No, Zodiac Taurus.
>
> Top, 9" Cut, Anything Goes, HIV Positive, Prefer meeting at: My Place.

This profile articulates and reflects a radical epistemology of Black gay sex that unabashedly highlights sexual pleasure and risk as co-constitutive. I consider this profile as a discursive move toward sexual autonomy in three ways. First, for this website, titling a profile with the proclamation, "I just wanna fuck raw . . ." is a radical claim because, while many men desire and engage in raw sex, many will not admit it.[24] He then reveals his positive HIV status. This is also nonnormative for these websites, as many men who are HIV positive either falsely represent themselves as HIV negative or occlude the status from their profile altogether because of the extreme stigma associated with HIV. This Black MSM (who is not out) is a sexual top, implying that he fucks bottoms raw and that he is into threesomes and group sex and not interested in a relationship (marked as romantic and monogamous). His claim to engage in this panoply of non-homosex-normative practices in the gay domain of this website can be viewed as a radical position and practice of sexual autonomy.

Second, when examining a profile like this, it is important to situate behavior within the larger context of Black gay identity and experience and grapple with its contradictions and complexities. For Black gay men who engage in raw sex, for example, sexual pleasure and desire are often in conflict with social norms and gay identity. In addition, while many men may engage in what is stated in the Black gay man's profile in practice, they are not willing to name and proclaim these practices publicly. It is very common for Black gay brothers to throw shade on other Black gay men who engage in raw sex and group sex, or who are HIV positive in public, while engaging in the same practices themselves in private. It is worth reiterating that non-homosex-normative Black gay men (bad sexual subjects) are not only stigmatized by larger society, particularly public health institutions; they are also stigmatized by other Black gay men.

Third, the social context in which this Black gay man, who is HIV positive, has raw sex is very informative. Because of his status, he lives with a multiple social disqualification: Black, gay, HIV positive, and has raw sex. This multiple disqualification constitutes the constraints under which he lives, and for him, the emphasis is placed on what he should not do sexually under the hegemony of safe sex. However, another dimension of his experiences is about his desire and pleasure—what he wants in terms of sex. Thus, the politics of desire that may inform this Black gay man's sexual pursuits can be seen as a sociopolitical resistance to the hegemony of safe sex that produces shame and self-hatred for those who do not comply. Of course, this is combined with the sensual and tactical pleasure of skin-to-skin sexual contact. Not only does skin-to-skin sex and catching nut feel better, as Vibe Issues and many other Black gay men in my research stated, but it also satisfies a craving for what I call a deep intimacy, a closeness and a "being desired and wanted" in a world in which Black gay men are rarely desired and wanted. One can assume that this is constrained by his HIV status, meaning that many people will not want to have any kind of sex with him, let alone raw sex, because he is openly HIV positive. Nonetheless, this Black gay man's profile represents a sexually autonomous articulation of Black gay sex that challenges the homosex-normativity logic that underpins dominant Black gay and HIV-prevention discourse.

Black Gay Sexual Spaces and Situations

How do Black gay men forge healthy sexual lives that, at least for some, no doubt, consist of "sexual situations," practices, and spaces that public health institutions consider to be high risk? What other means of sexual risk and pleasure do Black gay men explore? I am interested in how and where Black gay men have sex as a means of greater sexual pleasure and satisfaction, regardless of the stereophonic pronouncements against it. Below, I bring into focus some of the diverse ways through which they gain sexual pleasure by analyzing how one Black gay man describes his group sex (sex party) experience. The discussion of the social factors that create vulnerabilities for Black gay men rarely consider the ways in which space can be a structural limitation for Black gay men. Hence, if Black gay men have limited access to spaces in which to have sex, let alone engage in stigmatized sexual behavior, public/private sex venues and events become important sites and situations that often serve as a means of heightened sexual pleasure.

One way that Black gay men contend with their spatial, structural vulnerability is to create and participate in an underground sex party network, similar to the party described by Raheim. One study suggests that in HIV-prevention research more emphasis needs to be placed on the sexual situation as opposed to what public health scholar Patrick Wilson and his colleagues call the "personal level behavior," as predictors of risk. They go on to argue that these particular sexual situations are likely to involve sexual risk factors such as drugs and alcohol use and group and sex club situations.[25] While I am sympathetic to Wilson and his colleagues' argument, I would like to consider how risk and pleasure are co-constitutive for Black gay men in these sexual spatial situations, regardless of HIV status. In addition, substance use within a group sex context creates the conditions under which Black gay men can experience greater unbridled pleasure and the freedom to explore their complex sexualities in ways they would not be able to in their everyday lives due to the extreme surveillance, stigma, and condemnation they experience. Black gay men are often intentional about creating and participating in spaces and situations of mixed sexual pleasure and risk as an expression of sexual agency and autonomy.

Coby Miller is a Black gay man from Indianapolis who was HIV negative at the time of the study. He describes his experiences at an Anything Goes sex party, organized by a white gay man in a mansion on the south side of Chicago.

> I remember entering [the mansion] from a side door and I was kind of nervous because it was like the patio door from the other house faces the side door so I'm like oh, what do they think go on up here at this time but we went on in and—and it was a ten dollar cover charge which my boy was aware of. He had to show the text message in his phone which he in turn forwarded to me, so I was able to show it as well. Because if we didn't have any type of, you know, association with knowing about this party, we would have been turned around at the door pretty much. So we paid our ten dollars. We went in. Walked into like a dining room type of area from the side door. . . . It was a little light. It was like a blue light, blue or red light, party light type of stuff. So you was able to see, you know, little images and stuff like that. It was like three big ass bedrooms, like huge, you know? We walked in, got us a drink. Was passed a blunt or two. You know like I say I don't really do anybody's, you know, drugs like that unless it's my own personal. So I went on, you know, followed him in the room and stuff like that. There was a huge round bed. Yeah . . . like something I ain't never seen before. I thought it was a waterbed; it was so nice, and I was like wow! It had like velvet sheets on it in dark blue. A couple of candles were lit on a desk surrounding a bowl with condoms, some lube. Actually they had like a big-ass dispenser of lube.

In many ways, Miller's description of the space is consistent with Raheim's description and those of many other sex parties described to me, except for the white man's mansion part. A couple of points are important here. First, the Anything Goes parties organized within this underground network use similar strategies to protect from surveillance and unwanted intrusion, even when it occurs at a private home. The strategies described are also the ways in which the organizers regulate who and what kind of bodies and sexual positions they wanted to be present at the party. For instance, in his interview, Coby Miller described a required dress code based on color that represented sexual positions, either top, bottom, or versatile (or anything goes). The room in which the sex takes place is usually an open space with a bed or similar to a "buffet flat" set up in which all sexual acts and partners are, as it were, potentially on the table.[26] I take notice of the similar organization and arrangement of the spaces of Black gay sex parties, no matter whether they take place in a hotel suite or a mansion.

Coby Miller emphasized how he, his friend, and other gay men at the party were drinking, smoking blunts, and using other drugs to help them get and remain in "party mode." Coby also describes how he felt in this space and situation, a means through which he and his friend experience pleasure.

Yeah. It was like something I had never seen before, like, wow! Different experience from what I've seen so you know, everybody pretty much just do whatever. So it was just like amazing. So anyway it was a bed with like about a good—I wanna say like eight people on it. Yeah, about eight people. All of them naked. We walked into the orgy that was already in place. Mind you, before we walked in there was a table with brown bags for our garments. Didn't receive a number or anything. Just pretty much picked up a brown bag, put my clothes in. Once we walked in, you know—once we entered the room, I observed for a second. Finally I took my clothes off, still observed for a little bit. Sipped my drink a little bit. I grabbed some lube, jacked off a little bit, and I just kinda watched. I seen this cute little bottom dude become available, so I started kissing and messing with him.

Miller starts to fuck the "cute little bottom dude" and uses a condom with him and the next guy he fucks. However, as the night goes on Miller abandons the condoms.

Eventually me and this guy switched up, and I proceeded to fucking the boy on the couch with no condom. He was a thick, brown-skinned man who obviously liked dick with a fat ass, so I guess, you know, I just took it upon myself to just not use a condom, you know. I think I came in, you know, with the impression or with the intention to use a condom but I think once things get squared away, I kinda did away with the condom. You know, it was a lot going on. I seen some stuff in action, some bodily fluid action that I had never really seen before . . . like squirting out of butts and I was like, wow, it's kind of crazy.

According to Miller, he has oral and anal sex, as a top, with several Black men in the room, and later, he abandons condom use altogether, as do others in the room. Many of the bottoms at the party were fucked without condoms and tops busted nuts inside them. Clearly, the meticulous spatial arrangements helped facilitate the heightened experience of co-constituted pleasure and risk. And, as Wilson and his coauthors argue, it is the combination of drugs and alcohol use, the freedom to not use condoms, and the many Black gay men in the room engaging in sex that helps make up the sexual situation that also creates a high propensity for HIV and other STD transmission. However, the Black gay men are fully aware of all the dynamics involved and choose to participate anyway. And, for the most part, these are sexual spaces that Black gay men collectively create and situations in which they participate. Considering both what Miller and Raheim describe, Black gay men deploy and engage in sexual, spatial, and situational practices as a means of pleasure, and for some, risk is a pleasurable, deliberate, and autonomous endeavor.

The Anything Goes Party Part II

Returning to the Anything Goes Black gay group sex party, after Raheim takes off all his clothes, places them into a paper bag (with his handle written on it), and gives it to a guy working the party, he enters the dark back room. As soon as he enters he smells a mixture of sweat and cologne. He sees a king-size bed with dudes getting fucked all over it, some doggy style, up against the wall, and others on their backs on the bed, in every corner of the room. Everybody's fucking raw, and he neither sees nor feels condom packages on the floor. A dude comes up to Raheim, bends down in front of him and puts his dick in his mouth, and starts to suck it until it gets hard. Then he turns around and claims a corner of the bed. He bends over and toots his ass up, signaling to Raheim to enter him raw. Soon after Raheim starts to fuck him, the guy's ass is so tight and hot that after a few pumps Raheim feels like he is about to bust: "You gon let me cum in this booty . . . huh . . . You gon let me cum in this booty?" The guy moans and starts breathing really hard, as his thighs begin to shake intensely, "Yea bust that nut nigga; give me them kids."

Notes

The research for this essay was funded by the Center for AIDS Prevention Studies (CAP) in the Department of Medicine at the University of California, San Francisco, as part of the Visiting Professors Program. I would also like to thank my Raw Sex Project research team for assisting me with the data collection. A short portion of this chapter appears in my previously published essay "Black Gay (Raw) Sex."
1 This ethnographic vignette is taken from a 2004 paper based on my field research, "What I'm Told, What I Want, What I Do," presented at the Whose Beloved Community? Conference at Emory University. Johnson quotes and discusses this vignette at length in his introduction to *No Tea, No Shade*, 8–11.

Raheim is a pseudonym. I use pseudonyms throughout this ethnography to protect my interlocutors' confidentiality.

2   Herukhuti, "Whose Booty Is This?," 101.

3   Bailey, "Black Gay (Raw) Sex," 239–61.

4   MSM is a public health term used to refer to men who do not identify as gay but who nonetheless have sex with men.

5   Bowleg, "'Once You've Blended the Cake,'" 764.

6   Bowleg, "'Once You've Blended the Cake,'" 764.

7   Ford and Airhihenbuwa, "Critical Race Theory," 30.

8   Ford and Airhihenbuwa, "Critical Race Theory," 30. For more on intersectional HIV and what she calls intersectional stigma, see Berger, *Workable Sisterhood*.

9   Centers for Disease Control and Prevention, "HIV Prevalence, Unrecognized Infection."

10 Kaiser Family Foundation, "Black Americans and HIV/AIDS."

11 Centers for Disease Control and Prevention, NCHHSTP Newsroom, "Lifetime Risk of HIV Diagnosis."

12 Centers for Disease Control and Prevention, "Fact Sheet."

13 World Health Organization (WHO), "Defining Sexual Health," 5.

14 World Health Organization (WHO), "Defining Sexual Health," 1.

15 World Health Organization (WHO), "Defining Sexual Health," 1.

16 For more discussion of how some service providers treat HIV-positive clients, see Bailey et al., "HIV (STDs, STIs, and Viral Hepatitis)."

17 Robinson, "Queer Potentiality of Barebacking," 102.

18 Robinson, "Queer Potentiality of Barebacking," 102.

19 Rubin, "Thinking Sex."

20 Daniels, "Barebacking Is Never a Safe Bet." For another example of the stigma around raw sex, see Kennedy, "'They're Peddling Death.'"

21 McGruder, "Black Sexuality in the U.S.," 254.

22 Alexander, "Erotic Autonomy as a Politics," 64.

23 Alexander, "Erotic Autonomy as a Politics," 100.

24 This is also very radical and risky because in some states, particularly the one in which this person lives, "Duty to Warn" laws or compulsory disclosure laws require that anyone who is HIV positive must reveal their status before having sex with anyone, protected or not.

25 Wilson et al., "Drug Use, Interpersonal Attraction, and Communication."

26 Bailey, *Butch Queens Up in Pumps*, 11.

Bibliography

Alexander, M. Jacqui. "Erotic Autonomy as a Politics of Decolonization: An Anatomy of Feminist and State Practice in the Bahamas Tourist Economy." In *Feminist Genealogies, Colonial Legacies, Democratic Futures*, edited by M. Jacqui Alexander and Chandra Talpade Mohanty, 63–100. New York: Routledge, 1997.

Bailey, Marlon M. "Black Gay (Raw) Sex." In *No Tea, No Shade: New Writings in Black Queer Studies*, edited by E. Patrick Johnson, 239–61. Durham, NC: Duke University Press, 2016.

Bailey, Marlon M. *Butch Queens Up in Pumps: Gender, Performance, and Ballroom Culture in Detroit*. Ann Arbor: University of Michigan Press, 2013.

Bailey, Marlon M., Xavier Livermon, Joshua Thompson, George A. Kraus, Katie E. Dieter, and Patrick Battani. "HIV (STDs, STIs, and Viral Hepatitis) Prevention and Men Who Have Sex with Men (MSM) Needs Assessment." Indiana State Department of Health, Indianapolis, 2010.

Berger, Michele Tracy. *Workable Sisterhood: The Political Journey of Stigmatized Women with HIV/AIDS*. Princeton, NJ: Princeton University Press, 2004.

Bowleg, Lisa. "'Once You've Blended the Cake, You Can't Take the Parts Back to the Main Ingredients': Black Gay and Bisexual Men's Descriptions and Experiences of Intersectionality." *Sex Roles* 68, no. 11 (2013): 754–67. doi:10.1007/s11199-012-0152-4.

Centers for Disease Control and Prevention. "Fact Sheet: HIV and Gay and Bisexual Men." 2019. https://www.cdc.gov/hiv/group/msm/bmsm.html.

Centers for Disease Control and Prevention. "HIV Prevalence, Unrecognized Infection, and HIV Testing among Men Who Have Sex with Men—Five U.S. Cities, June 2004–April 2005." *Morbidity and Mortality Weekly Report* 54, no. 24 (2005): 597–601.

Centers for Disease Control and Prevention, NCHHSTP Newsroom. "Lifetime Risk of HIV Diagnosis." 2016. https://www.cdc.gov/nchhstp/newsroom/2016/croi -press-release-risk.html.

Daniels, Drew-Shane. "Barebacking Is Never a Safe Bet for Black Gay Men." *Mused*, July 2013.

Ford, Chandra L., and Collins O. Airhihenbuwa. "Critical Race Theory, Race Equity, and Public Health: Toward Antiracism Praxis." *American Journal of Public Health* 100, no. S1 (2010): S30–35.

Herukhuti, "Whose Booty Is This? Barebacking, Advocacy, and the Right to Fuck." In *Conjuring Black Funk: Notes on Culture, Sexuality, and Spirituality*, vol. 1, edited by H. Sharif Williams, 99–102. New York: Vintage Entity Press, 2007.

Johnson, E. Patrick, ed. *No Tea, No Shade: New Writings in Black Queer Studies*. Durham, NC: Duke University Press, 2016.

Kaiser Family Foundation. "Fact Sheet: Black Americans and HIV/AIDS." *HIV/AIDS Policy*, November 2010. https://www.kff.org.

Kennedy, Sean. "'They're Peddling Death': Profiting from Unsafe Sex." *Advocate*, August 29, 2006, 44–48.

McGruder, Kevin. "Black Sexuality in the U.S.: Presentations as Non-normative." *Journal of African American Studies* 13, no. 3 (2009): 251–62. doi:10.1007/s12111-008-9070-5.

Muhammad, Abdul-Aliy A. "Moralism, Plentiful in HIV Prevention, Is the Fuel of Stigma." *TheBody*, September 23, 2016. http://www.thebody.com/content /78454/moralism-plentiful-in-HIV-prevention-is-the-fuel-o.html?ap=1200.

Robinson, Brandon Andrew. "The Queer Potentiality of Barebacking: Charging, Whoring, and Breeding as Utopian Practices." In *A Critical Inquiry into Queer Utopias*, edited by Angela Jones, 101–30. New York: Palgrave Macmillan, 2013.

Rubin, Gayle. "Thinking Sex: Notes for a Radical Theory of the Politics of Sexuality." In *The Lesbian and Gay Studies Reader*, edited by Henry Abelove, Michèle Aina Barale, and David Halperin, 3–44. New York: Routledge, 1993. First published in *Pleasure and Danger: Exploring Female Sexuality*, edited by Carole S. Vance, 267–319. Boston: Routledge and Kegan Paul, 1984.

Wilson, Patrick, Rafael M. Díaz, Hirokazu Yoshikawa, and Patrick E. Shrout. "Drug Use, Interpersonal Attraction, and Communication: Situational Factors as Predictors of Episodes of Unprotected Anal Intercourse among Latino Gay Men." *AIDS and Behavior* 13, no. 4 (2009): 691–99.

World Health Organization (WHO). "Defining Sexual Health: Report of a Technical Consultation on Sexual Health." Geneva, 2006.

TEN HIV, INDIGENEITY, AND SETTLER COLONIALISM: UNDERSTANDING PTIS, CRISIS RESOLUTION, AND THE ART OF CEREMONY

Andrew J. Jolivette

This chapter attends to the structural, global, and regional ramifications of settler colonial narratives and laws on the sociocultural factors that produce, enable, and maintain HIV risk within Indigenous communities. Taking from theorizations of post-traumatic invasion syndrome (PTIS) in urban Indigenous communities, this chapter asserts that HIV crisis resolution must begin with movement away from individual to communal forms of healing, prevention, and disease management through the art of ceremony as a radical methodology to increase Indigenous self-determination and transformative HIV interventions.

According to the Centers for Disease Control and Prevention (CDC), HIV/AIDS affects American Indians and Alaska Natives (AIAN) in ways that are not always obvious because of their small population size. Studies indicate that AIAN have seen a 63 percent annual diagnoses increase over the last decade among gay and bisexual men.[1] Stigma, poverty, and high rates of sexually transmitted infections (STIs) each contribute to ongoing HIV risk within this population. In order to fully understand the syndemics of AIDS within urban Indian populations (as the epicenter of the crisis), we must analyze the impact of settler colonial narratives and laws that redefine, limit, and pervert Indigenous cultural practices and diverse gendered behaviors in favor of Western, colonial notions of normative behavior. To be more specific, when Indigenous communities are at the center of the planning, implementation, and assessment of their own cultural programs to address issues such as HIV/ AIDS, we are able to see a reduction in rates of infection, and there is also a close correlation between prevention and traditional wellness practices that include tribally specific ceremonies and intervention models.

Scholars such as Karina Walters (Choctaw) and Linda Tuhiwai Smith (Maori) have written extensively about the impact of using Indigenous-centered programs and methods for combating health and educational disparities.[2] AIAN have the third-highest rates of infection after African Americans and Latinos. According to the CDC, at least 75 percent of HIV infection cases in the Native American community involve men who have sex with men (MSM).[3] The CDC identifies several factors specific to American Indian communities that increase the chances for seroconversion (the threshold at which an antibody becomes detectable in the blood, confirming a change in viral infection status from negative to positive). American Indians have the second-highest rate of STIs among all ethnic groups; having an STI increases susceptibility to HIV infection. American Indians have higher poverty rates, complete fewer years of education, are younger, are less likely to be employed, and have lower rates of health insurance.[4] Each of these factors limits American Indian and Alaska Native access to high-quality health care, housing, and HIV-prevention education. High rates of alcohol and drug use, which lead to sexual behaviors associated with increased risk for infection, are other factors leading to increased rates of infection. Documentation of colonialism, intergenerational trauma, and anti-Indian wellness practices by the United States are thoroughly detailed in the research literature as the most salient factors for HIV transmission.[5]

HIV intervention models in Indigenous communities must recenter tribally specific as well as urban Indian regionally specific crisis resolution and intervention models that focus on communal as opposed to individual health promotion models. Settler colonialism as articulated by several scholars in Native American and Indigenous studies places both white and nonwhite settlers at the center of health crisis and anti-Indian sentiments.[6] I contend, however, that Indigenous communities must place much greater focus on issues of self-determination. As Indigenous communities attend to self-determination, they will oppose defining settler colonialism within a context that describes enslaved Africans as arrivants and marginalized immigrant groups (which include Indigenous immigrants from across the Americas) as settlers. Issues related to violence and cultural genocide are more properly placed within the context of white supremacist systems that deny legal rights to Indigenous people as well as to people of color.

If we aim to deal with global issues such as the AIDS crisis, turning to more local, specific, and applied interventions that speak directly to the needs and concerns of Indigenous communities must be placed outside the theoretical canon that does not necessarily serve the interests or daily lived experiences of AIAN in the United States. In other words, if we redefine and build upon settler colonialism within a specific context such as the law, it will make much more sense on the ground in Indigenous community organizing spaces. An exploration, however, of settler colonialism within the framework of PTIS allows us as researchers and community members to work collectively toward intervention models that embrace ceremony as a radical methodology for curtailing the ongoing impact of colonization on rates of HIV infection within Indigenous communities. In addition, PTIS within settler colonial states must contend with the problems of structural competency that are often lacking in systems of care, prevention, and treatment.

In *The Protest Psychosis: How Schizophrenia Became a Black Disease*, Jonathan Metzl introduces the term *structural competency* to challenge researchers and practitioners to move beyond simple notions of cultural competency in addressing larger macrolevel systems of change in order to practice effective health promotion.[7] Metzl and Helena Hansen assert that "the politics of the present moment challenge cultural competency's basic premise: that having a culturally sensitive clinician reduces patients' overall experience of stigma or improves health outcomes."[8] In a settler colonial state, structural factors ranging from income inequality and marginal housing coupled with cultural barriers prevent Indigenous populations from accessing the necessary care to reduce rates of seroconversion. Metzl and Hansen offer five core aspects for achieving structural competency: (1) recognizing the structures that shape clinical interactions, (2) developing an extraclinical language of structure, (3) rearticulating "cultural" formulations in structural terms, (4) observing and imagining structural interventions, and (5) developing structural humility. Of these five, the third aspect, rearticulating "cultural" formulations in structural terms, is the most striking for Indigenous communities seeking measurable reforms in health practices. At times, these practices end up engaging with settler colonial narratives and policies in a way that creates a "culturally sensitive model" where there is always already a "tragic Indian." Instead, what is needed is an emphasis on the importance of decolonizing Western medical systems that do not accept, recognize, or comprehend Indigenous medicine, science, and structural-tribal systems. Using patient navigation within the context of both cultural and structural competencies provides a more comprehensive framework for ensuring that practical steps are being taken to address inequities in HIV treatment among Indigenous communities deeply impacted by ongoing settler and illicit colonialism.

From Settler to Illicit Colonialism: A Genealogy
of Illegal Cultural Disintegration

Redefining settler colonialism as illicit colonialism provides both a theoretical and legal means of understanding the true impact of non-Indigenous colonial acts as felonious, illegitimate, and criminal in a global context. Illicit colonialism is a series of intentional and ongoing acts of disruption, removal, and destabilization through illegal means that work to destroy tribal-, clan-, and nation-specific forms of adjudicating health crises such as HIV/AIDS. All forms of colonialism are always already illicit in the very workings that seek to take by illegal means the land, rights, and means of self-governance and geopolitical self-determination of Indigenous peoples under global law. As Patrick Wolfe states of settler colonialism, "Land is life—or, at least, land is necessary for life. Thus contests for land can be—indeed, often are—contests for life." Wolfe further asserts that "settler colonialism destroys to replace" and as such it is "a structure not an event."[9] While settler colonialism focuses on a structure of erasure and displacement, it still at times neglects to examine the extralegal ways that cultural genocide continues to erode culturally specific practices that do not elide with oppressive global systems of colonization both within and outside the United States.[10] Moreover, settler colonialism at times surrenders the agency that many nations possess in defining and maintaining cultural autonomy even in the face of colonization.

As we disentangle both the dialectical and heuristic approaches to settler colonialism and link them more explicitly to the unlawful, we can unpack and simultaneously document a genealogy of illegal cultural disintegration, genocide, and an attempted dissolution of sovereign status and tribally specific cultural protocols for health promotion among many other areas of community life for AIAN in the United States. Illicit colonialism is thus an act of ongoing terrorism, illegal land seizure, and illegitimate foreign control over Indigenous nations in the United States. Illicit colonialism, however, remains contested by American Indian nations that refuse to surrender their self-determination and by extension their ceremonial practices. When we describe processes of colonialism, we must remember the differing experiences of each and every tribal community. Many nations did not experience the same form of conquest. Several others did not lay claim to their self-determination on the basis of federal recognition *granted* by an illegal foreign power.

I raise the issue of moving from settler to illicit forms of colonialism to underscore the history of cultural dissolution of Two-Spirit people within American Indian societies as not only a process of colonial settlement but an illegal crime, and a structural barrier to addressing state-sanctioned inequalities in health.[11] The refusal by many third- and fourth-gender people (known in contemporary society as Two-Spirits) to accept or participate in illicit colonialism offers important evidence of resistance while also providing a genealogy of queerness for contemporary Two-Spirit people seeking positive health promotion and a reduction in HIV/AIDS.

Contact with Europeans, with white Americans, and particularly with white American anthropologists has directly shaped the discordant and contested definitions of American Indian sexuality and gender for more than five hundred years. Early anthropological studies misunderstood the complex and diverse variations in gender and sexuality among Native American tribes and communities throughout the Americas.[12] The plethora of early anthropological studies on Indigenous sexuality and gender identities have reduced rather than expanded scholarly understanding of Native American culture, behavior, and social interaction within Native and non-Native communities. While these studies reduce the complexity of sexuality and gender among male Two-Spirits, they in large part ignore the roles and experiences of female Two-Spirits. In the case of both male and female Two-Spirits, "homosexuality" and the construction of the "berdache" identity are favored as ways of producing "deviant" "subcultures" within American Indian tribes and communities.[13]

Despite the acceptance and internalization of Western beliefs and values about the diversity of gender and sexual identities within some tribal and urban Indian communities, substantial scholarly evidence suggests not only that has there always been tremendous gender and sexual diversity in Indigenous communities in the United States but also that these identities are based upon much more than sexual behavior.[14] Furthermore, these roles and gender/sexual expressions were historically integrated, accepted, and valued in most cases. Sabine Lang asserts that "in many Native American cultures there existed—and in a number of cases still exists—three or four genders: women, men, two-spirit womanly males, and, less frequently, two-spirit/manly females. In each Native American culture that acknowledges multiple genders there also exists specific words to refer to people who are of a gender other than woman or man. Terms referring to two-spirit people in

Native American languages usually indicate that they are seen as combining the masculine and feminine."[15]

Today, effectively disentangling the discordant and contested meanings of Native sexuality and gender within the context of settler colonialism, illicit colonialism, and HIV means turning to historical figures that represent a resistance genealogy for Two-Spirit people. At stake in mapping alternative and diverse genealogies of American Indian gender and sexuality are questions of tribal sovereignty and community cohesion. How can a people so traumatically impacted by colonialism, genocide, and cultural disintegration remain if their own epistemological ways of being are continually policed, not just by non-Natives but by other Natives who adopt a Eurocentric mind-set? Two-Spirit dissolution produces colonial, non-Native approaches to health and wellness. For example, in my research with Two-Spirit people in the San Francisco Bay Area from 2010 to 2012, I documented a specific correlation between HIV seroconversion and intergenerational trauma. Many of the respondents in my study report a lack of cultural connection to their tribes and Native community support networks in general. Additionally, respondents also identify Native-specific organizations as beneficial in their modes of reducing stress and high-risk behavior for HIV/AIDS transmission. Native organizations are central in combating structural inequalities in health and are significant stakeholders for ensuring structural competencies. Ceremony has been used by many tribes as a form of medicine and healing for centuries, but because of religious, military, and government policies and practices there have been periods when ceremonial practices have been either lost or become less accessible to Indigenous peoples as an option for treating social, behavioral, and physical ailments such as HIV. The Western medical industrial complex does not always value or incorporate culturally appropriate methods for addressing risk factors for HIV. As Scott Morgensen's research argues, when we connect American Indian gender and sexuality with queer studies, we must understand how settler colonialism has impacted Indigenous and non-Indigenous perceptions of Two-Spirit people as well as the methods of resistance employed by Two-Spirit people throughout history.[16]

The story of We'Wah (1849–96), a Zuni Lhamana (third-gender, Two-Spirit individual), is an important starting point in considering the diversity of gender roles and ceremonial practices among many American Indian nations prior to and during the initial phases of illicit colonialism in the United States. We'Wah's refusal to submit to illicit colonial attempts to eradicate Two-Spirit traditional roles within Zuni Pueblo society represents a key moment in the genealogy of Two-Spirit history in the United States.[17] The Zuni "princess" We'Wha (pronounced WAY-wah), as local papers in New Mexico described her at the time, was very popular among US officials because of her artwork. She was also a major figure within the Zuni Pueblo Nation for her central role in maintaining traditional ceremonies in the face of colonization. During the spring of 1886, We'Wah spent a considerable amount of time mingling with politicians, government officials, and local elites in Washington, DC. She even became friends with the Speaker of the House and his wife. As a Two-Spirit, We'Wah represents a tradition of negotiating queer and nonqueer spaces as well as Native and non-Native worlds. Her ability to garner the attention of President Grover Cleveland as well as other public officials speaks to what Jodi Byrd describes as the "transit of empire" in that imperialist regimes have no problem making use of Indigenous peoples, themes, images, and general representations to create a particular narrative about American exceptionalism that readily replaces any trace of Native Americans.[18]

That someone who exhibited a gender "nonconforming" identity was able to represent her tribe and maintain the "respect" of anti-Indian colonists suggests that while gender diversity was not accepted among white Americans, there were unexpected exceptions through subtle acts of resistance. The case of We'Wah is significant in considering art as a form of resistance and intervention. For instance, how do we make the stories, artistic creations, and recorded memories of Two-Spirit individuals like We'Wah tangible and visible to young Two-Spirit people today? How might, for example, an exhibit on famous Two-Spirit people throughout history serve as an intervention to address issues of intergenerational trauma, and "high-risk" sexual behavior?

It is important that we also note that despite the relative acceptance of individuals like We'Wah in the genealogy of cultural disintegration of Two-Spirit people, there has also been a centuries-long process of dismantling Two-Spirit ceremonial practices and roles within illicit colonialism in the United States. In order to understand the contemporary implications of HIV/AIDS and seek resolutions, it is important that we first examine the ways that American Indian Two-Spirit people have been represented and erased throughout time through a process of what I term Two-Spirit cultural dissolution.[19]

The dissolution of Two-Spirit cultural practices is a direct result of the actions of religious missionaries and government officials who worked to erode, destroy, and reshape gender and sexual practices within Native communities throughout the Americas.[20] Today, many Indigenous communities have internalized and adopted some of these Western views of gender and sexuality. But there is a long history of Two-Spirit, third-gender, and fourth-gender military and religious leaders in tribes throughout the United States. The stigmas today attached to "nonnormative" gender behavior were non-existent in many tribal societies, as demonstrated by the story of Osh-Tisch (Finds Them and Kills Them), a traditional Crow *boté*, or third-gender male. According to Will Roscoe, the *boté*

> were experts in sewing and beading and considered the most efficient cooks in the tribe. According to one anthropologist, *boté* "excelled women in butchering, tanning, and other domestic tasks"; another reported that their lodges were "the largest and best appointed," and that they were highly regarded for their charitable acts. Indeed by devoting themselves to women's work, which included everything connected with skins and their use in clothing, robes, moccasins, various accessories, and lodges (or tipis) free of interruption from childbearing and rearing, *boté* were in effect full-time craft specialists.[21]

This account demonstrates the range of social and cultural spaces that individuals whom we today call Two-Spirit or LGBTQ traditionally occupied in daily practices, without any sense of moral judgment from fellow tribal members. Today interdependent relationships and complex definitions of third- and fourth-gender identities and practices are absent. If we do witness these practices, either through labor or ceremony, it is usually among those elders who still have knowledge, and marginal acceptance, of these precolonial practices of gender diversity.[22] The values and beliefs of European missionaries and colonists led to the demise of the Two-Spirit identity in some communities. The acceptance of non-Native values and epistemologies has left many contemporary LGBTQ/Two-Spirit American Indian people searching for community and cultural buffers to protect them in a world that sees them as aberrant both in mainstream and in internal ethnic group contexts. As Roscoe notes:

> The values of European and American observers, however, led them to single out and denounce Crow customs regarding sexuality and gender. In 1889, when A. B. Holder reported observations of *boté* made during his assignment as a government doctor at the Crow agency, he concluded, "Of all the many varieties of sexual perversion this, it seems to me, is the most debased that could be conceived of." In this century, anthropologist Robert H. Lowie described Crow berdaches as "pathological cases," "psychiatric cases," "abnormal," "anomalies," "perverts," and "inverts."[23]

Traditional tribal gender and sexual systems that were accepting of many different individual expressions of gender and sexual identity only begin to erode as a result of conflicts over morality with colonists. Military and government collusion to replace diverse Native sexuality and gender practices as well as traditional roles with Judeo-Christian models of heteronormative sexuality were made possible through legal and moral debasement of many Native American customs. The biological and the political were often merged with religious and military assaults on Native communities. All of this led to a process in which settler colonialism vis-à-vis illicit colonialism sought (and still seeks) to replace Indigenous ways of articulating gender and sexual identities and practices with European moral standards. As Scott Morgensen argues, "In the Americas and, specifically, the United States, the biopolitics of settler colonialism was constituted by the imposition of colonial heteropatriarchy and the hegemony of settler sexuality, which sought both the elimination of indigenous sexuality and its incorporation into settler sexual modernity."[24] The inherent contradiction of the imposition of settler sexuality narratives onto Indigenous peoples is that these narratives and interactions always sought to extinguish Indigenous sexual practices while also studying and/or participating in Indigenous forms of sexuality.

Post-traumatic Invasion Syndrome: Indigeneity and the Distribution of Crisis

Two-Spirit cultural dissolution is a major aspect of what I term post-traumatic invasion syndrome (PTIS).[25] By using the word *post*, I am in no way suggesting that the process is over but that the specific event of invasion has taken place and its ongoing impacts can be witnessed through an enduring legacy of trauma, weakened stress-coping mechanisms, and poor health outcomes in Native communities as a result of deeply embedded structural systems of racism in settler colonial health-care systems. After the initial European invasion in the Americas, a process began in American Indian tribal societies that continues to produce painful memories of a history that is seldom told but is very evident when we look at contemporary public health issues facing American Indians. These traumatic invasion and postinvasion experiences continue to threaten the well-being of Two-Spirit and queer American Indians, whose racial, gender, and sexual diversity make them one of the most marginalized groups in the United States. Because of their diversity and their perceived lack of authenticity, many contemporary Two-Spirit Natives are left isolated and looking for community support networks that will accept them for who they are regardless of their racial identification, or whether they identify as queer, transgender, or some other category.

One symptom of PTIS is the adoption of non-Native morals and values: when you change a people's cultural values and norms you change who they are as a people, often irrevocably. As Roscoe explains, prior to colonial invasion, every individual had a role and a purpose in tribal life—and the acceptance of Two-Spirit tribal members left the possibilities for contribution available to each individual fairly open; among the Crow, for example, "if some individuals did not accept or were unsuited for the usual role assigned to their sex, they could still contribute to the community."[26] In the wake of colonization, with its narrower views of social normality, the options open to Two-Spirit individuals were severely curtailed. These actions have also resulted in violence against Native Two-Spirit and transgender people on and off the reservation.

Today, American Indians continue to face issues related to both settler and illicit colonialism, and while some of the legal and religious mechanisms used to disintegrate cultural protocols and support networks in the face of PTIS are being combated by a return to ceremony and Two-Spirit practices, we must understand how health interventions in Native communities must center Native people themselves as the best "medicine" for eliminating HIV/AIDS.

The Art of Ceremony: A Radical Methodology of Healing

In 2015 something remarkable happened. Lakota medicine man Richard "Dickie" Moves Camp led a ceremony of return (Healing the Broken Spirit: Bringing Back the Two-Spirit/Wichapi Koyaka Tiospaye) for members of the San Francisco Bay Area American Indian community to welcome Two-Spirits back into the community and to offer them an apology for their treatment over the past centuries as a result of settler and illicit colonialism. Healing the Broken Spirit was held in Oakland, California, at the American Indian Friendship House and included a feed, music, and most importantly prayers and wishes for reconciliation. The ceremony is significant because it provides Two-Spirit and LGBTQ-identified Natives an opportunity to heal in very culturally specific ways.

As I discuss earlier, Two-Spirit cultural dissolution creates ruptures in the social, psychological, and political mechanisms of community support. Healing the Broken Spirit not only acknowledges these cultural ruptures; the ceremony also includes an apology from the broader Native American community for the many years of exclusion that Two-Spirit members have endured. The distribution of the AIDS crisis in global contexts is often explained by ongoing stigma and silence. Healing the Broken Spirit intentionally seeks to address silence around shaming and to restore a balance between all members of the San Francisco Bay Area urban Indian community regardless of sexual orientation, Two-Spirit identification, or HIV/AIDS status. The collective approach in the ceremony allows for both individual as well as community-centered conversations and plans for ongoing healing from the effects of intergenerational trauma. As an ongoing ceremony, there is an acknowledgment among community members that the problems associated with health disparities such as HIV/AIDS in Native communities cannot be addressed without continuity and consistency in the use of ceremony as an intervention tool specific to Indigenous peoples living in this territory.

The ceremony happened again in 2016 and is important in its focus on crisis reduction. Ceremony is an art. It requires balance and good intentions, and people who participate must be willing to move away from colonial perspectives that reduce the experiences of those at risk for HIV to Western constructs of heteropatriarchy. Healing the Broken Spirit is similar in nature to Drum-Assisted Recovery Therapy for Native Americans (DARTNA) in its use of ceremony and Indigenous cultural mechanisms to reduce substance abuse that continues to be a major contributing factor in the spread of HIV in American Indian and Alaska Native communities.[27] By making use of drumming and tribally specific mechanisms related to ceremony, both DARTNA and Healing the Broken Spirit focus on medicine and healing as more than physiological and biological. These ceremonial acts serve as important interventions into the social and psychological determinants of health related to substance abuse and HIV/AIDS.

While I have argued that we must look at HIV and the art of healing from a communal level in understanding structural competency, I also want to underscore the very real personal impact of this disease and how my own story as a professional and researcher was impeded by a medical system that blames the individual while failing to acknowledge how racial bias and homophobia continue to plague a best practices approach for supporting health and wellness within Indigenous communities. I thus want to intentionally offer a personal narrative to support critiques of medical systems based on my own lived experience.

My own entrance into the world of HIV/AIDS begins from a place of trying to understand what healing means and how the art of ceremony can be used to address HIV/AIDS in Indigenous communities. As a mixed-blood, Afro-Latin/French Creole (French, Black/West African, American Indian

[Opelousa/Atakapa], Spanish, Italian, and Irish) researcher, the experiences of Two-Spirit, gay, transgender, bisexual, and queer people resonates with my own life experiences in profound ways. In my previous research, I have argued that the concept of radical love can support a healthy process for addressing trauma and risks associated with the syndemics of HIV/AIDS.[28] Radical love asserts that as community members from the same ethnic group come together to share their experiences and vulnerabilities, they open up a space for transitioning from individual to collective wellness. My own journey toward healing was deeply impacted by a need not only for cultural understanding and competency but to transform how we actually address in practical, everyday ways the unequal treatment of Indigenous peoples within settler colonial nation-states.

I see my work as something that must demonstrate integrity and relational accountability. In fact, a key component in addressing structural competency depends upon researcher self-reflection and responsiveness. I came to the question of HIV/AIDS and questions of public health and queer theory relatively late in life. I came to these questions from the vantage point of a race theorist, not as a scholar of public health or sexuality studies. In the spring of 2003, as I was preparing to leave my position as the dean of middle school students and multicultural programs at Presidio Hill School in San Francisco, two professors in the biology department at San Francisco State who were the grandparents of one of my students asked if I would consider teaching a course on people of color and AIDS. I agreed.

Developing this course as someone with a mixed-race studies background allowed me to understand that there was an aspect of the epidemic that no one was really talking about in the academic literature. There was no substantial public health policy analysis of ethnicity, especially mixed-race ethnicity. There was also within ethnic studies a very limited discussion of public policy and health concerns from a mixed-race, queer, LGBT, or Two-Spirit perspective.

In the fall of 2002, I was the dean of students and multicultural programs at Presidio Hill School, I was lecturing at San Francisco State University, and I was finishing up my dissertation at the University of California, Santa Cruz. I was busy and in many ways on top of the world. In early October of that year I was feeling a little flu bug and started to have this terrible cough that just would not go away. I did not think much of it until one afternoon when I was walking up the hill from Julius Kahn Park in San Francisco with some of my middle school students and I could not breathe. But like so many of us often do, I ignored my breathing problems and chalked it up to the flu.

On Wednesday, October 8, I went in to see the doctor and he told me it looked like I had a bad case of asthma. So I went home with my inhalers in hand and the doctor told me he would call by Friday if anything showed up in my X-rays. He did not call so I assumed that everything was fine. That Friday, as my breathing worsened and I developed a fever, I decided I should just take the day off. I was never one to get a cold very often, and when I did, it never lasted very long. I also hate taking off from work, but this time my body seemed to do the deciding for me. I stayed over at my parents' home that afternoon and by Sunday with my parents' urging I considered going to the doctor again. It was about midnight Sunday night when I called my sister and told her that I had changed my mind and that I needed her to take me to the emergency room. I could not breathe in a resting position.

Once we arrived at Kaiser's emergency room, I felt much better and thought, *I should have just stayed home. I feel fine. They are going to think I am just wasting their time.* So as the nurse took my temperature, I fully expected to be going home. I was wrong. My temperature was 102 or 103 and my oxygen level was 87. She informed me that I was a very sick man. As I lay in a bed waiting for X-ray results, a doctor suddenly emerged and said she had some questions for me. She proceeded to tell me that I had pneumonia and that it was on the front and back of my lungs, something they usually only saw in the elderly and in people with HIV. My throat dropped into my stomach. She then rattled off several questions: When was the last time you had an HIV test? Have you had sex with men? Can we give you an HIV/AIDS test?

The room seemed to get very small; it also seemed to be moving ever so slowly until it was spinning. I looked at my sister and wondered what this was all about. Neither of us discussed HIV. I just shared with her what the doctor had said and informed her that I had had a test when I started dating my ex-boyfriend in 1998. It was negative, as were previous tests, and because I had only been with him and had only recently broken up with him, there was no way I could be HIV positive. I was confident and my declaration to my sister made me more confident because I could hear myself speaking the words out loud. I was never promiscuous, we were monogamous, and I was negative when I started dating him, so how could I have it? How could I have it? This is surely a question many living with HIV/AIDS must ask at one time or another. I was shortly informed after consenting to the HIV test that I would have to stay in the hospital overnight because of my oxygen level. That was a very sleepless night as I awaited the results of my test and whether or not I had a walking pneumonia (common to a lot of people) or pneumocystis pneumonia (PCP), an opportunistic form of pneumonia that only attacks people with weakened immune systems.

Later that morning, a doctor came into my room and told me to turn the television off. He then told me that they had the results of my test. The doctor remarked, "I'm afraid it's positive. You have HIV and we have already begun treating you for PCP, but the only way we can confirm the PCP is by giving you a bronchoscopy." I stopped, my ears began to swell, my stomach knotted up as he talked, and it was like I could not hear him anymore. I started thinking about my parents, about my brothers and my sister, and about my students at Presidio Hill School. I held firm as the doctor told me, "I have a friend who recently went through the same thing. Things are different. You can live a long time with the disease. We have been able to treat this as a chronic illness and not a terminal death sentence."

He asked me if I had any questions. I insisted that this was impossible— that I was recently tested and the only person I had been with since that test was negative. What did this all mean? He said, "There are two things we look for to monitor your progress: your CD4 or T-cell count and your viral load." Although I considered myself somewhat knowledgeable or "well educated" at least, I honestly was not sure what he was talking about. Of course I knew what T-cells were, but I was not sure what viral load meant. He proceeded to explain to me that the T-cells fought infection and that the viral load measured the amount of the virus in my blood. I was having an internal conversation with myself as I listened to him. Once I snapped out of it, I asked him what my count was. He told me that I had thirty-five T-cells. I asked him what was normal. He responded, "Five hundred to eighteen hundred. Anytime you have less than two hundred T-cells you become vulnerable for opportunistic infections, and the CDC defines AIDS as anyone who has or has ever had less than two hundred T-cells." "So I have AIDS?" I asked. The doctor responded in the affirmative. The doctor informed me that my viral load was over five hundred thousand copies per milliliter of blood. He told me that the closer one gets to one million, and the lower the T-cell count, the closer one is to death. "Is there anyone you can call?" he asked. I bit back my tears.

He told me they were going to run some more tests and he would be back to see me. I thanked him and no sooner had the door shut than I let out a yelp and the hot tears started streaming down my face. I was so overwhelmed by grief. I felt cold and so alone. I picked up the receiver and called my uncle Charlie. I was too afraid to call my parents first. They would be devastated and the only thing that would be worse than dying was hurting them. He picked up and I gave him the news. I burst out crying and could not really talk to my uncle. I decided to call him because he works in a hospice with cancer and AIDS patients, and because he had been out since he was fifteen years old, but mostly I called my gay uncle because he would understand that this was not inevitable, as so many parents sometimes tell their children when they first come out.

He listened, comforted me, and said that he would be right there and that until they could positively confirm the PCP, they could not tell me that I had AIDS. That gave me a little hope. I hung up the phone and could not contain my tears. I imagined dying and never seeing my brothers, my sister, my parents, or my students again. "Nobody wants to see their teacher die," "nobody wants to see their child die," is something I would repeat as I dealt with the news and shared it with family and friends. After being released from the hospital a few days later and twenty-five pounds lighter, I went to stay with my parents. I had already called and told my dad and mom. My dad had suspected AIDS all along when my cough would not go away. Before leaving the hospital, I had had so many conversations, so many tests, and needles poked in me. I was terrified but perhaps not as terrified as some of my nurse providers, who were noticeably careful but also noticeably afraid to touch me.

As I was awakened one night for blood tests, I heard the nurses talking in what I think was Russian and I knew that they were saying, "Be careful—he has AIDS" (I had already heard this once earlier that day). It was tough once I was released from the hospital not knowing what to do or what would happen. Would I finish my PhD? Would I ever work again? How long did I have? And how did this happen to me? After about three weeks I decided I needed to see my kids, so I went to Presidio Hill School for Halloween appropriately dressed as a medical doctor. It was good to see them. It gave me hope. It gave me energy. I decided I had to go back to work. I had spent three weeks going to the doctor for more tests and went through the scare of thinking I had liver failure. Disclosing my HIV/AIDS status to my friends and siblings was very hard, perhaps the hardest thing I have ever had to do. I blamed myself and did not know how they would react. Was God punishing me, I thought? Is this what I get? Is this what I deserve for being gay?

Every time I would see my two younger brothers and my older sister talking and laughing, I started to think one day I might not be here to hear their laughter, to share in the jokes, to see their children grow up. My family and friends were so good to me during that time. That period in my life taught me to slow down in terms of work and it also taught me to put myself first a little more often. I went back to work in early November and began my HIV antiviral medications as well as medicine for the PCP, which had been confirmed. No sooner had I returned to work than I got sick again. It was hard missing school and work. I only told a few people at work about my status. After dealing with being sick for another two weeks, in December I went back to work part-time in January and started finishing my dissertation. I thought, if I am going to die, I am going to finish what I started first, so I worked with a sense of urgency.

I sent my dissertation in to my committee that January and graduated in March 2003. Slowly I started putting my life back together. It was hard. I lived by myself and I had just broken up with my partner of almost four years a few months prior to my diagnosis. It turned out he was positive too. I wondered if I had infected him. My doctor told me that advanced HIV takes at least ten years to develop to the stage I was at, but as far as I knew this could not be possible because I was not sexually active at seventeen. I struggled to figure out if I infected him or if he infected me. Eventually these questions dissipated and I had no choice but to move on. I got my first lab results back that January and amazingly my viral load had dropped to about 1,200 and my CD4 count was an impressive 411 after only a month and a half on meds.

My numbers, however, would go up and down after this. But it was a card I received in the mail from my uncle Charlie after those first results that gave me the hope to keep living. He wrote on the inside, "God is everywhere even beneath the wings of a dove. Congratulations on your good health. Love Uncle Charlie." Since that time I have thought deeply about why this happened to me. I finally decided that this was not a death sentence, but the next big obstacle for me was learning to cope with my status and the issue of love. All I ever really wanted was to find love and to have my own family. This seemed impossible now. Who would want me? How would I tell anyone I met that I was positive? Right before getting sick, I had met a nice guy from Lebanon but once he found out why I had not called and that I had been in the hospital, I never heard from him again. My confidence and self-esteem around disclosure and dating were really low. I considered a reconciliation with my ex-partner but realized that we were not right for each other and that getting back together at this point would be self-destructive and for the wrong reasons. Since my diagnosis in 2002, I have had six very loving relationships, but the most important relationships that helped me cope with HIV/AIDS were found within the community.

I share my own personal story at length here to provide a mirror into the questions, struggles, and pathways to wellness for Indigenous people. Community wellness approaches in Native American communities must also consider the diversity of experiences, ranging from rural/reservation life to urban Indian living. I also share my own story here because it is an example of the stigma that HIV/AIDS can have for members of Native communities. For all the resources and advanced education I had at the time of my diagnosis, it was not until I engaged in ceremony that I was able to truly begin a process of healing. A few months after my release from the hospital, friends in the community organized a pipe ceremony for me with a mutual friend, Daniel Freeland, who is a medicine man for the Navajo nation. I can still hear Dan's words today: "You can't think of yourself as sick, Andrew. A lot of our people are going through what you are going through. They can't tell their stories. You can share your story and in doing that you can begin to heal yourself and you can also help with the healing of our communities, so that others will know this is part of the life cycle of challenges we face that can make us stronger." He went on to say, "Sharing your voice and your story can be its own form of ceremony because as each of us shares our story, we help someone else to feel stronger and more connected. We become medicine when we share our pain and in becoming that medicine and creating ceremony you become your own medicine and your brothers and sisters also become your best medicine." It is often hard to explain how ceremony can be medicine and vice-versa. However, in my own experience as a queer, Two-Spirit, mixed-race Native/Creole man, medicine means making use of something that will make us feel better. Sharing our painful stories through what I have termed radical love means that we can only understand medicine and ceremony when we open up and release all the stigma and emotional and physical suffering that we are experiencing. We must also acknowledge how these experiences differ from region to region and person to person while still respecting the fact that the differences are also what make Indigenous communities stronger.

The differences between rural, reservation, and urban Indian communities and HIV stem from issues related to access and tradition. In rural and reservation settings, there are limited resources and support mechanisms for people at risk for HIV, whether LGBTQ/Two-Spirit or heterosexual. There is also a tremendous amount of silence and taboo related to Two-Spirit people and HIV in rural reservation communities. As a result, many Two-Spirit people move to urban areas in the hopes of finding more support within a more ethnically diverse population. According to Irene Vernon, although use of alcohol and drugs is not itself a route of transmission for HIV, it plays a critical role in the AIDS epidemic: under the influence of substances, protective behaviors are often forgotten or ignored. Several HIV/AIDS-positive individuals within Vernon's research report that tribal communities not only deny that HIV/AIDS is a problem among American Indians but have also ostracized infected members. These actions create fear and mistrust, and therefore reluctance to obtain services. This social stigma also manifests itself in the context of risk behavior, as many displaced or marginal members of tribal communities who leave reservations and come to urban areas do not have the economic means, social networks, or access to vital services to receive adequate preventative services or adequate treatment after seroconversion. Many of these urban Indians unfortunately become homeless, turn to sex work, or become intravenous drug users (or a combination of all three), all of which put them at greater risk for contracting HIV.[29]

When issues of tribal displacement and relocation are combined with mixed-race identity, enrollment status, and queer identification, the result is greater levels of trauma and risk. The work of Karina Walters and her co-investigators, in the article "Keeping Our Hearts from Touching the Ground: HIV/AIDS in American Indian and Alaska Native Women," suggests that the sustainability of American Indian communities is based on the health of the women within them, who have been central to the survival of so many communities throughout history, both pre- and postinvasion.

> In traditional indigenous cosmologies, the feminine spirit is often regarded as that which sustains life. Even the earth, often referred to as "Mother Earth," is assigned a feminine identity who provides all that sustains human needs. Women and their bodies are representations of this life-sustaining force, and, in many indigenous cultures, women are regarded as agents of cultural and community preservation. As poetically articulated in the traditional Cheyenne proverb ... a nation cannot be vanquished while the women remain strong enough in body and spirit to carry and protect not only physical but also cultural and spiritual survival. As such, survival of American Indian and Alaska Native (AIAN) cultures can be seen as integrally linked to Native women and this reality frames the need to protect their overall health and wellness, which is currently in a state of crisis.[30]

I would argue that a similar assertion is true for Two-Spirit people. There have been attempts to fuse the past and the present as they relate to the practice of diverse gender and sexuality constructions, but I would suggest that we are still deeply entrenched in a decolonization project regarding both gender and sexuality. Until we can begin to move toward healing among all individuals within our communities—especially the most marginalized—we will continue to experience Two-Spirit cultural dissolution and a host of PTIS symptoms related to sexual violence, racial hybridity, and gender discrimination.

Ironically, even as Two-Spirit cultural dissolution creates divisions within Native communities, Two-Spirit identity/discourse is being put to use by non-Natives to appropriate a history associated with "authenticity" or "normativity" for their own same-sex relationships and political struggles. The use of precolonial Native and Indigenous religious, political, and cultural belief systems has long been available to non-Natives in ways that this same history is not readily accessible to the very people who descend from these traditions. These Native descendants have had these histories and practices taken away from them, only to be reused by non-Natives for their own political purposes. Morgensen notes that "U.S. queer projects define their integrity by appealing to the cultural status of an ethnic group or the legal status granted racial and national minorities, through 'racial analogy.' However, they have not asked how these normatively white and *non-Native* queer routes to 'race' play on indigeneity as a history or model of the authenticity they seek, while absenting Native people from the 'racial' queerness that secures citizenship."[31] Here, Morgensen argues convincingly that non-Native queer activists and scholars normalize their rights to "queer citizenship," based on racial entitlements attributed to Native peoples, whom they then deny "queer citizenship" on the basis of race.

To address the issue of "queer citizenship," which is ultimately about community inclusion, I return to the Healing the Broken Spirit / Wichapi Koyaka Tiospaye event that was held in 2015 and 2016. When we turn away from settler and illicit colonial narratives that erase, marginalize, and unsettle community cohesion, we can provide new opportunities for Indigenous peoples to make use of ceremony as a radical act of healing. In contemporary US society under Donald Trump as POTUS, we must be ever vigilant about creating sustainable intervention and prevention mechanisms that will lead to healing and a reduction in the transmission of HIV/AIDS in American Indian communities. Ceremonies that restore the cultural support networks within Indigenous communities can have a profound impact on the everyday practices of wellness that will one day eliminate the AIDS crisis around the world, but only when we also eradicate settler and illicit colonialism from the medical industry and society in general.

Notes

1 Centers for Disease Control and Prevention, "American Indians and Alaska Native Populations."
2 Walters, Simoni, and Evans-Campbell, "Substance Use among American Indians and Alaska Natives"; Smith, *Decolonizing Methodologies*, 19–23.

3 Centers for Disease Control and Prevention, "American Indians and Alaska Native Populations."

4 Centers for Disease Control and Prevention, "American Indians and Alaska Native Populations."

5 Vernon, *Killing Us Quietly*; Walters et al., "Keeping Our Hearts"; Jolivette, *Indian Blood*.

6 Wolfe, "Settler Colonialism"; Byrd, *Transit of Empire*; Morgensen, *Spaces between Us*; Simpson, *Mohawk Interruptus*, 387.

7 Metzl, *Protest Psychosis*, 25–30.

8 Metzl and Hansen, "Structural Competency," 126.

9 Wolfe, "Settler Colonialism," 387.

10 On cultural genocide, see Tinker, *Missionary Conquest*.

11 Two-Spirit people are tribal members who are gender nonconforming individuals who possess both female and male attributes and roles and often serve particular purposes in religious ceremonies.

12 Jacobs, Thomas, and Lang, *Two-Spirit People*; Roscoe, *Changing Ones*.

13 Jacobs, Thomas, and Lang, *Two-Spirit People*.

14 Jacobs, Thomas, and Lang, *Two-Spirit People*; Roscoe, *Changing Ones*.

15 Lang, "Various Kinds of Two-Spirit People," 103.

16 Morgensen, *Spaces between Us*.

17 "We'Wha the Revered Zuni Man-Woman."

18 Byrd, *Transit of Empire*.

19 Jolivette, *Indian Blood*.

20 Tinker, *Missionary Conquest*.

21 Roscoe, *Changing Ones*, 25–26.

22 Jolivette, *Indian Blood*.

23 Roscoe, *Changing Ones*, 26.

24 Morgensen, *Spaces between Us*, 34.

25 Jolivette, *Indian Blood*.

26 Roscoe, *Changing Ones*, 26.

27 Dickerson et al., "Drum-Assisted Recovery Therapy."

28 Jolivette, *Indian Blood*.

29 Vernon, *Killing Us Quietly*.

30 Walters et al., "Keeping Our Hearts," S261–65.

31 Morgensen, *Spaces between Us*, 106.

Bibliography

Byrd, Jodi. *The Transit of Empire: Indigenous Critiques of Colonialism*. Minneapolis: University of Minnesota Press, 2011.

Centers for Disease Control and Prevention. "American Indians and Alaska Native Populations." Accessed August 29, 2019. https://www.cdc.gov/hiv/group /racialethnic/aian/index.html.

Dickerson, Daniel L., Kamilla L. Venner, Bonnie Duran, Jeffrey J. Annon, Benjamin
Hale, and George Funmaker. "Drum-Assisted Recovery Therapy for Native
Americans (DARTNA): Results from a Pretest and Focus Groups." *American
Indian and Alaska Native Mental Health Research* 21, no. 1 (2014): 35–58.

Jacobs, Sue-Ellen, Wesley Thomas, and Sabine Lang. *Two-Spirit People: Native
American Gender Identity, Sexuality, and Spirituality.* Urbana: University of
Illinois Press, 1997.

Jolivette, Andrew. *Indian Blood: HIV and Colonial Trauma in San Francisco's Two-
Spirit Community.* Seattle: University of Washington Press, 2016.

Lang, Sabine. "Various Kinds of Two-Spirit People: Gender Variance and Homosexuality in Native American Communities." In *Two-Spirit People: Native
American Gender Identity, Sexuality, and Spirituality,* edited by Sue-Ellen Jacobs,
Wesley Thomas, and Sabine Lang, 100–118. Urbana: University of Illinois Press,
1997.

Metzl, Jonathan. *The Protest Psychosis: How Schizophrenia Became a Black Disease.*
Boston: Beacon, 2010.

Metzl, Jonathan, and Helena Hansen. "Structural Competency: Theorizing a
New Medical Engagement with Stigma and Inequality." *Social Science and
Medicine* 103 (2014): 126–33.

Morgensen, Scott. *Spaces between Us: Queer Settler Colonialism and Indigenous
Decolonization.* Minneapolis: University of Minnesota Press, 2011.

Roscoe, Will. *Changing Ones: Third and Fourth Genders in Native North America.*
1998. New York: St. Martin's Griffin, 2000.

Simpson, Audra. *Mohawk Interruptus: Political Life across the Borders of Settler States.*
Durham, NC: Duke University Press, 2014.

Smith, Linda Tuhiwai. *Decolonizing Methodologies: Research and Indigenous Peoples.*
Dunedin, NZ: Otago University Press, 1999.

Tinker, George. *Missionary Conquest: The Gospel and Native American Cultural
Genocide.* Minneapolis: Fortress, 1993.

Vernon, Irene S. *Killing Us Quietly: Native Americans and HIV/AIDS.* Lincoln:
University of Nebraska Press, 2001.

Walters, Karina, Tessa Evans-Campbell, Ramona Beltran, and Jane Simoni.
"Keeping Our Hearts from Touching the Ground: HIV/AIDS in American
Indian and Alaska Native Women." *Women's Health Issues* 21, no. 6 (2011):
S261–65.

Walters, Karina, Jane Simoni, and Teresa Evans-Campbell. "Substance Use among
American Indians and Alaska Natives: Incorporating Culture in an 'Indigenist'
Stress-Coping Paradigm." *Public Health Reports* 117 (2002): S104–17.

"We' Wha the Revered Zuni Man-Woman." *Two Spirits* (blog), February 15, 2011.
http://twospirits.org/http:/twospirits.org/blog/wewha-the-revered-zuni-man
-woman/.

Wolfe, Patrick. "Settler Colonialism and the Elimination of the Native." *Journal of
Genocide Research* 8, no. 4 (2006): 387–409.

ELEVEN ACTIVISM AND IDENTITY IN THE RUINS OF REPRESENTATION

Juana María Rodríguez

Our scholarship on AIDS must be located at the crossroads of art and politics, life and art, and life and death.—Alberto Sandoval-Sánchez, "Response to the Representation of AIDS"

Activism is an engagement with the hauntings of history, a dialogue between the memories of the past and the imaginings of the future manifested through the acts of our own present yearnings. AIDS has surrounded us with the living memory of familiar ghosts, faces that haunt our intimate realities of being infected/not yet infected, sick/not yet sick, alive but not yet dead. As we wait for passage to the other side, we plan our revenge and chart strategies of resistance to head off the silence. Identity politics, as an organizing tool and political ideology, has historically had specific investments for marginalized groups in this country. Political groupings based on identity categories, however, have become highly contested sites, splintering ever further into more specialized and discrete social and political units, based on more precise yet still problematic categories of identification and concomitant modes of definition. As a lived practice, strategic essentialism (and the policing of identity) that often defines it has become a messy and contentious organizing strategy that ultimately reveals the limits and problematic assumptions of identity politics. Identity politics formed in resistance to state power thus remains implicated in the perpetuation of the narratives upon which it is founded, specifically the conflation of identity, ideology, and political practices and the lived ramifications of the constructed and problematic duality of insider/outsider. Yet for many, it becomes impossible to conceive of political organizing without explicative narratives or definitive social positions.

This chapter asks: What possibilities for political and social intervention are opened up outside the discourse of identity politics? How can we deploy power creatively and consciously in the service of radical justice? And how effective are these strategies for bringing about individual and social change?

Projecting Life

This chapter uses the example of one social service agency in San Francisco, Proyecto ContraSIDA por Vida (PCPV), founded in August 1993, to analyze how it has negotiated and reimagined the discursive terrain of identity politics to respond to the social crisis that surrounds the AIDS pandemic.[1] Its name indicates both what it is working against, ContraSIDA (against AIDS), and what it is working for, Por Vida (for life). Through an examination of the agency's programming and cultural production, I document how it employs various creative strategies of organizing and intervention to enrich the cultural and political climate in the service of radical social change. Rather than relying on personal interviews of clients, volunteers, or staff to document the work being conducted at the agency, I examine the existing representations of Proyecto that have already made their way into the public sphere through flyers, brochures, promotional materials, public speaking engagements, and published accounts. This methodological decision stems from my interest in bringing into focus the ways these subjects are continually involved in speaking back to contest and reimagine subjectivity through individual and collective self-representation. Furthermore, by using archival materials generated by the individuals and groups I seek to present, I demonstrate in practice a methodological shift that foregrounds previously marginalized cultural production.

The focus of this chapter is on analyzing the ways Proyecto represents and names itself and the communities it serves in the public arena, and how these practices of self-representation circumvent some of the pitfalls and limitations of identity politics. I argue that Proyecto is involved in forging a new type of identity project based on ideas, affiliation, and alignment rather than on static categories of race, gender, culture, or sexuality. Its organizing and outreach strategies speak to the creative, transformative powers of reading and writing language and images as symbolic codes. Its texts engage the possibilities of refusing explication, without abandoning the political significance of inscribing subjectivity. In the process, it is challenging cultural, social, and state apparatus conceptualizations of sexuality and culture in the postmodern wreckage of a metropolis crumbling under the weight of capitalist gentrification, racialized dis-ease, and social inequity.

San Francisco has been an epicenter of queer Latina/o organizing and resistance since the 1960s, as well as a focal point of the AIDS pandemic. Proyecto ContraSIDA por Vida emerged through the threads of the many groups that preceded its existence: the United Farm Workers (UFW), the Gay Latino Alliance (GALA), the Mission Cultural Center, Community United in Responding to AIDS/SIDA (CURAS), Mujerío, the National Task Force on AIDS Prevention, La Familia at UC Berkeley, and the strands of other groups and influences as numerous and diverse as the individual personal and political histories of its founders.[2] The texture of its political and social ideology has been shaped through the traces of Black and Chicano nationalism, third world feminism, queer liberation, AIDS activism, immigrant rights movements, the third world peoples' strike at San Francisco State University and at Berkeley, Freirian models of consciousness raising and education, and the Birmingham school of social education and organizing.[3] Individuals, texts, and ideas from Ciudad de México, Los Angeles, La Habana, New York, Miami, the California Central Valley, and elsewhere have traversed the social and political landscape of San Francisco, creating established lines of motion that have facilitated and informed local organizing efforts.

Proyecto is not the only queer Latina/o organization in San Francisco; many other groups and agencies also serve and represent the diverse configuration known as the San Francisco queer Latino community. The combined force of three ideological components differentiates Proyecto from other Latina/o community organizing projects: its commitment to multigender organizing, its declared posture of providing sex-positive programming, and its commitment to harm reduction as a model for prevention and treatment.[4] Proyecto ContraSIDA por Vida is neither representative of other organizing efforts nor a unique exception; however, its strategies for effective resistance and creative survival offer a window into the possibilities of local organizing in the ruins of representation.

Proyecto ContraSIDA por Vida is located at Sixteenth and Mission, a busy intersection in the heart of San Francisco's Mission District, an area generally figured as a Latino neighborhood. This street corner and its vectors have a long history as a magnet for queer Latinos, having been the site of two gay Latino bars, Esta Noche and La India Bonita, and a short-lived Latina lesbian bar, Sofia's.[5] Yet the multiethnic, multicultural Latina/o majority of the Mission shares this geographic space with Arabs, Asians, Anglos, African Americans, and others, as well as a thriving criminalized drug culture and prostitution trade, elements that all come into play in Proyecto's self-representation. Proyecto's offices are street level; there are couches and magazines; music plays in the background. Its walls are papered with flyers and art produced by students, volunteers, and supporters; a basket of condoms sits at the reception desk, generally staffed by one of Proyecto's many volunteers. Sex workers come in to pick up free condoms before running off to work, newly arrived immigrants come to find out about the intricacies of creating green cards and social security numbers, multihued transgenders and intravenous drug users stop by for information on needle exchanges for drugs and hormones, the queer neighborhood homeboys and girls come by to flirt or hang out with familiar faces. Sandra Ruiz, Proyecto's youth health educator, comments, "All kinds of people stop and look in our windows, including grandmothers, cops and kids. . . . They ask, 'What is this place?' Well, this is a place where I can be everything I am."[6] Proyecto's target audiences are gay, lesbian, bisexual, transgender, and questioning Latinas/os, yet those who walk through its doors and avail themselves of its many services reflect the ethnic and sexual diversity of the neighborhood and the complexities of social and biological families.

Proyecto's mission statement combines the elements of a radical social analysis and visionary political conviction with a poetic urgency that demands our attention and merits its full citation.

> Proyecto ContraSIDA Por Vida is coming to you—you joto, you macha, you vestida, you queer, you femme, you girls and boys and boygirls and girlboys de ambiente, con la fe and fearlessness that we can combat AIDS, determine our own destinies and love ourselves and each other con dignidad, humor y lujuria. Nos llamamos "a multigender, sex-positive, neighborhood-based Latina/o lesbian, gay, bisexual and transgender HIV service agency." *Multigender* because we believe as the gay poet Carl Morse states, ". . . I want at least 121 different words to describe gender. Because there are at least that many ways of having, practicing, or experiencing gender." Different nombres, different cuerpos, different deseos, different culturas coming together to form a community dedicated to living, to fighting the spread of HIV disease and the other unnatural disasters of racism, sexism, homophobia, xenophobia and poverty.[7] *Sex-positive* quiere decir positively sexual and shameless, profoundly perverse and proud. Queremos romper el silencio y represión among our pueblos who for 500 years have been colonized/catholicized/de-eroticized. In the tradition of lesbian and gay liberation creemos en our gente's right to desire as we please, to buscar placer when, how and with whom we choose. We believe that deseo transformará el mundo. We also understand that in

order to examine our sexualities we must first participate in groundbreaking discussions of diverse sexual practices: butch y femme, leather, bisexuality, etc. *Neighborhood-based* means we work within the barrio most identified with Latina lesbianas, gays, bisexuales y vestidas—the Mission as it is bordered by the Castro. Our current location at 18th and Dolores and street-front offices allow for easy access, for off-the-street clientele and keeps our programming en el pulso of our target population.[8] All of the programming we provide here at PCPV attempts to continue to expand these notions and develop new ones. Our definitions are not rigid but rasquachi, our position playful, our efforts at empowering done with grace in the face of so much dolor.[9]

This mission statement, which is also referred to by its title, "Así somos" (This is how we are), begins with the deconstruction of binary sexual and gender terms, a direct address to a multiply constituted constituency. It articulates these multiple enactments of identities through naming: "you joto, you macha, you vestida, you queer, you femme, you girls and boys and boygirls and girlboys de ambiente." The piece is published without indicating an originating author; however, Ricardo Bracho, the Chicano poet and playwright and Proyecto's health education coordinator, is responsible for its composition, which grew out of a group writing exercise he developed for his coworkers at Proyecto. In a memo to this author, Bracho records how in this piece he intended to use the process of interpellation to effect hailing from a "non-dominant dialogic voicing." He writes, "the althusserian model of interpellation posits the hegemonic hailing of the subject—the cop who screams 'hey you' thus giving the you a you to be—a state-derived identity, the subject for the (dominant) other in hegelian terms. I wanted to hail without such dominance. Hence you joto macha which not only reads the reader into the text but asks the reader to read the author(ity) within such signs of degradation."[10] Asking the reader to read both the author and the authority of hailing calls into focus the constitutive context in which discursive resignification operates. Through the process of interpellation, the text validates the existence of a subject that had previously been constituted through degradation. In the context of a promotional text for a social service agency, this hailing offers "jotos and machas" not only a linguistic space to occupy but a physical site as well: the space of Proyecto. Yet these words bring with them the haunted histories of these names and the memories of their previous enunciation. The narrative shadows of *joto*, *macha*, and queer carry with them traces of violence, familiar rejection, and cultural alienation even as they confer social existence and oppositional validation. As troubling as this discursive resignification is to some, for others it becomes a rallying point for a discursive autonomy, which, while fictive, becomes a tool through which narratives of shame, violence, and alienation are verbalized and countered.

Shifting the pronoun from the "you" in "you joto, you macha" to the "we" in "we believe" recontextualizes these linguistic memories by situating them in a framework of a shared philosophy of sexual liberation: "deseo transformará el mundo" (desire will transform the world). Yet it also maps the contested grounds of community: "Different nombres, different cuerpos, different deseos, different culturas coming together to form a community dedicated to living" (Different names, different bodies, different desires, different cultures . . .). Bracho's text reaches for the political valency of community without imposing an adherence to preexisting identity categories; instead identity and community are constituted through political commitment and action. It asserts desire and the expression of desire as basic human rights and advocates dialogue on sexual practices as a necessary strategy in order to counter silence and repression. The focus is on sexual liberation rather than gaining "equal rights" under the existing regimes of state power. Furthermore, the text and the mission of Proyecto remain open, playful, continually in process.

Neither the Spanish nor the English is italicized or visually marked as "different" in the text, creating a visual seamlessness as it moves from one language to another. The insistence on code-switching from English to Spanish, as well as from street vernacular to political theory, blurs the boundaries of these discourses. Words such as *xenophobia* or *rasquachi* may not be equally accessible to all readers, yet the aim is not to create a text based on the lowest common denominator of language, but rather one that provides a diversely literate audience a point of entry into the text.

Proyecto's Spanglish poem–manifesto–mission statement reflects a disinvestment in static concepts of language, culture, and gender and mirrors the agency's irreverent style of community organizing and education. Rather than focusing on AIDS as a discrete disease or as a single and primary health priority, Proyecto focuses on understanding and addressing the multiple social, economic, cultural, and spiritual dimensions that contribute to individual and collective health and well-being. Proyecto's approach to HIV prevention and service affirms its belief that as we near the fourth decade of the AIDS pandemic, handing out condoms and brochures is simply not enough. Instead, its work addresses the underlying issues of sexual and cultural shame and alienation, gendered and racialized social and sexual repression, and the historical consequences of colonialism and political disenfranchisement. Underlying Proyecto's prevention agenda is the belief that giving people a reason to want to live, survive, and resist erasure is imperative if we are to combat the spread of HIV and promote health in our diverse communities. Its work challenges basic assumptions that have guided much of mainstream AIDS prevention, namely, that all people want to live, that all of us are equally capable of negotiating sexual contracts, and that all of us benefit equally from health maintenance.

In addition to more traditional prevention and support services, such as street-level outreach, treatment and prevention counseling, and in-service training to schools and other social service agencies, Proyecto's prevention programming aims to tackle the ways health, disease, social and sexual power relations, and individual agency are socially and culturally constructed. Events have included a community forum series titled "Escándalo" (Scandal), a multicultural transgender support group, diverse multilingual rap groups, organized retreats, career guidance workshops, a soccer team for young women called Las Diablitas (The Little Devils), and an ever-changing offering of creative educational courses organized as part of Colegio Contra-SIDA. These activities target the conditions necessary for social health and well-being: self-esteem, meaningful social bonds, individual and collective consciousness through dialogue and education, personal and political empowerment skills, and the tools of critical inquiry.

Las Diablitas, for example, began as a Colegio class and later became established independently under the economic sponsorship of the bar Colors. Initially, under Proyecto, it was geared toward *jotas* twenty-five years of age and under; since then the parameters of membership have been expanded to include players ages sixteen to thirty, lesbian, bisexual, questioning women, an FTM transgender, and players of diverse ethnic backgrounds. It is one of the youngest and most inexperienced teams in the Golden Gate Women's Soccer League. The vast majority of its members had never played soccer before joining and it is the only team in the league made up exclusively of women of color. The emphasis of the team is on "promoting young women's physical and mental health." One team member, Lisa Arellanes, writes, "Rather than sitting in a support group, having to 'check in,' introduce yourself, or worry about being put on the spot, all we do is play soccer, hang out, and build familia. If they need support later, they have seventeen fellow soccer players to turn to."[11]

Some of these events are configured around gender, age, language, HIV status, or culturally specific audiences; some are organized exclusively by

Proyecto; others are presented in collaboration with other community organizations.[12] Proyecto has not abandoned the idea of creating identity-specific spaces as a means to interrogate the complexities of subjectivity; most of its programming is still designed by and for various configurations of queer Latinos. By continually shifting the terms around which these spaces are conceptualized, however, and by also creating spaces constructed only by a common interest or political agenda, its programs and events creatively circumvent some of the limits and exclusionary practices of other identity projects.

Proyecto's monthly informal community dialogues, "Escándalo," are open to anyone interested in the topic and draw very different crowds from one event to the next. These have included "¿Y Tu Abuela Donde Está?" (And Where Is Your Grandmother?) in celebration of Black History Month, an event that brought together a panel of participants to talk about the legacy and lived realities of African culture, history, and identity in the Americas.[13] Another discussion, "Sex: What's Age Got to Do with It? A Discussion on Relationships between the Ages," tackled the relationship between age, agency, desire, and power, a highly charged and controversial issue in most queer communities. This flyer used an image of the Mexican comedian Cantinflas with the US comedian Buster Keaton, with the heading "What's Too Young? Too Old? Jail Bait or Chicken Hawk."[14] Queer and questioning youth form one of Proyecto's primary target audiences; these are individuals whose sexual agency is currently criminalized by existing age-of-consent laws.

One of the most controversial and well-attended roundtables was titled "Cracking On! A Roundtable and Community Dialogue on Amphetamine (Crystal) Use and Misuse." The flyer depicted an image of a superhero cartoon figure surrounded by the phrases "Trick or Treat? partying hard? super stud? feeling powerful and alert? what's the date? coming down? need some sleep? did you eat? safer sex? what a tweak." Under the agency's address and contact information are the words "Confidentiality Assured." This particular roundtable attracted one of the largest and most diverse audiences, illustrating the lack of information and nonjudgmental dialogue on drug "use and misuse." It also raised considerable opposition from several drug treatment providers in attendance because its premise, that not all forms of drug use are equivalent to abuse and that harm reduction is an effective and necessary model for addressing risk, directly challenged the established biomedical discourse on drug use and treatment.

The images used to advertise these events are as intellectually sophisticated and visually complex as the ideas they represent. As part of Proyecto's

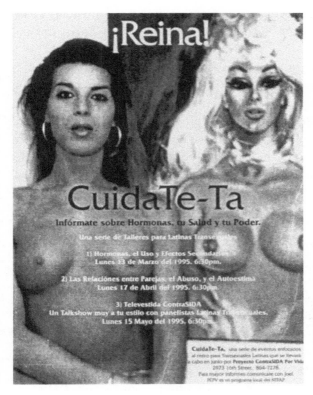

FIGURE 11.1. Flyer produced by Proyecto ContraSIDA por Vida, 1995. Design by Joel Reyna.

outreach to transgenders, another flyer reads, "¡Reina! CuidaTe-Ta: Infórmate sobre Hormonas, tu Salud y tu Poder" (Inform yourself about hormones, your health and your power) (figure 11.1). The language combines the word *reina*, an endearment meaning "queen," and *CuidaTe-Ta*, a wordplay that combines *cuídate* (take care of yourself) with *teta*, or tit. It lists a series of three workshops that present a glimpse of the range of services directed toward transgenders: "Hormonas, el Uso y Efectos Secundarios" (Hormones, Their Use and Secondary Effects); "Las Relaciones entre Parejas, el Abuso, y el Autoestimo" (Relationships, Abuse and Self-Esteem); and "Televestida ContraSIDA: Un Talkshow muy a tu estilo con panelistas Latinas Transexuales" (Televestida ContraSIDA: A talk show, very much your style, with Latina Transsexual panelists). *Televestida* plays on the word *tele*, from television, and *vestida*, a popular word for drag queens. The three different events in the series reflect the multiple strategies of intervention offered by Proyecto: providing concrete information about health and risk factors; addressing the underlying issues of sexual power and agency in relationships necessary to negotiate sexual and emotional contracts; and providing a public forum in which to perform, celebrate, and discuss lived experiences and theories of living.

The accompanying image is of a naked male-to-female transsexual standing in front of a portrait of herself, in which her hair, makeup, and dress are exaggerated. The image plays on a kind of doubling, where the "real" and the "representation" are set side by side. By providing a forum where the contradictions, implications, exaggerations, and lived consequences of identity, behavior, and affiliation can be explored, Proyecto creates a social, aesthetic, and critical context where questions of difference and divergence advance, rather than stifle, collective dialogue. The images and language used in these flyers are as thought-provoking as the events they advertise. In fact, their dissemination and visual presence in various citywide venues serve the function of providing a common cultural text that sparks interrogation and dialogue as it furthers the cause of propagating self-defined representations.

One of the most innovative and vibrant features of Proyecto's programming has been its Colegio ContraSIDA offerings. These are free multiweek classes taught by local artists, activists, and community residents. They have included makeup, sewing, and drama classes for Latina drag queens called "AtreDivas," a neologism that plays with the words *atrevida* (daring one) and *diva*; Tai Chi classes; "girl-colored," a photo-sculpture class for lesbian and bisexual women of color under twenty-five; various writing classes organized along and across language and gender; a multigender photography class titled "Jotografía," a combination of *joto* (faggot) and *fotografía* (photography); and a video production workshop for young Latinas titled "Shoot This." Here, the distinctions between students, clients, volunteers, and staff break down the entrenched categories of "victims, volunteers and experts" evident in many AIDS service organizations.[15] But the movement is not linear or progressive. Past employees now attend classes; paid Colegio teachers become unpaid volunteers. There is a continual exchange, movement, and circulation of money, knowledge, and resources.[16]

¡Imagínate!

Many of these courses have been focused on or resulted in creative manifestations of self-representation through autobiography and self-portraiture. Whether it is within the intimacy of these small classes or through the public persona of Proyecto's promotional materials, Proyecto is continually engaged in the process of creative individual and collective representation. Its programming is directly involved in addressing the themes of desire, pleasure, fear, and humanity to remap the theoretical and aesthetic terrains of sexuality and culture. These themes constitute the psychic excesses of structuralist categories of identity that often elude, or are excluded from, mainstream discourses on HIV infection and AIDS.

The course offerings through Colegio ContraSIDA have also valued the role spirituality plays in healing and cultural activism. One such class, "Retablos del Retrovirus," appropriates a culturally specific art form to meet the needs of gay Latinos living with "the heartbreak that is the AIDS epidemic." In México *retablos*, or *ex-votos*, have historically been used as a form of visual prayer, painted on tin, and often combining both a visual representation of the spiritual or physical crisis and a textual accompaniment asking or giving thanks for divine intervention. This class, taught by the Chicana artist Celia Herrera Rodríguez, combined a culturally specific art therapy with self-determined spiritual expression as a means of coping with the loss, alienation, grief, and spiritual anxiety associated with AIDS. The flyer advertising the class used an established retablo image and situated it within a new interpretive context that complicates the form's relationship to Catholicism and culture. It is the image of a man turning away from the priests at the hour of his death, facing instead the image of his desire in the hands of the devil. The accompanying text from the flyer reads:

> Retablos have been used for centuries by Latinos to speak of faith, suffering and miracles. PCPV's Retablos del Retrovirus continues this tradition within the Latino Gay and Vestida communities and our heroic response to the heartbreak that is the AIDS epidemic. This series of visual art workshops will allow participants to discuss and draw the losses and grief they have experienced in the AIDS crisis, as well as illuminate moments of divinity and outrage.

The following three images are examples of the retablos produced in the class that were reproduced in Proyecto's first promotional calendar.[17] In the first, the artist, Daniel Genara, writes, "Le pido al Sagrado Corazón de Jesús que oiga mis ruegos y me ayude en mi pelea contra este vicio" (I ask the Sacred Heart of Jesus to hear my pleas and help me in my fight against this vice) (figure 11.2). The solitary figure facing us sits with three bottles of beer and a lit cigarette. The bar slopes down onto the figure, as the Sacred Heart rests on a separate horizon flanked by Grecian columns, suggesting a heavenly plane. The bar depicted conforms to the visual layout of La India Bonita and is reminiscent of many Latino nightclubs. It appears as a kind of altar,

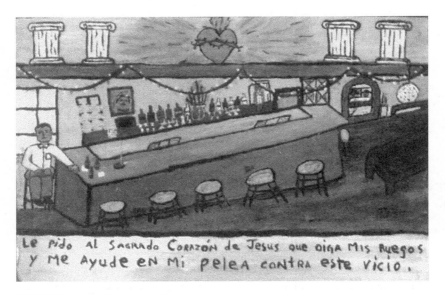

Le pido al Sagrado Corazón de Jesus que oiga mis ruegos y me ayude en mi pelea contra este vicio.

FIGURE 11.2. Daniel Genara, retablo, 1993.

complete with an image of the Virgin, flowers, and a picture nestled between bottles, glasses, and packages of chips. The "vice" in question is never named, yet the image allegorizes the alienation associated with the bar culture prevalent in many queer and Latino communities.

In the second image, the artist, Juan Rodríguez, writes, "Sto. Niño de Atocha que me has protegido y cuidado desde el día que nací, te pido por mi salud en mi lucha contra el SIDA" (Santo Niño de Atocha who has protected and cared for me from the day I was born, I ask you for my health in my struggle against AIDS) (figure 11.3). Floating above the horizon are two seemingly celestial images connected along a curved path. At one end is a church marked "Plateros" and at the other the smiling figure of El Santo Niño de Atocha encased in a white and gold aura. Plateros is the site of the sanctuary dedicated to El Santo Niño de Atocha, a small village in the area of Fresnillo, the artist's birthplace. At a reception for the artists, Juan recalled his childhood memories of making the pilgrimage on foot with his family to Plateros to visit the shrine of El Santo Niño. The image is marked by three dates, two incorporated into the image, and the other, in red, marking the date of signature. The first, Sept. 1964, appears next to a man and a woman carrying a child almost midway along the path, and suggests birth. The July 1989 date is situated below the path next to two images, one turned away from us with

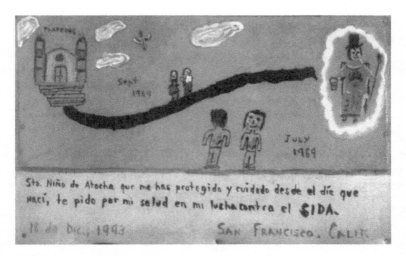

FIGURE 11.3. Juan Rodríguez, retablo, 1993.

the letters HIV and the other, crying figure facing the viewer, with the initials VIH emblazoned across his chest. Here the artist uses both the Spanish and English initials for human immunodeficiency virus to denote a possible date of diagnosis, although it is noteworthy that the image marked in Spanish, VIH, is the one facing us. These red letters physically mark the body, in the same way that an HIV diagnosis marks one physically, socially, and spiritually.

In the third image, the artist, Angel Borrero, rather than relying on the words that usually accompany *retablos*, uses a combination of symbols to construct his prayer (figure 11.4). These eclectic icons—yin and yang, the Sacred Heart, the Bible, the moon, an ankh, the symbol of infinity, a butterfly, and others—hover above a weeping naked red figure. Borrero redraws the precolonial ideographic codices to produce a new postcolonial, transcultural imaginary landscape. To his right an image of a conquistador stands above two dark statues spewing yellow and white liquids, possibly urine and semen. These seem to be creeping into the blue water-like surface below the reclined figure as sources of contamination. The "bodily fluids" depicted in this *retablo* also include the tears of the figure and the red bloodlike color of the body.[18] The recessed window peering out into a dark blue sky, situated in the center of the image, suggests the infinity of an afterlife, as the figure lies in a space between life and death.

This workshop and the images produced attempt to address the question posed by Alberto Sandoval-Sánchez, "What is the question of identity

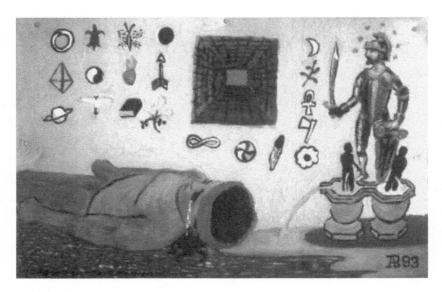

FIGURE 11.4. Angel Borrero, retablo, 1993.

for a person with AIDS? After the diagnosis and continuous symptoms and diseases, how is a new speaking-subject constituted, articulated, and configured?"[19] These artists are "speaking" their subjectivity through a visual language, but the medium and the context in which these articulations are produced respect both the process and singularity of individual subjectivity. This workshop and others like it reach toward an understanding of difference and affinity, of individual inscriptions of subjectivity within a larger political context of collective action and resistance.

"de(a)dicated to the one i love," a flyer advertising a reading from Bracho's Chicano gay writing workshop "(t)he (w)rites of mourning," transforms the lyrics of the oldies classic and juxtaposes it with an image of a fallen revolutionary hero, who lies bleeding, wrapped in the mantle of the Mexican flag (figure 11.5). The image/text plays with and against romanticized visions of Mexican nationalism and heterosexual romantic martyrdom, by situating them in a queer Latino context. In this refiguration of nationalism, as Bracho put it in his presentation, "dying for the nation" also becomes intermingled with "dying for love" in the age of the AIDS pandemic. It is the text, "de(a)dicated to the one i love," that calibrates the image within this new appropriated context. Yet that new queer reading is dependent on a particular kind of previous diasporic literacy, in this case the iconography

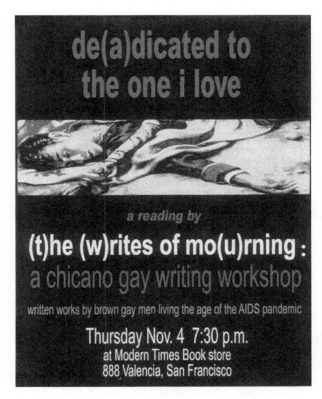

de(a)dicated to
the one i love

a reading by

(t)he (w)rites of mo(u)rning :
a chicano gay writing workshop

written works by brown gay men living the age of the AIDS pandemic

Thursday Nov. 4 7:30 p.m.
at Modern Times Book store
888 Valencia, San Francisco

FIGURE 11.5. Flyer designed by Ricardo Bracho and Willy B. Chavarria, 1993.

of Mexican independence and the relevance of sixties pop music to urban Chicano culture.[20]

Similarly, the flyer for a sex-positive women's retreat employs a 1927 photograph by the Peruvian Alberto Chambia titled *La Señorita Torera* to draw in the imagination of its audience (figure 11.6). The use of an image from the twenties with a sexually ambiguous figure serves to situate the Latina butch as part of a historical cultural iconography, to reclaim a queer Latina past. Again the framing text attempts to answer "what is it?" with the words *Tetatúd* and *el deseo es la fuerza* (the desire is the power), responding to questions about both the image and the idea of a sex-positive retreat. The term *sex positive* inverts the negative connotations of being "positive" in a queer context and resignifies it as a statement of resistance against the imposed sexual abnegation evidenced in much mainstream AIDS prevention. The word *tetatúd*, assembled from the phrase *actitud con tetas* (attitude with tits), was coined by Marcia Ochoa and Nancy Mirabal.

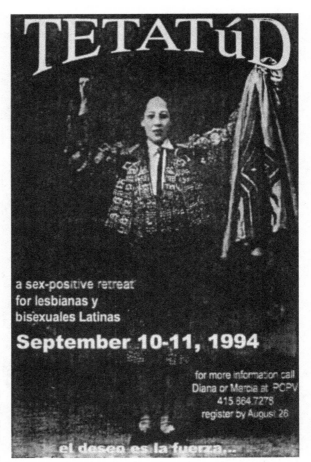

FIGURE 11.6.
Flyer produced by
Proyecto ContraSIDA
por Vida, 1994. Design
by Marcia Ochoa.

It is one of several neologisms employed in Proyecto's promotional materials and resonates with power and sexuality. Equally important, it was a catchy phrase, the significance of which traveled quickly throughout the communities it was intended to reach and beyond. Initially, the word *tetatúd* functioned as an intentionally imprecise translation for sex positive, evidencing the need to re-create or "trans-create" a sexual language in Spanish. Redefining the words that have been used to silence or shame us, reinterpreting them within a new queer cultural context that values sexual expression and sexual self-determination, subverts the hegemony of linguistic and cultural codes and uses language itself as an expression of agency.

¿Y Qué?

Recently, Proyecto has produced several new bilingual promotional brochures targeting specific audiences as part of its social marketing campaign.[21] The idea behind social marketing is to use traditional marketing tools "to 'sell' healthy behaviors to target audiences."[22] Proyecto's reconceptualization of social marketing extends this concept to confront community norms and values. Rather than simply using advertising to advocate condom use or promote its services, Proyecto's promotional materials invite the audience to challenge ideas about sexuality, culture, representation, and communities. One such brochure, titled *What's the T?* is geared toward transgenders. It is small, bright, colorful, and seductive. The opening text reads, "Pues, tú sabes, we the T. Transgenders, that is. Oh, so who exactly are transgenders? Well, that's anyone experimenting with their biological sex. This includes a whole lot of folks, so it's safe to say anyone who calls themself a transgender is one." "What's the T?" is San Francisco queer barrio-speak for what's up? new? hot? happening? The text directly engages the reader and responds to a question, "What's the T?" but shifts it into a new context of meaning. Inside appear the words *Props, Respeto, Riesgo, Risk, Presence, Presencia, Rhythm, Ritmo, Magic,* and *Magia.* Though these words include the repetition of translation, there is no attempt to make them equivalent or even parallel. The word *Respeto,* for example, is translated as *Props,* borrowing from an intersecting queer and urban lexicon.

The front image is of a papaya, already charged as a visual and linguistic female sexual signifier for many Latinos/as, sliced both vertically and horizontally and situated so the pieces fit together to suggest a female sex (figure 11.7).[23] Inverted, it becomes a small penis and the circular hole dripping with shiny black seeds becomes an anus, suggesting the rich complexity of organic forms, magic, and incisions as a metaphor for transgender realities. A group picture included in the flyer depicts a diverse set of individuals consciously posing for the camera (figure 11.8). A frequently stated or unstated response to this photograph is the question, "Are they all transgenders?" An equally charged question might also be, "Are they all Latinos?" It is the question rather than the answer that produces the moment of critical intervention, forcing a confrontation with assumptions about transgender identities and communities. Rather than relying on authorial strategies of representation or explicative narratives, the image draws in the viewers' faculties of interpretation.

In a flyer geared at youth, *¡Y QUE! Young, Queer & Under Emergency,* photographs, images, and text work together to lure and entice, to make action, *vida,*

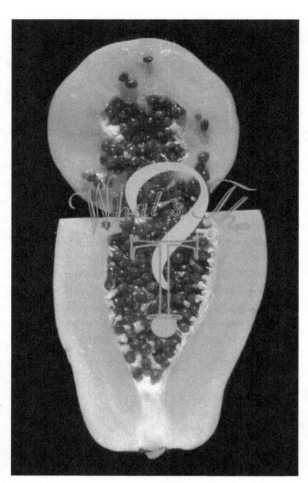

FIGURE 11.7.
Flyer produced by
Proyecto ContraSIDA
por Vida, 1997. Design
by Jill Bressler, Pail of
Water Design. Photo-
graph by Patrick "Pato"
Hebert. Text by spikxil-
dren kolectiv.

and learning desirable and even sexy (figure 11.9). It is a message of exploring options, of figuring it out together, of doing something for yourself and
for others. The language is sweet and *picante* at once; layers of barrio youth
Spanish and English rub and play together. As in the flyer *What's the T?* the
text appears in both English (heavily spiked with Spanglish) and a more
standard but still colloquial Spanish. The opening "English" text reads, "Was-
sup mujer? Qué onda homeboy? What's up with your young, fine Latina/o
lesbian, gay, transgender, bisexual or just curious self? If you got questions
about coming out, dealing con tu familia, friends and your sweet thang, and
how you can help stop the spread of HIV en tu barrio y entre tu gente. . . .
Pues, then you gots to come check out ¡Y Q.U.E.!" Inside it offers youth a

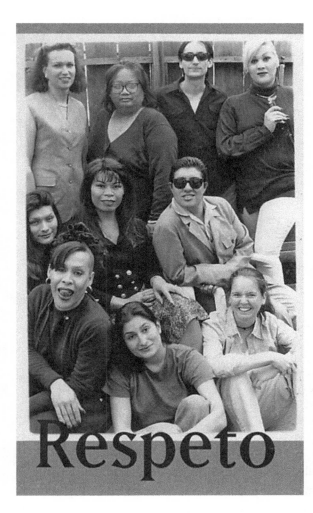

FIGURE 11.8. Flyer produced by Proyecto ContraSIDA por Vida, 1997. Design by Jill Bressler, Pail of Water Design. Photograph by Patrick "Pato" Hebert. Text by spikxildren kolectiv.

whole range of opportunities for self-discovery and self-expression, from resume writing and participation in one of Colegio ContraSIDA's many youth-specific classes or rap groups to learning street outreach and tabling. It also tells them that Proyecto is a place where you can come by and just "kick it on the couch with your friends."

¡Y QUE! (so what? or literally, and what?) functions as a response to the hailing of the subject, a response to the names *jota, macha, vestida*. It is a statement against the totalizing implications of interpellation. By responding to the injurious name with a question, rather than an explanation, a counterattack, or a claim to misrecognition, it shifts the focus back onto the author and

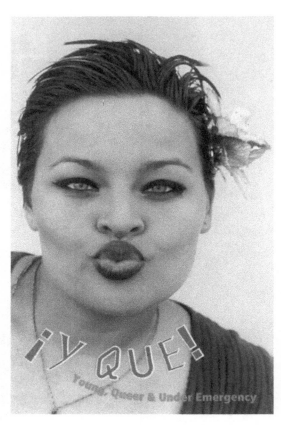

FIGURE 11.9. Flyer produced by Proyecto ContraSIDA por Vida, 1997. Design by Jill Bressler, Pail of Water Design. Photograph by Patrick "Pato" Hebert. Text by spikxildren kolectiv.

the authority that hails. *¡Y QUE!* forces an interrogation of the constructed significance of those names. It deflects the power of naming away from the singularity of the hailed subject and restates it as an indictment of heteronormative authority to name and thus define.

Included in the brochure are two panels that echo the words of what other youth think about *¡Y QUE!* Some of the quotes read, "Me siento en casa" (I feel at home), "Me di cuenta de mi misma y mi comunidad" (I became aware of myself and my community), and "I'm going to become an advocate for lesbian safe sex."[24] These responses capture the multiple levels of empowerment and discovery available through Proyecto's programming and presence—creating a space of safety and support, offering a space for conscious and critical learning about ourselves and our relationship to the world, and serving as a springboard for collective and individual action. In fact, many of the queer youth affiliated with Proyecto as volunteers, clients, or staff have gone on to gain employment in other community-based service and arts organizations, testifying to the material benefits of the formal and informal job skills (public speaking, teaching, community outreach, public relations, computer skills, and direct service) gained through their association with Proyecto.

The prevalence of Spanglish in Proyecto's textual self-representation suggests its dynamism as a powerful language of *activismo*. Yet the ability to make sense of linguistic codes is also constructed by age, geography, culture, and experience; each constitutes an important vector of analysis in social mappings of insider/outsider. Linguistic and cultural codes, however, create permeable borders that can be traversed through knowledge and affiliation. Understanding how these borders are constructed and mediated also gives us another way to understand and appreciate the cultural phenomenon of US African American *santeros*, Filipina artists constructing altars for El Día de los Muertos, or barrio-bred Anglo *cholos* cruising the Mission in their low-riding Impalas. A shared cultural and spiritual heritage, a mutual colonial religion, or a common city block create the organic conditions for the expression of these cultural affinities to emerge. Very often, however, conscious attempts to learn about a culture only serve to reveal the intricacies, complexities, and depth of cultural codes. The process of cultural affiliation, appropriation, and transformation occurs interethnically, but it also takes place within ethnic groups. Particularly for Spanish speakers, participation in the multiethnic, multicultural, multinational, multigenerational Latino community of San Francisco necessitates a willingness to learn and adapt to new cultural idioms, regional synonyms, and local vernacular.

On a political and collective level, this multilingualism becomes an acquired skill used to navigate different discursive spaces in order to achieve specific goals: to reach and inspire different constituents; to get and maintain funding; to learn about viral counts, double blind studies, and the language of pharmacology; to manipulate the intricacies of the legal system; or to access the resources of the social service sector. Understanding the ways communities are structured linguistically assumes paramount importance in creating promotional materials that speak the languages of their target audiences. Part of Proyecto's success has been its ability to speak and respond in multiple registers of language in order to reach different constituents. In addition to the interlingual mission statement cited earlier, Proyecto also has a more "traditional" monolingual mission statement directed toward its various funding sources, and has recently produced Spanish and English

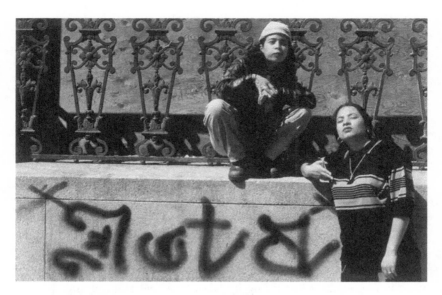

FIGURE 11.10. Photograph taken on set by Patrick "Pato" Hebert, from *Sabrosura*, directed by Janelle Rodríguez, 1996.

versions of a newly conceived mission statement directed at a more general audience.

The final text for consideration is the three-minute public service announcement for Proyecto titled *Sabrosura* (Tastiness), directed by a young Puerto Rican filmmaker, Janelle Rodríguez.[25] This fast-paced, colorful collage of moving images is set to the sizzling sounds of salsa and relies almost exclusively on visual language to promote its message. In her comments following the film's screening, Rodríguez noted that the film involved twenty-three separate location shoots and the collaborative work of eighty individuals. Most of the film is shot in the bright light of day and draws heavily on the local color of the urban geography. It intercuts scenes depicting young *cholos* and *cholas* flirting against a backdrop of one of San Francisco's many vibrant murals, wrestling in grass, dancing on the steps of Mission High School, masturbating in the dim light of a bedroom, marching down Market Street, kissing on street corners, hanging out in Dolores Park, and cruising through *el barrio* (figure 11.10).

Advocating and eroticizing safer sex forms part of the message. In one scene a fierce femme blots her lipstick through a dental dam; in another a young cholo flashes a rainbow collection of condoms; in still another a lounging Diane Felix, Proyecto's program director, slowly slides a condom down a banana. *Cultura* is everywhere, but it is the cultural hybridity of San Francisco's Latino community that is evident rather than any specific national or regional culture. Leana Valencia, wearing a traditional multilayered Mexican dress, spins her skirt to the soundtrack of a Caribbean salsa beat; another shot captures a zoot suiter flashing the twists and turns of a veteran *salsero*. In one scene, reminiscent of a gang jumping in ceremony, a topless Ruben Carillo, Proyecto's intake specialist, is held down and sprayed with a hose in slow motion as he playfully resists. Proyecto is about *familia*, but it is also about a new gang of urban warriors "fighting the spread of HIV disease and the other unnatural disasters of racism, sexism, homophobia, xenophobia and poverty." The message of the film is that belonging to a community is life-affirming, safer sex is sexy, that activism is about reclaiming the streets where you live and play. The film is meant to turn you on; the rhythm and energy of the music and images are contagious, they make you want to join the party, join the gang, join the movement. The film is not about explaining or translating experiences or culture. It is representation without explication. The individuals who appear in the footage may not all be Latina/a or queer. Some of them may be sex workers or academics, some of them may shoot drugs and others may be celibate. There is no attempt to make representation and identity equivalent. Yet in the final scene they all come together under the banner of Proyecto ContraSIDA por Vida: "a community dedicated to living."

Proyecto's willingness to address the issues of desire and difference, fear and power, evidenced in representations of subjectivity, respects and fosters the deployment of agency as a tool for individual and collective empowerment. Its programming, cultural production, and critical practices function as missiles of resistance against the hegemonic structures that demand our conformity or erasure. Proyecto's strategies for survival and resistance creatively engage and transform ideas of visibility, identity, representation, community, and activism within the ruins of postmodern representation. In the process, Proyecto has also succeeded in impacting the lived realities of some of the most disenfranchised members of queer Latina/o communities: immigrants, youth, IV drug users, sex workers, transgender people, and people living with HIV and AIDS. Toward that end, Proyecto has trained and supported a new generation of artists, activists, thinkers, and community workers to respond to the state of emergency that constitutes queer life *en el barrio* and in the world. Proyecto creates spaces where not only individual "subjects-in-process" emerge but where the collective subject of "community-in-process" is also given an open venue for expression, self-representation, and self-discovery.

Unlike other plagues and pandemics, the nightmare of AIDS has been used by activists as an attempt to bring diverse sectors together to talk about the ways death and sex are represented in our diverse communities, to begin to understand how our fears and desires unite us. AIDS itself creates a community of ghosts, linked through transmission. Bracho writes, "Given that it takes one to infect one, in aids heaven there is a relationality, a collectivity that undoes the individuated singularity of Western morbidity."[26] Perhaps the ironic collectivity that we share in death will serve as the occasion for our collective will to creatively circumvent the systematized divisiveness that haunts our organizing efforts, an homage to our shared ghosts enacted through our daily practices of survivance and resistance.

Postscript: Los Jodidos/The Fucked Peepo

OCTOBER 7, 2017

If there is an afterword to the activist legacy of Proyecto ContraSIDA por Vida and the kind of community engagement that it inspired then, that word is *gentrification*. Proyecto closed its doors in 2005, and the scant remaining energies left in its wake were poured into its successor, El/La Para Trans-Latinas, which opened in 2006 and has been struggling to survive ever since with a much smaller budget and a more focused mission. As housing prices have risen in the Mission District, poor, working-class people of color have moved out, and white, more educated, and wealthier people have moved in, riding the tumultuous waves of the tech boom and housing market that have left San Francisco one of the most expensive cities in the United States. By 2015, 60 percent of all leases in San Francisco were for technology companies, making it hard for nonprofits to compete but also driving up rents for local residents and driving away the club spaces, art spaces, and community venues that had created such a vibrant, multicultural scene in the first place.

Like AIDS, the ghosts of gentrification perform their own slow death of disappearance and erasure. In the 1980s and 1990s, queer Latinx immigrants to San Francisco, whether arriving from the agricultural towns of California's Central Valley or as sexiled refugees from Havana, Mexico City, or San Salvador, thought they had arrived at the promised land—a place to live and die together; a land of queer salsa, hunky vaqueros, and multilingual sexcapades. But increasingly, the thriving multigendered, multicultural, multigenerational community that helped bring Proyecto into existence has slowly slid off the map. With the arrival of PrEP and new kinds of retrovirus cocktails, HIV infection and AIDS have become manageable conditions for those who can manage, where managing is often a code for being white, educated, employed, and connected to the dominant gay male scene in the city. But Proyecto was always about more than just responding to HIV and AIDS; it was a project of community health and healing from the "unnatural disasters of racism, sexism, homophobia, xenophobia and poverty," and that work remains crucial to our collective survival.[27]

Today, as we fight back against state-sanctioned and increasingly emboldened attacks against immigrants and queers; against the undocumented, the homeless, the poor and the disabled; against transgender peoples' right to pee or sex workers' right to work; against Black, Brown, and Native peoples' ability to walk, drive, protest, or just live free from police violence, the risks facing our communities are just as life threatening and our collective work is just as urgent. Having survived the AIDS pandemic (if only for now), those of us still committed to a "community dedicated to living" are struggling to keep the spirit of community and the space of utopian possibility that Proyecto embodied alive. But, if "activism is an engagement with the hauntings of history," much of the queer Latinx activism now is also about mourning the loss of what used to be.[28]

Few if any of the original crew of Proyecto can afford to live in San Francisco anymore. Today, when and if we are called back to the city from our new disparate locations spread across Oakland, Richmond, San José, and other more affordable and less picturesque localities, we are the ones who now haunt the hipster corridors of a city that no longer has a place for us. But one summer evening in 2017, we were called back to witness the gentrified remains of the city that made the vision of Proyecto possible. Performance artist Xandra Ibarra, née La Chica Boom, invited us—the queer-, trans-, Latinx-plus community—on a walking tour of the Mission district for a piece she called "The Hookup/Displacement/Barhopping/Drama Tour." This mobile public performance functioned as a moving funeral procession commemorating the death of a neighborhood that we once called our own, a chance to publicly mourn all that we have lost in recent years. In her description of the event, Ibarra wrote:

> I can still hear the music, feel los dedos, smell the sobacos and see the drag queen mugre on the walls of our old neighborhood haunts EVEN after they resurfaced as sterile establishments. I KNOW you can too ... you just need a little motavation.
>
> Let's invade, resurface, and imprint our titties, besos sucios, and pleasures on the phantom walls of our adored queer nightlife venues!

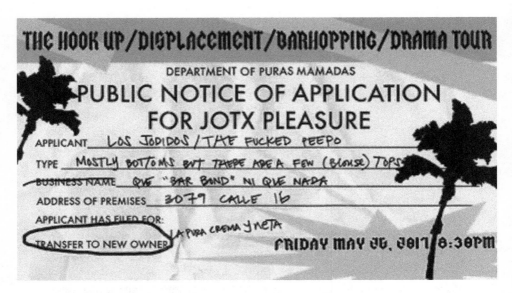

THC HOOK UP/DISPLACCMCNT/BARHOPPING/DRAMA TOUR

DEPARTMENT OF PURAS MAMADAS

PUBLIC NOTICE OF APPLICATION
FOR JOTX PLEASURE

APPLICANT ___LOS JODIDOS / THE FUCKED PEEPO___

TYPE ___MOSTLY BOTTOMS BUT THERE ARE A FEW (BLOUSE) TOPS___

~~BUSINESS NAME~~ QVE "BAR BOND" NI QVE NADA

ADDRESS OF PREMISES ___3079 CALLE 16___

APPLICANT HAS FILED FOR:
LA PURA CREMA Y NETA
TRANSFER TO NEW OWNER   FRIDAY MAY 26, 2017 8:30PM

FIGURE 11.11. Xandra Ibarra, performance permit. Courtesy of the artist.

> Join me as I barhop to 5 former beloved queer Latino and Lezzi historic sites in the Mission!!!"[29]

An homage to what once was, the performance piece also enacted an insistence on the radical potential of exerting our continued presence. Like so many of Proyecto's own published texts, Ibarra's language intentionally code switches to perform a playful localized urban vernacular, hailing those participants who know how to interpret the linguistic codes presented. In a swipe at the need for the city to authorize the use of public space, Ibarra created her own permissions from the Department of Puras Mamadas, a "Public Notice of Application for Jotx Pleasure," listing the applicants as "Los Jodidos/The Fucked Peepo" (figure 11.11).[30]

The event assembled a ragtag band of aging Latinx memory seekers hugging old friends and fellow survivors, an equal number of younger queer performance artist types, many newly arrived to a city they had dreamed of making their own, and anyone else who wandered into the fray. The first stop was the iconic Esta Noche (1979–2014), the last queer Latinx bar to close in the Mission. Of the numerous sites on the Drama Tour, Esta Noche was the longest lived and its closure was most deeply felt. In his essay "The Dirt That Haunts: Looking at Esta Noche," Iván Ramos describes it as "an explicitly working class Latino gay bar that catered to a queer Latino microcosm of culture, adoration, and desires."[31] There in the alley, against the wall where so many of us had grinded our queer desires onto the crotches of strangers, Ibarra projected excerpts from the 1994 film *¡Viva 16!*, directed by Valentin Aguirre and Augie Robles, a visual reminder of the vibrant club and street scene that had once existed at the corner of Sixteenth and Mission. The film's projection onto the walls of the alley, screened onto the bodies of those of us in attendance, created a kind of virtual communion with the dead—allowing us to dance, mingle, and flirt, if just for a moment, with the floating presence of friends now gone, with younger versions of our own aging bodies, and with a community that is being forcibly disappeared. As the procession traveled to the five spots designated on Ibarra's Drama Tour—La India Bonita (1970s–1996); Amelia's (1978–91); the Lexington Club (1997–2015); and Osento's Bathhouse (1979–2008)—participants stopped to make out on the streets, shout at the new skinny blond residents in Spanish, snap selfies, and refresh our motivation. As a group, we responded as best we could to Ibarra's demands to keep it *bien sucio*, real dirty. The event description stated that "sexual activity with the architecture of our old haunts and/or people is encouraged."[32] At each location, participants set up altars in the nearby alleys, leaving behind flowers, carnival beads, dildos, and empty condom wrappers, chalking up the sidewalks with pink and purple messages of our love and hate. All the spaces of *jotería* in the Mission are gone, but so are all of the "Lezzie" spaces, the bookstore, the bars, the bathhouse, erased from the newly sanitized city made safe for tech workers and their bright white families of urban pioneers.

So much of the affective work of Proyecto was about teaching us how to deal with the loss and devastation that surrounded the AIDS pandemic, creating a space where we could mourn, dream, and create—together. Being together, being in close physical proximity to the places and the people that affirmed our right to exist, made so much of that work possible. Today, the white supremacist state is trying to make an example of California, punishing our sanctuary cities, trying to dismantle our public education system, and making access to health care more impossible while unchecked development fuels the never-ending needs of the tech sector for more yoga studios and vegan burritos. Forced evictions, skyrocketing rents, and a lack of community services combine with the notoriously racist, sexist, ageist hiring practices of the tech sector to feed a growing income gap and opportunity gap for those displaced and shut out of the new "bro"-based economy that has taken over the city. But that night, on Ibarra's Drama Tour, some of us managed to "expose avenues of pleasures buried away under the sign of tech progress."[33] Like ghosts summoned from the great beyond, those of us close enough to answer Ibarra's call showed up for ourselves, each other, and a vision of another way of living and loving—making a fleshy spectacle of our broken hearts, smearing our disease- and trauma-stained fluids over the power-washed sidewalks of a city we once called home, our stubborn commitment to survive serving as the ultimate revenge against those who plot our erasure.

Notes

Adapted from Juana María Rodríguez, "Activism and Identity in the Ruins of Representation," in *Queer Latinidad: Identity Practices, Discursive Spaces* (New York: New York University Press, 2003), 37–83. © 2003 Reprinted by permission of NYU Press.

1 In its promotional materials, it is variously referred to by its full name, by the initials PCPV, or as Proyecto. I refer to it as Proyecto throughout the body of the text.

2 Origin stories are always fraught with controversy. Nevertheless, it seems appropriate to offer a narrative that accounts for the genesis of Proyecto. It emerged from the National Task Force on AIDS Prevention (NTFAP), where Jesse James Johnson and Juan Rodríguez worked at the time; they would be the first director and assistant director. The first national gay men of color HIV organization, NTFAP was also Proyecto's first fiscal agent from 1993 to 1998. The initial founders of Proyecto included Ricardo Bracho, Diane Felix, Jesse Johnson, Hector León, Reggie Williams, and Martín Ornellas-Quintero.

3 The order cited is not intended to present a chronological, linear, or developmental progression. Many of these groups and movements emerged simultaneously and there exist both significant overlap and divergence relative to individuals, ideology, and social context.

4 The Harm Reduction Coalition, with offices in Oakland, California, and New York City, states in its promotional brochure: "Harm reduction accepts, for better and for worse, that licit and illicit drug use is part of our world and chooses to work to minimize its harmful effects rather than simply ignore or condemn them." Proyecto's reformulation of harm reduction extends this philosophy toward the practices of safer sex, stressing reducing risk whenever possible rather than simply condemning or ignoring unsafe sexual practices.

5 See the 1994 film *¡Viva 16!*, directed by Valentin Aguirre and Augie Robles.

6 Ferriss, "Mission Meets Castro," A12.

7 The phrase *unnatural disaster* is borrowed from Yamada, "Invisibility Is an Unnatural Disaster."

8 Proyecto began at Eighteenth and Dolores, then moved to its storefront offices at Sixteenth and Mission.

9 PCPV, "Calendar of Events," promotional calendar, 1994.

10 Ricardo Bracho to Juana María Rodríguez, August 8, 1997.

11 Lisa Arellanes, to Juana María Rodríguez, September 4, 1997.

12 Among the many community-based programs Proyecto has worked with in the past are Mission Neighborhood Health Center, Haight Ashbury Free Clinic, Institute for Community Health Outreach, Asian and Pacific Islanders Wellness Center, New Leaf, Lavender Youth Recreation and Information Center (LYRIC), Young Brothers Program, and Tenderloin AIDS Resource Center. Arts organizations Proyecto has collaborated with include Galeria de la Raza, Folsom Street Interchange for the Arts, Mission Cultural Center, the Mexican Museum, Artists Television Access (ATA), Cine Acción, San Francisco Cinemateque, and Brava for Women in the Arts.

13 This popular refrain is often credited to "¿Y tu agüela a'onde ejtá?," a poem written in the local Afro-Antillian vernacular by the Afro–Puerto Rican poet Fortunato Vizcarrondo. It is a reference to the practice of negating dark-skinned ancestors or relatives.

14 Unless otherwise indicated, all the flyers were produced in-house at Proyecto without credits, using appropriated images from a variety of sources. This disinvestment in authorial ownership seems particularly significant as an expression of collective subjectivity and a commitment to collective representation.

15 Patton, *Inventing AIDS*, 5.

16 The instructors for Proyecto's classes are too numerous to cite individually; however, I feel compelled to name several of the instructors who formed part of the Proyecto village: Patrick "Pato" Hebert and Marcia Ochoa co-taught the "Jotografía" class; Jaime Cortez, the comic book artist, writer, and editor of *A la Brava: A Queer Latino/a Zine*, taught "La Raza Cósmica Comix"; the writer and playwright Jorge Ignacio Cortiñas taught the writing class "Bemba Bilingüe: Double Tonguing"; the visual artist Wura-Natasha Ogunji taught "girl-colored"; the photographer Laura Aguilar and Patrick "Pato" Hebert taught "Diseños del Deseo: Sexual Self-Imaging in Photography"; Horacio Roque Ramírez taught "Te Toca la Tinta"; Marcia Ochoa and Lebasi Lashley taught "Cyberspace for Women"; Ana Berta Campos taught a Spanish-language video class for women; and Al Lujan taught "Altarations," an altar-making workshop. Other instructors are mentioned throughout the text.

17 PCPV, "Calendar of Events."

18 All three of these artists died from AIDS shortly after these images were produced; they are remembered with love.

19 Sandoval-Sánchez, "Response to the Representation of AIDS," 183.

20 This class was funded by NTFAP and preceded Proyecto; however, it served as an inspirational and organizational model for Colegio and brought together individuals who would later become significant in the genesis of the organization, including Juan Rodríguez, Jesse Johnson, Valentín Aguirre, Augie Robles, Loras Ojeda, and Willy B. Chavarria, to name a few.

21 These two flyers were funded by the Department of Public Health-AIDS Office.
22 San Francisco HIV Prevention Planning Council and Department of Public Health AIDS Office, *San Francisco HIV Prevention Plan*, 402.
23 In certain cultural circles, particularly in many parts of Cuba, papaya is a reference to vagina.
24 Unless otherwise noted, all translations are my own. In this portion of the flyer that records participants' responses, the quotes are not translated and instead appear in the languages in which they were recorded.
25 *Sabrosura* never aired as a PSA on local television stations but was shown at various national and international film festivals.
26 Bracho to Juana María Rodríguez, August 8, 1997.
27 PCPV, "Calendar of Events," promotional calendar, 1994.
28 Rodríguez, *Queer Latinidad*, 37.
29 La Chica Boom, "Hook Up." My translation notes are decidedly imprecise. *Dedos* are fingers; *sobacos* are armpits; *mugre* is filth; *motavation* is a neologism that draws on one of the many Spanish-language terms for marijuana, *mota*; *besos sucios* are dirty kisses.
30 *Puras mamadas* refers to pure bullshit, but *mamada* also refers to blowjobs. Los Jodidos is accurately translated as "The Fucked Peepo." The new owners are listed as "La pura crema y neta," which could be translated as the cream of the crop; *neta* can be used to signify something wonderful but also to signal the truth of something.
31 Ramos, "Dirt That Haunts," 135.
32 La Chica Boom, "Hook Up."
33 Ramos, "Dirt That Haunts."

Bibliography

La Chica Boom. "The Hook Up/Displacement/Barhopping/ Drama Tour." Accessed September 5, 2017. https://www.facebook .com/events/168340807031647/?acontext=%7B%22action _history%22%3A%22null%22%7D.
Ferriss, Susan. "Mission Meets Castro." *San Francisco Examiner*, June 1, 1997, A12.
Patton, Cindy. *Inventing AIDS*. New York: Routledge, 1990.
Ramos, Iván A. "The Dirt That Haunts: Looking at Esta Noche." *Studies in Gender and Sexuality* 16, no. 2 (2015): 135–36. doi:10.1080/15240657.2015.1038195.
Rodríguez, Janelle, dir. *Sabrosura*. Proyecto ContraSIDA por Vida (PCPV), San Francisco, 1996. https://www.youtube.com/watch?v=kDsPB8IfPzY.
Rodríguez, Juana María. *Queer Latinidad: Identity Practices, Discursive Spaces*. New York: New York University Press, 2003.
Sandoval-Sánchez, Alberto. "A Response to the Representation of AIDS in the Puerto Rican Arts and Literature: In the Manner of a Proposal for a Cultural

Studies Project." *Centro: Journal of the Center for Puerto Rican Studies* 6, nos. 1–2 (1994): 181–86.

San Francisco HIV Prevention Planning Council and Department of Public Health AIDS Office. *San Francisco HIV Prevention Plan, 1997.* San Francisco: Harder and Company Community Research, 1996.

Yamada, Mitsuye. "Invisibility Is an Unnatural Disaster: Reflections of an Asian American Woman." *Bridge: An Asian American Perspective* 7, no. 1 (1979): 11–13.

TWELVE DISPATCHES FROM THE FUTURES OF AIDS

A Dialogue between Emily Bass, Pato Hebert,
Elton Naswood, Margaret Rhee, and Jessica Whitbread,
with Images by Quito Ziegler and an Introduction by Alexandra Juhasz

I am going to switch to the first person here. It's Alex. It's not me smoothed over or mixed in with my coeditors, a gesture and approach that has heretofore signaled our solidarity, compromise, listening, and respect. Those commitments have not left me—not in the least—but I need to write this last introduction from my perspective alone for two reasons. First, I'm not sure how Nishant and Jih-Fei feel about the future right now, as I write this in the summer of 2018, as we wrap up this collection and as the world falls ever more precipitously from beneath our feet, but with every passing day we seem to notice this less—or is it more?—and is that an I or a we? It's hard for me to tell. So, I won't speak of the present for them or on our behalf because the future (of AIDS in and of our world, at least looking out from the besieged and besieging United States in 2018) seems uncertain, yet again, and also violent and desperately sad; and because of this, I can only write about my reading of my colleagues' dispatches about the "Futures of AIDS" with the feeling and honesty that I find, and need, and learn from them, modeled below. Our writers deserve this reciprocity; they gave us their words written in 2017 (and time-stamped, marking these realities of crises) as just this sort of gesture of individual-in-community.

Who are these amazing individuals that you are about to read, how did we find them, and why did they join us? As is true of all the dispatches, and for the collection more generally, to find our contributors, Jih-Fei, Nishant, and I shared and grew our personal connections in the field, keeping our eyes on the significant array of talents, perspectives, locales, and approaches that create and sustain us.

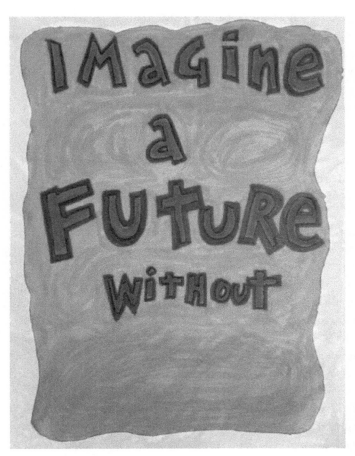

FIGURE 12.1.
Created by
Quito Ziegler.

For this last round of introductions, I would like to take a little time to explain how we came to this particular grouping. My introductions to these contributors follow the circuits by which they came to me (not their order in the text that follows). I know no better way to honor how intellectual, artistic, and activist communities are actually born, shaped, and sustained. Taking time is one way that we claim a hold on our futures. When we find (the time) and work with each other, in any place of crisis, we push against the "dystopian collapse" that Margaret Rhee felt so strongly in 2017. Even if this is only in temporary or rushed engagements—there are so many more places to run, as Emily Bass suggests—or even if we only get to stay still momentarily, rubbing shoulders when we share words on a page. We make space and time for our others. There and then, we remind ourselves that we cohabit our crises, together, for each other.

Anthologies, asynchronous dispatches, and other places where we fabricate connection evidence our courageous efforts to aspire to and speak together about a difficult present and perhaps a better future, particularly in times and places of fear and despair. I think this defines a good deal of how we have lived through the long and varied lives of HIV/AIDS: our political, communal, and personal responses seem to take all of our effort and mutual commitment in any one moment; and yet, somehow, we find both more time and more of ourselves to give each other later. Critically, these rough but sustaining efforts are often volunteered. This is especially true for the several activists, people with HIV and/or AIDS, and artists in these dispatches for whom writing for us here is not part of any scholarly portfolio. We do this to stay politically alert, to learn from what others have taken the time to learn and make and share, and to invest in the hope "that acts of kindness are stronger than acts of fear and that strong, united hearts can overcome the inequalities of this world," as Jessica Whitbread writes here.

I know Jessica through her contributions to Visual AIDS, an organization with which I, too, often partner, volunteer, and engage. She is also a friend and collaborator of my friend and collaborator Theodore (Ted) Kerr, whom I met when he was working there. Jessica Whitbread often uses her own body and experience as a queer woman living with HIV as the primary site of her work. She puts strong words onto images, like her plastic cross-stitch collaboration with Allyson Mitchell: FUCK POSITIVE WOMEN.

"It is not a silence but a linguistic sliding that is happening," writes Emily Bass about current changes and cuts to international AIDS efforts. Ted also introduced me to Emily. I read her "How to Survive a Footnote: AIDS Activism in the 'After' Years" (Fall 2015) when Ted circulated it for his PDF club, a loose group of readers who came together to read and discuss selected writing about HIV/AIDS. Her health-related journalism circulates widely, and at the same time, she travels in similar social and activist circles to me. Emily is an advocate, communicator, and strategist with twenty years of experience focusing on a rights-based response to HIV prevention and treatment.

"What is powerful is our refusal for unidirectional directions, and our preference for difference and participatory conversation and making," writes Margaret Rhee. I met Margaret when she reached out to me, refusing unidirectionality, because she wanted to engage together around her HIV prison media activist/academic work (her doctoral and activist research and art making), which she connects to the activism and scholarship I conducted during my own doctoral research on AIDS media decades before. A feminist experimental poet, new media artist, and scholar, her research focuses on technology and its intersections with feminist, queer, and ethnic studies. I have learned about, and together practiced, such "dynamic ways that grass-roots organizing is cultivating a world where AIDS need not overwhelm our very ability to flourish and be free," as Pato Hebert writes here, with many friends and colleagues. Pato and I, too, are longtime collaborators who met first as college teachers but aligned forever through our shared commitments to AIDS activist art making inside and crossing between the academy and AIDS service organizations. He is an artist, educator, and organizer whose work explores the aesthetics, ethics, and poetics of interconnectedness. From this I have benefited, learning from him about the porous boundaries between disenfranchised people, the possibility of their voice in the right circumstances, and our capacities to hear.

Speaking of circumstance needing to be heard, Pato introduced me to his colleague Elton Naswood when they were both at AIDS Project Los Angeles. Jih-Fei also knows Elton through their friend R. Benedito Ferrão. Pato and I had invited Elton to engage with us in a shared art project years ago about activism on the internet. His contributions were steady, eloquent, knowledgeable, and deeply in the space of HIV that is held by Native Americans. According to his bio on the website for the fourteenth Circle of Harmony HIV/AIDS Wellness Conference, he "is of the Near to the Water People Clan, born for the Edge Water People Clan, his maternal grandfather's clan is of the Mexican People, and his paternal grandfather's clan is of the Tangle people, this is how he is Navajo, *Dine*."[1] I was saddened when he couldn't speak for himself about his view of the future, but I am certain that his silencing will speak some of the volumes we need to and can hear even so: "Repeal of the ACA will lead to AI/ANs having less access to health services, less options for care, worsening health disparities, increased unnecessary suffering, and an increase in preventable deaths."

Expanding possibilities for care in the face of diminished health supports inspires Quito Ziegler to draw their vision of the future in pen and ink: "Imagine a World without Prisons." Imagine no prisons of silence or walls, no prisons of an industrial complex that monetizes suffering and racism expanding and producing the circumstances for the movement and pain of AIDS. I met Quito through their anti-Trump activism and New York–based curatorial projects focusing on gender-nonbinary and trans art and activism with a feminist, antiracist heart. Online, Quito explains many of their interests that brought me to request their artwork for this effort: "They are particularly fond of collective movie-making, organizing an annual intergenerational retreat for queer artists who are surviving or have survived transience, and dreaming up the trans-feminist world of the future."[2] We see images of their openhanded imagining here. I reached out to them because I had seen these images and thought they might raise all our spirits. I needed that.

Over the two or more years we have been making this book, I have led and read and edited this section many times. I read it again today, in the summer of 2018, right after rereading Cindy Patton's eloquent foreword and our own stately introduction. Writing and reading books, while not crises in the least, are other methods and places for asynchronous, fractured time and place, disruptions of the best kind. Along these lines, the dispatches were written in 2017, my introduction in 2018, and this book will be released in 2020. The crises we name change. We do not see the world, or our actions in it, as one. Nor are we sages; we can only guess what the future will be. But we are educated, decent people who can learn from history, and each other, about how humans can and do strive to contribute to one of the many futures we might desire. There is always the possibility for hope, or at least action, or words, even as I might feel despair and fear about Trumpism and its powerful steamrollering over what we have already done, and the course of what HIV might be in the future. We are willing to try even so, to imagine, and work, for us I suppose, for nothing more than the reality and hope of us.

All of the many authors of this anthology have done this: worked hard to see and share the violence that has already happened in the past and is being magnified in this present; the fine work that we have done that is being distorted and torn apart; the new work that we will continue to do, even so.

Patton ends her foreword: "Is it happening?" I think it is. All of it: the "capitulation(s)" in "increments and acceptable diction shifts" that Bass saw in 2017 and anticipates more of; the suicides that Whitbread suffers as the brutal AIDS deaths of her day-to-day life; the fact that Naswood cannot speak about and during this administration; the beauty of these efforts, even so. Emily reminds us that "how we speak will pave the road that lies ahead." And Jessica asks, *"How can I focus in on you being as open and amazing and wonderful as possible?"*

The "shadow gestures" of callous cruelty can be met by our words of overt honesty, intelligence, and self- and communal care. To "Live the Future Now" means to write and read as we want to live, with the furor, fear, pain, and honesty of our time and place, with disruption but without its crisis.

—*Alexandra Juhasz*

Prompt 1

Alexandra Juhasz: The recent election of Donald Trump and his era of Trumpism endangers our future health as humans and as a society. In your first answer, can you reflect upon how current health-related policies and commitments of the current administration affect your/AIDS futures or that of your work/organization (i.e., the repeal of the Affordable Care Act; attacks on reproductive health and Planned Parenthood; the removal of HIV/AIDS from the White House website; impacts on mental health care, access to substance abuse treatment, and/or disabled populations who rely on Medicaid for independent living, etc.)? What are you doing, what can be done, to insure our ongoing health?

Jessica Whitbread: As a community organizer, artist, activist, academic, and at times a "professional," I am interested in doing work that creates spaces for dialogue about social justice and social change. I do this through public installations, consciousness raising, workshop development and facilitation, engaging in direct action, policy review, research, and any other method that allows a variety of stakeholders to engage in a diversity of ways. I believe that acts of kindness are stronger than acts of fear and that strong, united hearts can overcome the inequalities of this world.

I think that the first thing that needs to be agreed upon is that health is a right and not a privilege. It's been interesting watching the nightmare unfold. My understanding of the impact of the many, many (isn't there some kind of limit to the amount one can have?!) executive orders comes from a global perspective as someone working in sexual and reproductive health and rights in Canada. The impacts of the constant attacks on women, through the global gag order and the proposed defunding of Planned Parenthood, are devastating to any progress made in recent years. Millions of women will lose essential reproductive health services due to these bad policies developed and signed off by rich white men. It's completely gross. This also has a larger impact on women's economic rights that is often underdiscussed. All bodies are under attack under the conservative administration: women's bodies, trans and gender nonconforming bodies, Black and Brown bodies, poor bodies, differently abled bodies, Indigenous bodies, Muslim bodies, HIV positive . . . so many bodies. But the good news is these bodies are becoming conscious and uniting to push back against systemic violence. While not always perfect, shifts are being made to work in collaboration to create bridges of understanding about the ways in which we share similar experiences and the ways

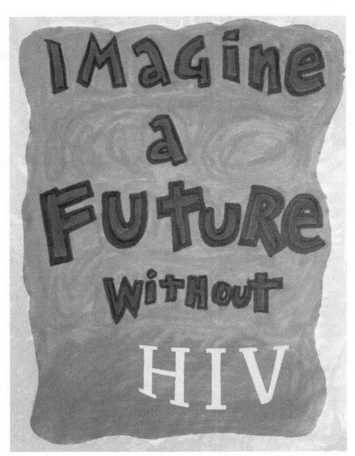

FIGURE 12.2.
Created by
Quito Ziegler.

that it has been different. It's been and is going to continue to be tough work but I think that it can be done.

Margaret Rhee

FROM THE CENTER

The removal of HIV/AIDS from the White House website is one of many shadow gestures in our postelection times. In the shadows of the Trump administration, these gestures prompt a "whitelash" from larger publics, and a flood of anti-immigrant, anti–health care, anti-Brown, anti–healthy bodies dystopian responses that are antithetical to justice and the work for justice of From the Center (FTC).

From the Center is a community-based program in partnership with HIV & Integrated Services (HIVIS, formerly known as Forensic AIDS Project) at the San Francisco Department of Public Health. Established in 1983, HIVIS was the first HIV service provider in a California jail/prison. As part of Jail Health Services, a division of the San Francisco Department of Public Health, HIVIS has successfully implemented HIV prevention and care programs/services in the San Francisco (SF) county jails for over twenty years.

From the Center has a threefold participatory model: pedagogical, technological, and artistic. In our project, incarcerated women utilize low-cost production technologies to create their own short digital stories, involving images and sound, to highlight how their lives are impacted by HIV/AIDS. These stories, in the form of short, narrated moving images or visual collages, serve as powerful educational tools inside and outside the jail setting. The process demonstrates the importance of centering incarcerated women as advocates, researchers, and storytellers of their own lives and communities. From the Center produces today's activist practices—what activist and scholar Alexandra Juhasz outlines in her 1995 book, *AIDS TV: Identity, Community, and Alternative Video*, as "the alternative AIDS media" and what scholar Priscilla Wald discusses as the stakes of storytelling and HIV/AIDS and inequality.[3]

For example, one of the FTC storytellers created a powerful story titled "Miracle." In her story, Helen Hall insists that the story of Black women and HIV/AIDS is collective: the story of "Ruth," an HIV/AIDS advocate and mother living with HIV/AIDS "is one of them. This is Ruth's story. Which is my story. And your story too."[4]

While we did collaborate with the San Francisco Department of Public Health, our work with FTC can be considered more than "localized." Our collaboration was sporadic and haphazard but also highly organized and powerful: a community of incarcerated, formerly incarcerated women, and academics, or what we prefer to term "inside researchers" and "outside researchers." As a feminist collective, we did not have institutional backing or funding. We found ourselves in allegiance with the parts of institutions—universities, research centers, government sectors—that relayed solidarity to our collective feminist vision.

What is powerful is our refusal for unidirectional directions, and our preference for difference and participatory conversation and making. Collaborative was our logics and optics. This comfort in difference and collaboration also shaped our vision for a healthy AIDS future that aimed to protect and centralize women of color.

Although From the Center was primarily local, gestures from the national administration under Obama had helped solidify our focus on new media technologies. In the summer of 2010, my collaborator Isela Ford (formerly González) and I were working hard to implement the first workshops in the jail setting. One summer day, we paused from our weekly meeting at the Forensic AIDS Project offices to watch the Obama administration's announcement of the first national comprehensive HIV/AIDS campaign. The formal announcement was livestreamed online.

The formal announcement was a gesture.

The gesture symbolically pushed our own work forward.

The national HIV/AIDS campaign included testimony by then secretary Kathleen Sebelius that pointed to racial and gender inequalities of HIV/AIDS statistics, particularly for women of color: "We've been very successful at keeping HIV/AIDS incidence low for some populations. If you are a white heterosexual woman, like me, your chances of being infected by HIV and AIDS are very low, 1 in 50,000. But if you're a black female, who is also an injection drug user, your chances of being infected are more than a thousand time higher than mine, 1 in 35."[5]

Under the Obama administration, Sebelius offered a particular national story. She pointed out her own raced and gendered body as privileged. The inclusion of race and gender within Obama's national campaign was a gesture that unfolded online, and that seemed to imbue within it our visions of FTC. Obama's campaign and our own inspired from it reside in stark contrast to the current administration's removal of HIV/AIDS from the White House website.

Our work—utilizing new media technologies to advocate and express feminist HIV/AIDS futures—is affected by Trump's regime in a variety of ways.

The removal of HIV/AIDS from the national website is a gesture of a dystopian collapse.

If dystopia is a story of a hopeless future, the present may be a collapse of the future into the past.

Yet I am reminded of Helen Hall's artist statement for "Miracle": "Because I want to help women know that it is okay to go through things like that, this life."

The removal of HIV/AIDS from the White House website shows us the stark reality of bodies and their images who are deemed not valuable to the current regime's optics.

FIGURE 12.3.
Created by
Quito Ziegler.

At the same time, removals reveal the edges of resistance, story, and life to be continually forged.

With darkness comes moonlight
flickering digital screens, this life.

Pato Hebert: I started working in HIV in 1994, and spent some fifteen years engaged in local and national HIV work with queer communities of color in San Francisco, Los Angeles, and New York. But my more recent efforts have been primarily transnational, and it is through this prism that I want to consider our AIDS futures, both the threats afoot as well as the dynamic ways that grassroots organizing is cultivating a world where AIDS need not overwhelm our very ability to flourish and be free.

My thinking is profoundly indebted to my colleagues at the Global Forum on MSM & HIV (MSMGF) and our hundreds of partners at local, country, regional, and transnational levels who are working together to deepen a global movement for the health and human rights of queer men, transgender people, sex workers, people who use drugs, and the other communities who are most impacted by HIV/AIDS. Vibrant and evolving, these global networks and their regional and local members are changing HIV responses all over the world. Often known as "key populations" in international HIV advocacy efforts, these communities are more organized and coordinated than ever before. This is exciting, and increasingly crucial.

In late February 2017, US president Donald Trump put forward a preliminary budget plan that would drastically cut funding for USAID and the State Department. These entities oversee the most important US resources for international HIV/AIDS initiatives, including funding for the United States President's Emergency Plan for AIDS Relief (PEPFAR) and the Global Fund to Fight AIDS, Tuberculosis and Malaria. Community activists and networks around the world have long lobbied for governments, including that of the United States, to contribute their fair share to the international HIV response and work with local movements to uphold normative guidance grounded in evidence-based, rights-affirming harm reduction, and community-led action. Local movements, in turn, leverage these resources to hold their national governments accountable and strive to ensure that HIV responses are targeted to and shaped by the communities who are disproportionately impacted by HIV.

If Trump and his team succeed in cutting the budget as proposed, tens of thousands of people living with HIV will struggle to access the life-saving treatment they deserve, and prevention initiatives will atrophy, thus causing infection rates to once again accelerate. Trump could dangerously set back our achievements at exactly the moment when we should be strengthening and expanding our response to ensure long lives, lower costs, and greater effectiveness worldwide. Statist solutions will never be enough to ensure our well-being and pleasure. But the scale of HIV-related challenges cannot adequately be addressed without governments playing their part to ensure nondiscriminatory legal frameworks, build accessible and effective health systems, and honor the invaluable role of community guidance and leadership.

It is refreshing, inspiring, and challenging to work alongside activists from around the world whose urgencies are not primarily determined by US politics. Although many of the structural impediments are shared across contexts, it is worth remembering that locally defined priorities, tactics, strategies, and implementation must always take precedence over either top-down or one-size-fits-all approaches. Trump's turbulence may exert great pull, but we cannot be distracted or deterred from the kinds of models being developed in unison at the grassroots global level.

In July 2016, at the International AIDS Conference in Durban, South Africa, the IRGT: A Global Network of Trans Women and HIV worked in partnership with other transgender regional organizations and networks to organize the first ever pre-conference on HIV and transgender people. Titled "No More Lip Service, Trans Access, Equity and Rights, Now!" the historic gathering was so popular that it maxed out its attendance capacity during registration. Now the IRGT is mobilizing trans-identified people to serve as technical advisors in support of trans-led organizing efforts happening regionally in Asia and the Pacific, Sub-Saharan Africa, and Latin America and the Caribbean.

The Global Network of Sex Work Projects (NSWP) has been supporting grassroots peer education efforts between sex workers from across the Global South. Sex workers run their own week-long academy, which offers peer-led workshops, site visits to community-led interventions, and art advocacy sessions. The academy is based in Kenya and convenes teams of sex workers from across Africa and increasingly from other contexts in the Global South, whereby local movements nominate peers for attendance and participation. This is an exemplary popular education model that is shaping the way sex worker movements strengthen and grow across the world. These initiatives include peer paralegal services for sex workers lobbying for their rights in India, and the engagement of sex workers–led organizations in Global Fund processes in Central Asia and Eastern Europe.

The International Network of People who Use Drugs (INPUD) has recently energized its leadership and deepened its work with members to better fight repressive drug policies. It is doing so through improved coordination of the voices and experiences of people who use drugs from around the word. As part of this process, INPUD has developed and launched the Drug User Peace Initiative (DUPI), a series of guiding documents that challenge harmful dogmas related to human rights, the stigmatization of people who use drugs, and the war on the health of such communities. The DUPI instead foregrounds clear and compelling harm-reduction strategies that counter criminalization and social control with progressive approaches to equity and empowerment.

At the Global Forum on MSM & HIV (MSMGF), we are working with colleagues to challenge the slide toward calcification that can so often occur as social movements congeal into organizations and then institutions. This is one of the great ironies and challenges of organizing—that we not simply succumb to shoring up the survival of NGOs or long-standing figureheads and gatekeepers but instead engage and follow the vision of new waves of leadership by transgender people and gay and bisexual men who are coordinating across the Global South in their response to HIV. We helped convene dozens of community leaders and stakeholders to develop the MSMIT (men who have sex with men toolkit), a practical guidance for collaborative interventions that can implement comprehensive HIV and sexually transmitted infection (STI) programs for gay men and other men who have sex with men (MSM).

What works well in one context or movement may not work elsewhere, but we can continue to learn from one another's efforts, tactics, struggles, strategies, and breakthroughs. All around the world, community members have been pushing for a greater role in determining the direction of their countries' responses to HIV/AIDS. A jointly vibrant and equitably distributed future is not guaranteed. We have much work to do, around scaling up testing and treatment initiatives led by communities, debating, prioritizing and resourcing our approaches to prevention, countering stigma and discrimination, and coordinating our responses to co-infections with tuberculosis and especially hepatitis.

As repression rises and resources shrink, there is pressure to take an overly narrow and conventional public health approach. Yet we would be wise to remember the sociocultural dimensions of our work, the structural inequities that challenge it, the criminalization of our lives, the liberation and effectiveness of harm-reduction and sex-positive approaches, and the crucial role that community must continue to play. Trump and his aftershocks will be with us for longer than we care to imagine. But together we must conjure other futures full of possibilities and wellness.

Emily Bass: Since the election, I have been thinking nearly every day about a problem that Madeline Levine, the English translator of Miron Białoszewski's *A Memoir of the Warsaw Uprising*, describes in her introduction. The book is Białoszewski's account of a sixty-three-day revolt against Nazi occupation in 1944. It is relentlessly plain spoken: "I went here, I went there." Levine's problem is that there are so many ways that Białoszewski used variations on the verb "to run." She writes that she strained to capture the nuances of the words he used to describe the movement of panicked rebels under assault and in flight.

In 2017, how many ways are there to run? Several days a week I go to stand down in Lower Manhattan—hurry to this corner or that one. I get to the

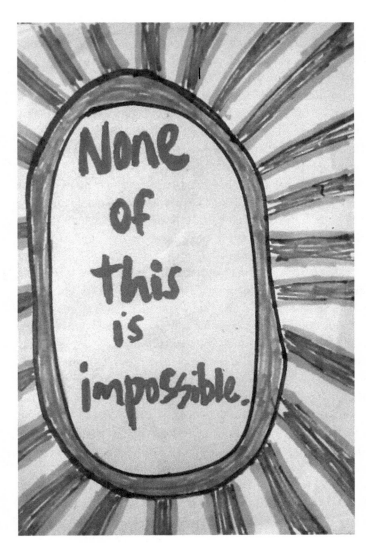

FIGURE 12.4.
Created by
Quito Ziegler.

corner. Sometimes there's just a few people; sometimes there's a crowd. A few weeks ago, a friend got so tired of carrying signs that she went to a protest with a piece of hot pink duct tape over her mouth. On Tuesdays, I grab food and run down to the ACT UP–infused and –informed Rise and Resist meeting—a new direct action group that was meeting in the old LGBT center until we outgrew its space and moved to the church across the street.

Speaking of that duct tape, my friend wore it on International Women's Day to protest the Global Gag Rule, a bipartisan binary piece of policy: an on-off switch that Dems and Republicans toggle on their first or second day in office. Up until now, it has prohibited foreign NGOs receiving US foreign assistance dollars from talking about, providing, referring, for or advocating for the legalization of abortion. You can't do these things even if you're doing them with other funds. Prior to 2016, the gag rule was last turned on under President George W. Bush. Then, groups that provide trusted, high-quality health care to women lost their funding; they had to close their doors. Women had to go find contraception elsewhere—or go without. Unplanned pregnancies went up; so, too, did unsafe abortions.

The Global Gag Rule has always been a nasty, hypocritical bit of policy. I expected Trump to reinstate it. But I hadn't expected that he would direct the State Department to apply it to all global health spending—including the $4 billion and change that we spend every year on global AIDS.

How many ways are there to run?

Old ACT UP dies hard—and long may it run. But in the health-care break-out group for Rise and Resist, where folks I've known for years and people I've never met sit in circles and try to find a common language across the generational divides of divergent histories and new technologies—"When we did the Wall Street action . . ." and "Wait, what's a Slack?"—I'm struck by the struggle to get women's sexual and reproductive health to matter. We do an action about TrumpCare and the phrase *family planning* gets plopped into the media brief. "Nope," I say, "that's not enough." A revision happens. The next action is on Medicaid Block Grants—it's a gas. Trump's ACA legislation dies and we feel great. But I keep waiting for the moment when the Global Gag Rule—I give an update about it at the Rise and Resist meeting every time I'm there—will become the next fight.

Is the Global Gag Rule narrow and femme-oriented? Is birth control too unqueer? Or is it because the Global Gag Rule always happens when Republicans are in power—people have said this to me—so it feels impossible to change?

I caucus with my duct-tape-wearing friend and other women and we decide not to form a women's health caucus for now. Meanwhile, in my day job directing strategy for an advocacy group focused on HIV prevention and dedicated to working in solidarity with women in East and Southern Africa whose bodies and families are daily impacted by the gag rule, we debate what to do about the portion of our own funding that comes from the US government. To accept the money is to accept the policy; to refuse it is to lose resources for the women who are our allies. We don't directly work on abortion anyway, so our actual work wouldn't be affected, we reason. It's better

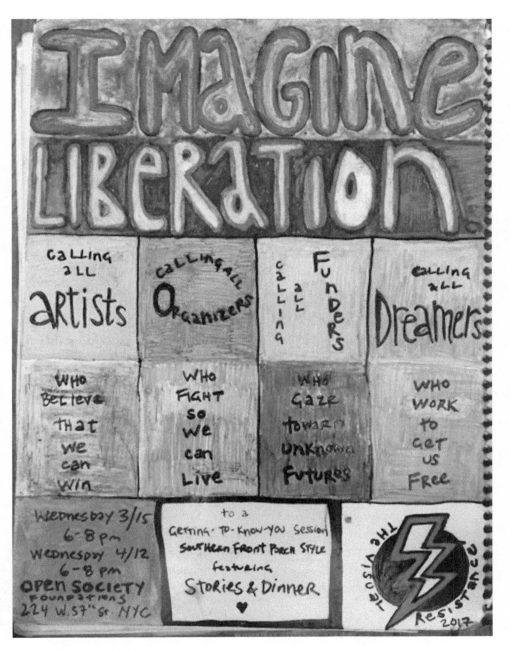

FIGURE 12.5. Created by Quito Ziegler.

to have the resources and use them well than to take a stand and lose them. But when do we make the first decision that is capitulation, collaboration? Do you know it at the time? I'm scattered here—and that's the point. It's an uprising under assault. Everybody run. We're doing what we remember—ACT UP rules of order apply at Rise and Resist—and we're trying to figure out when to split off into smaller groups, and when to hide. I don't have the answers yet about what health looks like now in 2017 and under Trump. My duct-tape friend just started an affinity group of Rise and Resist women to work on the global gag. I've skipped the last few weeks. I'm tired. As for health? Well, PEPFAR's been maligned for its faith-based initiatives and it's a sick patriarchal biblical reading that's driving Vice President Mike Pence, who's undoubtedly behind the gag rule expansion. And I have begun balancing my AIDS work with local work on immigrant justice. I have been running toward meetings in churches by people who are literally running for their lives. I find myself walking into these basements hoping someone might show me how to pray.

Elton Naswood: Unfortunately, I'm not able to respond to the prompt as it is a political question and in my current position as a federal government contractor, I'm not able to give a response. However, below is the summary of the ACA repeal response from the National Indian Health Board and a link to the entire report.

"IMPACT OF ACA REPEAL ON AMERICAN INDIANS AND ALASKA NATIVES," HTTPS:// WWW.COMMONWEALTHFUND.ORG/PUBLICATIONS/ISSUE-BRIEFS/2017/JAN/ REPEALING-FEDERAL-HEALTH-REFORM-ECONOMIC-AND-EMPLOYMENT

SUMMARY

Repealing the ACA presents risks beyond access to health services. Analysis recently released by the Commonwealth Fund shows that dire impacts to states will result from repeal, including losses in 2019 of $140 billion in federal funding to state budgets, a loss of 2.6 million jobs across all states, with only a third of those jobs being in health care and the rest in other industries as ripple effects.[6]

In Indian Country, it is common that federal programs providing federal services to AI/ANs [American Indians and Alaska Natives], of which health care is a major component, are one of the primary sources of employment for Tribal people. Federal jobs, in many cases, stimulate and grow the local

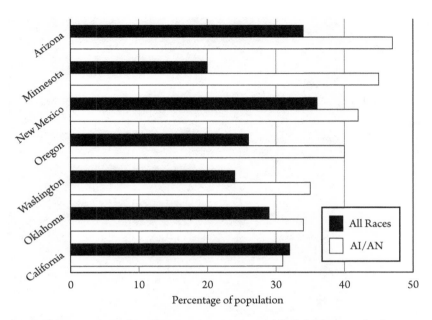

FIGURE 12.6. Percentage of population under 138 percent of the federal poverty level, by state.

economy by providing a rare source of income from the outside. As a result, the impacts on local Tribal economies would likely be even more severe—and come at a time when recent improvements from health care reform were starting to take root. Repeal of the ACA will lead to AI/ANs having less access to health services, less options for care, worsening health disparities, increased unnecessary suffering, and an increase in preventable deaths. The issue of repealing the ACA, therefore, should be examined through the lens of treaty responsibilities, social justice, and civil rights. Any attempt to repeal and replace the ACA should leave in its place programs and options that will increase access to direly needed health services, not further limit care for Indigenous Americans.

Prompt 2

Juhasz: I'd like you to speak to any or many of these following interventions from your colleagues, in a second, brief vision statement about AIDS futures.

- Removals reveal the edges of resistance, story, and life to be continually forged. (Margaret Rhee)
- We would be wise to remember the sociocultural dimensions of our work, the structural inequities that challenge it, the criminalization of our lives, the liberation and effectiveness of harm-reduction and sex-positive approaches, and the crucial role that community must continue to play. Trump and his aftershocks will be with us for longer than we care to imagine. But together we must conjure other futures full of possibilities and wellness. (Pato Hebert)
- I find myself walking into these basements hoping someone might show me how to pray. (Emily Bass)
- Repeal of the ACA will lead to AI/ANs having less access to health services, less options for care, worsening health disparities, increased

unnecessary suffering, and an increase in preventable deaths. The issue of repealing the ACA, therefore, should be examined through the lens of treaty responsibilities, social justice, and civil rights. Any attempt to repeal and replace the ACA should leave in its place programs and options that will increase access to direly needed health services, not further limit care for Indigenous Americans. (Elton Naswood)

– But the good news is these bodies are becoming conscious and uniting to push back against systemic violence. While not always perfect, shifts are being made to work in collaboration to create bridges of understanding about the ways in which we share similar experiences and the ways that it has been different. (Jessica Whitbread)

– Any of Quito's images.

Bass: Hello from South Africa, and the far side of a week spent within the US government PEPFAR program. It's an annual gathering to review the plans that each country makes for its coming year. These are called Country Operational Plans or, nearly universally, COPs, so that when you say where you are going— as you head toward the Rosebank Hyatt in Johannesburg, with its pinky-purple art photos of townships—you say you are going to the COP review. This is how America's global AIDS program works: there is an annual gathering to make decisions about how to spend US money—which accounts for a full two-thirds of the investment in "global" AIDS, a phrase that here means AIDS in Black and Brown bodies living with and at risk of HIV beyond our borders. Perhaps because it is beyond our borders, there is no irony and no wincing that we call this caucus on how to keep Black people healthy the cop review.

Let's look at those COPs/cops. Or no, let's not, because the fact that we use this language without wincing or even noticing means that we are doing what America does so well so often: *let's look away*.

Looking away can mean ignoring; it can also mean seeing and dismissing. It can mean deciding that even with a rose-colored filter, a photo of the shanties is still a document of suffering and not innocuous wall art. Let's look away, then, from the apparent victories sustained since I last wrote. The fact that the head of PEPFAR appointed under Obama is still running the program, the fact that the program is still running, that it hasn't lost its funding at all. Let's look away from that and past, through, toward, something else: the price of these "wins," which is not unlike the price—untallied, maybe even unnoticed—of working on an American-funded program that is more diligent and focused about saving foreign Black lives from AIDS deaths than any work happening on HIV within our borders.

What I need you all to know is that to preserve the space that PEPFAR has carved out for working with and for adolescent girls and young women—beautifully and sometimes even close to revolutionarily—another language is underway. I wrote something similar last time concerning the Global Gag Rule, which eliminates all speech about abortion, but this is different. It is not a silence but a linguistic sliding that is happening.

The head of PEPFAR is one of the last Obama-era presidential appointees—if not *the* last such appointee—still at her post under the Trump administration. She is playing a high-stakes game to keep her job and keep the program running, and often she makes me want to stand and salute. But in these days, patriotism is shot through with desperation. The better route is looking away from the performance. So I must report on her diction shift, which has her now mentioning, in every single speech, the extreme prevalence of "first-sex-as-rape" among African girls. It is true and it is horrifying; it also forecloses a sex-positive conversation about girl's bodies and women's bodies that engages support by foregrounding pleasure. But pleasure has no place in the new talk that forefronts sex through depictions of an eleven-year-old girl who is raped by an older man. While there is abhorrent truth to this illustration, there is more owed to that girl as an adult or a teen: a place where she can reclaim her body, its strength and sensation, for herself after such abuse. The news from the COP review is that hers is not that world. Not right now.

AIDS funding will survive, I believe, by turning to old tropes of geographic instability and atrocities in countries far away—no more piles of bodies and coffin shops but now the violated girl child. What do we do when the language selected is true but insufficient? When the means to survival is to speak horror because it plays well with congressmen who consider themselves devout? Is this caring for that girl or is it adding, in some infinitesimal way, to her pain? Find your own version of this question. It is about capitulation, increments, and acceptable diction shifts. Ask it and then see what words your answer takes. How we speak will pave the road that lies ahead.

Whitbread: I won't lie; sex-positive approaches are kinda my thing. So, when I read Pato's statement, all I could think about was hanging out with my lovers at the bathhouse (why yes, they do have woman and trans bathhouse nights in Toronto) and inviting all the amazing activists I know for an extended period—a really extended period (COME!). Then, I thought that was selfish and gets into that whole queer island thing and that excludes many folks I care about, making me feel bad (or good, if for a day or two).

When we talk about wellness, where do self-care and self-preservation fit in? I have known way too many community activists that have left too soon because they were beaten down. About a year or so ago, I realized that everyone I knew who had died of AIDS had committed suicide. At that same time, I also thought, *How come I haven't tried yet?*

Mental health is underrepresented in our discussions. I don't think that people actually know how tough it is to keep on keeping on living and breathing this work. It is easy to get together with your pals, laugh it up and join a one-off protest, but then what? In some ways, I envy the people who can turn their social justice rah-rah on and then turn it off—Facebook repost and I've done my daily duty—ha! As if?!

How can movements better work together and understand the layers and layers of personal and societal hurt? There doesn't seem to be much space within our current activist culture for rest and healing. I don't know if it is because I just had twins, but I look at them and think, *How can I focus in on you being as open and amazing and wonderful as possible? And how do I do this at the same time as all the other stuff on almost no sleep?*

Rhee:

AIDS Futures: A Poem in Response

This blood, my veins, our AIDS Futures, I listen to you:

"I find myself walking into these basements hoping
someone might show me how to pray." (Emily Bass)

Show us, as we hold our hands collectively because
"None of this is impossible." (Quito Ziegler)

See the circular in the drawing, along with
sun beams radiating out,
outlines our eyes, and makes visions.
For a world of limitless care for Indigenous people,
we fight for care, resist the cutbacks, and the incarceration.
(Elton Naswood)

"I believe acts of kindness are stronger than acts of fear."
(Jessica Whitbread)

Your words are kindness. So I release, fear. Fear runs as
we organize, convene, disseminate,
". . . and follow the vision of new waves of leadership . . ."
   (Pato Hebert)

Say, I am listening to you
"Imagine Liberation."
It's a song I repeat.
After you, and over again.
Our chant
teaches us
how to pray.

Notes

1   "Elton Naswood."
2   Quito Ziegler, "If You Must," accessed August 10, 2018, https://quitoziegler.com
    /bio/.
3   Juhasz, AIDS TV; Wald, *Contagious*.
4   These stories are available to the public at From the Center's Vimeo site,
    https://vimeo.com/user7696400. From the Center is a public humanities proj-
    ect, and the digital stories are screened in jails and prisons. For more about the
    project, see https://ourstorysf.wordpress.com/.
5   Sebelius, "National HIV/AIDS Strategy."
6   Ku et al., "Repealing Federal Health Reform."

Bibliography

Bass, Emily. "How to Survive a Footnote: AIDS Activism in the 'After' Years." In "As
    If," special issue, *n+1* 23 (Fall 2015). https://nplusonemag.com/issue-23/annals
    -of-activism/how-to-survive-a-footnote/.
Białoszewski, Miron. *A Memoir of the Warsaw Uprising*. Translated by Madeline G.
    Levine. New York: New York Review Books, 2015.
"Elton Naswood." *Circle of Harmony*. Accessed September 12, 2019. http://
    www.aaihbcircleofharmony.org/index.php/planning-committee/planning
    -committee/elton-naswood/.
Juhasz, Alexandra. *AIDS TV: Identity, Community, and Alternative Video*. Durham,
    NC: Duke University Press, 1995.
Ku, Leighton, Erika Steinmetz, Erin Brantley, and Brian Bruen. "Repealing Federal
    Health Reform: Economic and Employment Consequences for States."
    Commonwealth Fund, January 2017.

Sebelius, Kathleen. "The National HIV/AIDS Strategy." Presentation, Washington, DC, July 13, 2010. Excerpted in Frank James, "Obama Unveils First National HIV/AIDS Strategy." NPR: *The Two Way*, July 13, 2010. https://www.npr.org/sections/thetwo-way/2010/07/13/128494452/obama-unveils-first-national-hiv-aids-strategy.

Wald, Priscilla. *Contagious: Cultures, Carriers, and the Outbreak Narrative.* Durham, NC: Duke University Press, 2010.

AFTERWORD
ON CRISIS AND ABOLITION

C. Riley Snorton

It is difficult to know, but perhaps unlikely, that Stuart Hall and his collaborators would recognize the prescience of *Policing the Crisis: Mugging, the State, and Law and Order* for thinking about HIV/AIDS. The introduction to their highly influential study begins with a series of writerly confessions. The authors note, "This book started out with 'mugging,' but it has ended in a different place. . . . Indeed if we could abolish the word [*mugging*], that would have been our principal—perhaps our only—'practical proposal.' It has done incalculable harm—raising the wrong things into sensational focus, hiding and mystifying the deeper causes."[1] As they argued, "mugging," as it came to be known in Britain in the 1970s, was a social phenomenon. Rather than a study of criminals or even criminality, they confessed that what followed was a sustained analysis of a carceral state. The "remedy" to the "mugging" crisis could only therefore be abolition.[2]

The initial circulation of *Policing the Crisis* coincided with a lesser-known node in HIV history. Treated at the London Hospital for Tropical Diseases before his death in 1978, a Portuguese man named Senhor José was memorialized in medical records as the first confirmed case of HIV-2.[3] While José typically receives only the briefest description in AIDS historiographies, some accounts also include that "he was believed to have been exposed to the disease in Guinea-Bissau in 1966."[4] One of the two main types of HIV, HIV-2 is generally regarded to be less common and less pathogenic than HIV-1. In a curious reformulation of the "West" and the "Rest," HIV-2 is spatially correlated to West Africa. In scientific literature, the strain is attributed to the virus jumping species between sooty mangabey monkeys and humans, precipitating a series of questions, including: What precipitated this encounter? Was he a soldier, or perhaps a colonial bureaucrat visiting Portuguese-occupied Guinea during the Guinea-Bissau War of Independence? And how can causality be so casually described? Here medico-scientific and historio-graphic discourses barely conceal a narrative about colonialism and power, in which the first documented case of HIV-2 in the West emerges from an encounter with decolonial insurgency. Incidentally, José began presenting symptoms in the year of Guinea-Bissau's formal independence (1974).[5]

If the mention of the last detail feels conspiratorial, it also rejoins and echoes what the authors of *Policing the Crisis* wrote about the prevailing ra-tionale of the carceral state: "the belief that conspiracy must be met with conspiracy."[6] Indeed, they argued that the legal framework for policing a cri-sis began with the idea of conspiracy—of secret plans and plots propped up by silence. Power-knowledge not only names what can and cannot be said (permissible speech and political silence) but moves according to what *feels* plausible.

To indulge briefly in the seductions of analogy, the HIV/AIDS patient and the mugger would come to share a number of characteristics: spectacular-ized, criminalized, and typified according to a number of identitarian ru-brics, they became the fodder-cum-rationale for the invention of new and different strategies for carceral containment or extinction. The response to both figures produced further investitures in security and securitization as the premier tools of late modern capitalist governance. The mugger and the HIV/AIDS patient would evince the imperceptible difference between figu-rations of the criminal and the criminally ill.

Speaking sometime later at a conference on the topic of cultural studies and its theoretical legacies, Hall described AIDS as an example of a question that compels research as a political praxis. He explained:

> The question of AIDS is an extremely important terrain of struggle and contestation. In addition to the people we know who are dying, or have died, or will, there are the many people dying who are never spoken of. How could we say that the question of AIDS is not also a question of who gets represented and who does not? AIDS is the site at which the advance of sexual politics is being rolled back. It's a site at which not only people will die, but desire and pleasure will also die if certain metaphors do not survive, or survive in the wrong way. [7]

The question of AIDS was in fact many questions that brought to the fore the condition of making theory in the midst of innumerable forms of loss. Writ-ing about the early era of AIDS, Dagmawi Woubshet refers to this calculus of grief as a "poetics of compounding loss," as a "leitmotif of inventory taking; the reconceptualization of relentless serial losses not as cumulative, but as compounding."[8] Yet one must also contend with other deaths—of the idea of desire or pleasure and of language for their survival. For Hall, attending to "the question of AIDS" also underscored the "modesty of theory," which I take as a caution to mind theory's political limits. Put differently, to engage in critical analyses of HIV/AIDS means to refuse the terms on which AIDS has been given; to refuse its biopolitical and necropolitical machinations; to refuse the representational structures that present some deaths as the requirement for the optimization of life itself; and to insist on different vocabularies for living, which involves asking more and better questions as well as laying claim to the survival of the damned.

AIDS is not the only metaphor for premature death. So is the prison, or living under occupation, or in underdevelopment, or living while Black, while trans, while undocumented, while poor. Many folks living with AIDS are also living with a combination of the aforementioned conditions. But if one believes that AIDS, and its precipitating and attendant crises, are structural and ideological, then one must consider how those very spatiotemporal formulations also forge abolitionist strategies and imaginaries. As Che Gossett notes,

> In contrast to the antifuturity institutionalized via domestic warfare, mass incarceration, deportation, and so forth, on the one hand, and nonfuturity evidenced by the well-resourced forward momentum of "LGBT" neoliberal "diverse/multicultural" nonprofitization in the name of "progress" and "feminism" from which sex workers, homeless people, street youth, trans women of color, those living with HIV/AIDS, and (dis)abled are evacuated on the other, radical queer and trans liberationist, AIDS activists of color have imagined queerly utopian alternatives. Ortez Alderson, black queer liberationist and antiwar and AIDS activist, and many others have fought to bring into being radical queer erotic lifeworlds that were also resolutely determined in constant struggle against forces and forms of antiqueer, antitrans, and antiblack violence.[9]

Displacement is rarely romantic, but it is nonetheless another place from which to do one's work. Gossett's historical example once again provokes the questions of the survival of desire and pleasure in relation to AIDS. The description of Alderson's "radical queer erotic lifeworlds" forged in struggle makes clear that pleasure is not freedom from violence. And as Saidiya Hartman writes with regard to the possibility of forms of pleasure in relation to the violence and unfreedom of chattel slavery that might serve as "figures of transformation": they would entail a "protest or rejection of the anatomo-politics that produces the black body as aberrant. More important, it [pleasure] is a way of redressing the pained constitution and corporeal malediction that is blackness."[10] In one sense, one might read Hartman's theorization of transformative pleasure as a kind of abolition akin to what Sylvia Wynter described as the goal of Frantz Fanon's *Black Skin, White Masks*: "to effect the black man's extrication from his very sense of self, from his identity."[11] But identity is not the problem; it is the fact of identity as an index of one's exposure to premature death that is at issue. And this is the material from which transformational pleasure is formed: in the insistence on the jouissance of survival ballasted by death.

So how does one abolish the HIV/AIDS crisis? It is not an uncommon (albeit ill-informed) opinion that if the crisis is not over, it is nearing its conclusion. But that apocryphal ending can only be narrated in terms of containment—an investment in pharmaceutical management (and even prevention), the relative invisibility of human suffering, a deeper linking of disability with criminality. In other words, the end of HIV/AIDS has only meant the redistribution of crises. Not to belie the tensions across the volume, each entry makes clear how crisis begets more crises. And perhaps this book aims to produce another kind of crisis—*a crisis of meaning*—that rejoins what the authors of *Policing the Crisis* hoped for their book: to be read "as an intervention—albeit an intervention in the battleground of ideas."[12] As Jih-Fei Cheng, Alexandra Juhasz, and Nishant Shahani note in the introduction to this volume, crisis is a spatiotemporal formulation that elucidates what AIDS is made to mean / is revealed to be / is in relation to myriad times and places. And in these contestations with the term, its representations, its histories and historiography, affects and effects, itineracies, one might find another kind of pleasure—of knowing the fight is not over.

Notes

1 Hall et al., *Policing the Crisis*, vii.
2 Hall et al., *Policing the Crisis*, x.
3 Bryceson et al., "HIV-2-Associated AIDS."
4 Regional HIV/AIDS Connection, "History of HIV/AIDS," 3.
5 Albion Centre: Partnerships in Health, "HIV/AIDS Timeline," 4.
6 Hall et al., *Policing the Crisis*, 285.
7 Hall, "Cultural Studies," 284–85.
8 Woubshet, *Calendar of Loss*, 4.
9 Ben-Moshe et al., "Critical Theory," 268.
10 Hartman, *Scenes of Subjection*, 58–59.

11 Wynter, "Towards the Sociogenic Principle," 11.
12 Hall et al., *Policing the Crisis*, x.

Bibliography

Albion Centre: Partnerships in Health. "A HIV/AIDS Timeline: Emphasising the Australian/New South Wales Perspective." January 2012. https://www.acon.org .au/wp-content/uploads/2015/04/History_of_HIV_5th-Edition.pdf.

Ben-Moshe, Liat, Che Gossett, Nick Mitchell, and Eric Stanley. "Critical Theory, Queer Resistance, and the Ends of Capture." In *Death and Other Penalities: Continental Philosophers on Prisons and Capital Punishment*, edited by Geoffrey Adelsberg and Lisa Guenther, 265–95. New York: Fordham University Press, 2015.

Bryceson, A., A. Tomkins, D. Ridley, D. Warhurst, A. Goldstone, G. Bayliss, J. Toswill, and J. Parry. "HIV-2-Associated AIDS in the 1970s." *Lancet* 2, no. 8604 (1988): 221.

Hall, Stuart. "Cultural Studies and Its Theoretical Legacies." In *Cultural Studies*, edited by Lawrence Grossberg, Cary Nelson, and Paula A. Triechler, 277–85. New York: Routledge, 1992.

Hall, Stuart, Charles Critcher, Tony Jefferson, John Clarke, and Brian Roberts. *Policing the Crisis: Mugging, the State, and Law and Order*. London: Palgrave Macmillan, 1978.

Hartman, Saidiya. *Scenes of Subjection: Terror, Slavery, and Self-Making in Nineteenth-Century America*. New York: Oxford University Press, 1997.

Regional HIV/AIDS Connection. "A History of HIV/AIDS in North America and the World." 2012. http://www.hivaidsconnection.ca/sites/default/files /images/RedScarf/A%20History%20of%20HIV%20AIDS%20in%20North%20 America%20and%20the%20World.pdf.

Woubshet, Dagmawi. *The Calendar of Loss: Race, Sexuality, and Mourning in the Early Era of AIDS*. Baltimore: Johns Hopkins University Press, 2015.

Wynter, Sylvia. "Towards the Sociogenic Principle: Fanon, the Puzzle of Conscious Experience, of 'Identity' and What It's Like to Be 'Black.'" 1999. http://coribe .org/PDF/wynter_socio.pdf.

CONTRIBUTORS

Cecilia Aldarondo makes deeply intimate, personal films that telescope outward onto broader social and existential issues, including sexuality, bigotry, family, and religion. Aldarondo's films have been supported by ITVS, HBO, A&E, the Sundance Institute, Cinereach, Tribeca Film Institute, the Jerome Foundation, and many others. Her feature documentary *Memories of a Penitent Heart* had its world premiere at the 2016 Tribeca Film Festival, was called "exceptional" by the *Village Voice*, and was broadcast nationally on the acclaimed documentary series POV in 2017. Her 2017 film *Picket Line* was commissioned by Laura Poitras and Stanley Nelson for the Field of Vision/ Firelight Media series "Our 100 Days" and screened at AFI Docs and the Metropolitan Museum of Art. Her writing has been published in *World Records*, *Performance Research*, and *The New Inquiry*, among other venues. She is a 2019 Guggenheim Fellow, an alumna of IFP's Documentary Lab as well as Sundance Institute's Edit and Story Lab, a 2017 Women at Sundance Fellow, a two-time MacDowell Colony Fellow, a recipient of a 2019 Bogliasco Foundation Residency, and one of *Filmmaker* magazine's "25 New Faces of Independent Film." She teaches at Williams College.

Pablo Alvarez is a first-generation Chicanx from Pico Rivera, California. He holds a BA in English and Human Development from Cal State Long Beach and an MA in Chicanx Studies from Cal State Northridge. He is a PhD candidate in Cultural Studies at the Claremont Graduate University. His essay "Gil Cuardos's 'AZT-Land': Documenting a Queer Chicano Literary Heritage" appears in *Queer in Aztlán: Chicano Male Recollections of Consciousness and Coming Out*. His archive "Queer Latinidad: A History of HIV/AIDS Art Consciousness in Los Angeles" was exhibited in 2012 at the Vincent Price Art Museum on the campus of East Los Angeles College and in 2014 at the University of La Verne. He is a member of Writers at Work, Los Angeles, and is committed to archiving the impact of AIDS in Latinx communities.

Marlon M. Bailey is Associate Professor of Women and Gender Studies in the School of Social Transformation at Arizona State University. He is a former Visiting Professor at the Center for AIDS Prevention Studies (CAPS) at the University of California, San Francisco. Bailey's 2013 book, *Butch Queens Up in Pumps: Gender, Performance, and Ballroom Culture in Detroit*, was awarded the Alan Bray Memorial Book Prize by the GL/Q Caucus of the Modern Language Association and was a finalist for the

Lambda Literary Book Award in LGBTQ Studies in 2014. Bailey has published in *American Quarterly*; GLQ; *Signs*; *Feminist Studies*; *Souls*; *Gender, Place, and Culture*; *Journal of Gay and Lesbian Social Services*; AIDS *Patient Care & STDs*; LGBT *Health*, and several book collections. His essay "Black Gay (Raw) Sex" appears in *No Tea, No Shade: New Writings in Black Queer Studies* (2016), edited by E. Patrick Johnson. Bailey is the coeditor, with Darius Bost, of "The Black AIDS Epidemic," a special issue of *Souls: A Critical Journal of Black Politics, Culture, and Society*. Bailey holds a PhD in African Diaspora Studies with a designated emphasis in Women, Gender, and Sexuality from the Department of African American Studies at the University of California, Berkeley.

Emily Bass has spent more than twenty years writing about and working on HIV/AIDS in America and East and Southern Africa. Her writing has appeared in numerous publications, including *Esquire*, *The Lancet*, *Ms.*, *n+1*, *Out*, *POZ*, and *Slice*, and she has received notable mention in Best American Essays. For the past thirteen years, she has worked at AVAC, a New York–based advocacy organization where, as director of strategy and content, she helps build powerful transnational activist coalitions that campaign for AIDS accountability and change. She was the 2018–19 Martin Duberman Visiting Research Fellow at the New York Public Library. Bass has been a Fulbright journalism scholar in Uganda and received scholarships from the Norman Mailer Writer's Colony and the Vermont Studio Center; she has served as an adviser to the World Health Organization and was lead rapporteur for human rights at the 2018 International AIDS Conference. She is a member of the What Would an HIV Doula Do collective. *The Plague War*, her history of on America's war on AIDS in Africa, will be published by PublicAffairs Press in 2021.

Darius Bost is Assistant Professor of Ethnic Studies in the School for Cultural and Social Transformation at the University of Utah. His first book, *Evidence of Being: The Black Gay Cultural Renaissance and the Politics of Violence* (2018), is an interdisciplinary study of Black gay arts movements in Washington, DC, and New York City during the early era of the AIDS epidemic in the United States. His research has been supported by the Woodrow Wilson Foundation; the Center for the Study of Race, Ethnicity, and Gender in the Social Sciences at Duke University; the President's Office and the Office of Research and Sponsored Programs at San Francisco State University; the Martin Duberman Visiting Scholars Program at the New York Public Library; and the Provost's Office at the University of Pennsylvania. Related research has been published or is forthcoming in *Criticism, Journal of American History, Souls, The Black Scholar, Palimpsest, Journal of West Indian Literature, Occasion*, and several edited collections.

Ian Bradley-Perrin is a PhD student in Sociomedical Sciences and History at Columbia University and has been living with HIV since 2010. He has been an activist on issues related to HIV/AIDS such as criminalization and public health policies like Track and Treat. He was the Pedro Zamora Public Policy Fellow at AIDS United in Washington, DC, as well as the coordinator for the HIV/AIDS project at Concordia University from 2013 to 2015. His current work explores the relationship between the pharmaceutical industry and the history of AIDS mobilization through the industry's involvement in HIV/AIDS organizations and advocacy, and he writes on topics such as PrEP, stigma, and pharmaceutical marketing.

Jih-Fei Cheng is Assistant Professor of Feminist, Gender, and Sexuality Studies at Scripps College. He has worked in HIV/AIDS social services, managed a university cultural center, been involved in media production and curation, and participated in queer and trans of color grassroots organizations in San Diego, Los Angeles, and New York City, addressing health, immigration, houselessness, gentrification, police brutality, and prison abolition. Cheng's research examines the intersections between science, media, surveillance, and social movements. His first book project examines the science, media, and politics of AIDS since the late twentieth-century emergence of finance capitalism in relation to the colonial history of virology, which developed during the period of late nineteenth-century industrial capitalism. His published writings appear in GLQ; *Catalyst: Feminism, Theory, Technoscience; WSQ;* and *Amerasia Journal;* among others.

Bishnupriya Ghosh teaches postcolonial theory and global media studies at UC Santa Barbara. After publishing two monographs, *When Borne Across* (2004) and *Global Icons* (2011), on the elite and popular cultures of globalization, in the last decade, Ghosh has turned to contemporary modes of speculative knowledge. Her current projects are a coedited collection with Bhaskar Sarkar, *The Routledge Companion to Media and Risk* (2018); and a monograph, *The Virus Touch: Theorizing Epidemic Media,* which spans comparative epidemic media in South Asia, South Africa, and the United States.

Roger Hallas is Associate Professor of English at Syracuse University. He specializes in documentary media, LGBT studies, and visual culture. His two books have examined how visual culture performs mediated acts of bearing witness to historical trauma. *The Image and the Witness: Trauma, Memory, and Visual Culture* (2007), which he coedited with Frances Guerin, analyzes how different visual media inscribe acts of witnessing and how the image itself can serve as witness to historical trauma. *Reframing Bodies: AIDS, Bearing Witness, and the Queer Moving Image* (2009) illuminates the capacities of queer film and video to bear witness to the cultural, political, and psychological imperatives of the AIDS crisis. He is currently working on a book about the relationship between photography and documentary film.

Pato Hebert is an artist, teacher and organizer. Hebert has worked in HIV-prevention initiatives with queer communities of color since 1994. He continues these grassroots efforts at the local and transnational levels, working with social movements and community organizations to develop innovative approaches to HIV mobilization, programs, advocacy, and justice. His recent work focuses on Latin America and Central Asia. He also curated exhibitions and led creative initiatives at the International AIDS Conferences in Vienna (2010), Melbourne (2014), Durban (2016), and Amsterdam (2018). Hebert's creative work explores the aesthetics, ethics, and poetics of interconnectedness. He is particularly interested in space, spirituality, pedagogy, and progressive praxis. His projects have been presented at Beton7 in Athens, PH21 Gallery in Budapest, the Centro de Arte Contemporáneo in Quito, the Ballarat International Foto Biennale, the Songzhuang International Photo Biennale, IHLIA LGBT Heritage in Amsterdam, and the Kunsthal Charlottenborg in Copenhagen. In 2015 he was an artist-in-residence with the Neighborhood Time Exchange project in West Philadelphia. In 2016 he was a BAU Institute/Camargo Foundation Residency Fellow in Cassis, France. Hebert's creative work has been supported by grants from the Rockefeller Foundation, the Creative Work Fund, the National Education Association, and a Mid-Career Fellowship for Visual Artists from the California Community Foundation. In 2008 he received the Excellence in Photographic Teaching Award from Center in Santa Fe. He is currently Associate Arts Professor in the Department of Art and Public Policy at Tisch School of the Arts, New York University.

Jim Hubbard has been making films since 1974. In 2012 he completed *United in Anger: A History of ACT UP*, a feature-length documentary on the AIDS activist group. The film grew out of the ACT UP Oral History Project founded by Sarah Schulman and Hubbard. A total of 102 interviews from the ACT UP Oral History Project were seen in a fourteen-monitor installation at the Carpenter Center for the Arts, Harvard University, as part of the exhibition *ACT UP New York: Activism, Art, and the AIDS Crisis, 1987–1993*, held October 15–December 23, 2009, and at White Columns in New York, September 9–October 23, 2010. Along with James Wentzy, Hubbard made a nine-part cable access television series based on the project. Among his nineteen other films are *Elegy in the Streets* (1989), *Two Marches* (1991), *The Dance* (1992), and *Memento Mori* (1995). His films have been shown at the Museum of Modern Art, the Berlin Film Festival, the London Film Festival, the San Francisco Jewish Film Festival, and the New York, San Francisco, Los Angeles, Tokyo, London, Torino, and many other lesbian and gay film festivals. His film *Memento Mori* won the Ursula for Best Short Film at the Hamburg Lesbian and Gay Film Festival in 1995. He cofounded MIX NYC: Queer Experimental Film and Video Festival. Under the auspices of the Estate Project for Artists with AIDS, he created the AIDS Activist Video Collection at the New York Public Library. He curated the series *Fever in the Archive: AIDS Activist Videotapes from the Royal S. Marks Collection* for the Guggenheim Museum in New York. The eight-program series took place on December 1–9, 2000. He also co-curated the series *Another Wave: Recent Global Queer Cinema* at the Museum of Modern Art in New York in July and September 2006. In 2013–14 he curated an eight-program series of AIDS activist videos from the collection of the New York Public Library to accompany their landmark exhibition *Why We Fight: Remembering AIDS Activism*.

Andrew J. Jolivette is Professor of Ethnic Studies and Senior Specialist in Native American and Indigenous Studies at the University of California, San Diego. A former Ford Foundation Postdoctoral Fellow, he is the author or editor of eight books in print or forthcoming, including *Indian Blood: HIV and Colonial Trauma in San Francisco's Two-Spirit Community* (2016; Lambda Literary Award finalist for best book in LGBTQ Studies) and *Louisiana Creoles: Cultural Recovery and Mixed-Race*

Native American Identity (2007). He is currently working on a new book, *Queer In-digenous Citizenship: Against Settler Violence and Anti-Blackness* (forthcoming). He is the former tribal historian for the Atakapa Ishak nation and the Indigenous People's Representative to the United Nations on HIV and the law.

Julia S. Jordan-Zachery's scholarship focuses on critical policy analysis dealing with race, gender, and sexuality. Her first book, *Black Women, Cultural Images and Social Policy* (2009), examines the racial and gendered processes of policymaking; how these affect the imageries, public attitudes, and discursive references about Black womanhood; and the impacts of these on the lives of African American women. She is also the author of *Shadow Bodies: Black Women, Ideology, Representation, and Politics* (2017), a book that explores the political and cultural representations of the Black woman's body and the implications for effective Black women's political organizing. In addition to these two important books, she has coedited three books and published several peer-reviewed articles exploring the intersectionalities of race, gender, citizenship, and social policy.

Alexandra Juhasz is Chair of the Department of Film at Brooklyn College. She has been making and thinking about AIDS activist videos since the mid-1980s. She is the author of *AIDS TV: Identity, Community, and Alternative Video* (1995) and a large number of AIDS educational videos, including *Living with AIDS: Women and AIDS* (1987, with Jean Carlomusto), *We Care: A Video for Careproviders of People Affected by AIDS* (1990, the Women's AIDS Video Enterprise), and *Video Remains* (2005). Most recently, she has been engaging in online cross-generational dialogue with AIDS activists and scholars about the recent spate of AIDS imagery after a lengthy period of representational quiet, including co-curating the art shows EVERYDAY and its Day With(out) Art video program: *Compulsive AIDS Video* (with Jean Carlomusto and High Ryan) for Visual AIDS and *Metanoia: Transformation through AIDS Archives and Activism* (with Katherine Cheairs, Theodore [Ted] Kerr, and Jawanza Williams).

Dredge Byung'chu Kang-Nguyễn, PhD, MPH, is Assistant Professor of Anthropology and Global Health at the University of California, San Diego. His research focuses on race, class, gender, sexuality, and nationality as they intersect with beauty, love, sex work, HIV, and structural violence from Thai, Korean, and US perspectives. Before becoming an academic, Dredge was a baby activist and worked for more than a decade in AIDS organizations, including prevention, testing, care, capacity building, and research.

Theodore (Ted) Kerr is a Canadian-born, Brooklyn-based writer, organizer, and artist whose work focuses on HIV/AIDS, community, and culture. Kerr's writing has appeared in *Women's Studies Quarterly, New Inquiry*, BOMB, CBC (Canada), *Lambda Literary, POZ Magazine, The Advocate, Cineaste, St. Louis American, IndieWire, Hyper-Allergic*, and other publications. Kerr earned his MA from Union Theological Seminary, where he researched Christian ethics and HIV. At his graduation, he spoke about the queer everyday in surviving. Currently, Kerr teaches at the New School. Kerr was the programs manager at Visual AIDS, where he worked to ensure social justice was an important lens through which to understand the ongoing epidemic. He also served as the programs manager at the Institute for Art, Religion and Social Justice at Union Theological Seminary. In 2016–17 Kerr performed ten interviews for the Smithsonian's Archives of American Art's "Visual Arts and the AIDS Epidemic: An Oral History Project." Kerr received his oral history training from Suzanne Snider as part of the Oral History Summer School. He was a member of the New York City Trans Oral History Project. Working with the Brooklyn Historical Society, Kerr indexed their AIDS oral history project. Kerr is a founding member of the What Would an HIV Doula Do? collective, a community of people committed to better implicating community within the ongoing response to HIV/AIDS. Creating post-cards, posters, stickers, and collages, Kerr's art practice is about bringing together pop culture, photography, and text to create fun and meaningful shareable ephem-era and images. Collaboration is a big part of Kerr's art practice. He has made work with Zachary Ayotte, L. J. Roberts, Chaplain Christopher Jones, Niknaz Tavakolian, Bridget de Gersigny, Malene Dam, and others. He has been in exhibitions curated by Kris Nuzzi, Sur Rodney (Sur), Danny Orendorff, and others. Two of his works, in collaboration with Shawn Torres and Jun Bae, are part of DePaul Art Gallery's permanent collection. His website is https://www.tedkerr.club.

Catherine Yuk-ping Lo is International Postdoctoral Teaching Fellow at University College Maastricht, Maastricht University. She was awarded her PhD in Security Studies from the University of Hong Kong. She specializes in international relations and health security with an Asian focus. Her current research interests include HIV/AIDS in China and India, infectious disease responses in Northeast and Southeast Asian states, antimicrobial resistance (AMR) challenges in the Asia-Pacific, and global health governance. She is the author of *HIV/AIDS in China and India: Governing Health Security* (2015). Her book has been awarded the 2017 International Studies Association (ISA) Global Health Section Prize for the best book. Her works appear in such journals as *Australian Journal of International Affairs*, *Health and Policy Planning*, *Globalization and Health*, and *Journal of Global Security Studies*.

Cait McKinney is Assistant Professor in the School of Communication at Simon Fraser University. Their research looks at the politics of information in queer and feminist social movements, emphasizing digital technologies, archiving practices, and the media histories of queer information activism. Recent publications appear in GLQ and *Continuum: Journal of Media and Cultural Studies*. They are the co-editor of *Inside Killjoy's Kastle: Dykey Ghosts, Feminist Monsters, and Other Lesbian Hauntings* (2019), and their first book on lesbian feminist information histories is forthcoming from Duke University Press in 2020.

Viviane Namaste is Full Professor at the Simone de Beauvoir Institute, Concordia University, Montreal. She is the author of *Savoirs créoles: Leçons du sida pour l'histoire de Montréal* (2019), *Imprimés interdits: L'histoire de la censure des journaux jaunes au Québec, 1955–1975* (2017), and *Oversight: Critical Reflections on Feminist Research and Politics* (2015).

Elton Naswood is Senior Program Analyst, Capacity Building Division, at the Office of Minority Health Resource Center, a nationwide service of the Office of Minority Health. He previously was Capacity Building Assistance Specialist at the National Native American AIDS Prevention Center (NNAAPC) and was formally Founder and Program Coordinator for the Red Circle Project, AIDS Project Los Angeles (APLA). He is currently a member of the Community Expert Advisory Council for the Indigenous HIV/AIDS Research Training (IHART) program at the University of Washington and the US Representative Leader for the International Indigenous Working Group on HIV/AIDS (IIWGHA). Naswood received his Bachelor of Arts in Sociology and American Indian Justice Studies from Arizona State University and attended the Graduate Degree Program in American Indian Studies at the University of California, Los Angeles.

Cindy Patton is Professor of Sociology and Anthropology at Simon Fraser University, in Vancouver, Canada. An early AIDS activist in Boston, she holds a PhD in Communications from the University of Massachusetts, Amherst. After inaugurating her academic career at Temple University (Rhetoric and Community) and Emory University (Graduate Institute of the Liberal Arts), she accepted a Canada Research Chair in Community, Culture and Health at Simon Fraser (2003–15). In that capacity, she worked with more than two dozen groups to develop small community-driven projects related to HIV/AIDS, housing, social welfare, mental health, and achieving, culminating in the creation of the Community Health Online Digital Research Resource, a cataloged, open-access, full-text collection of the materials from those groups (www.chodarr.org). Her academic publications span the social study of medicine, especially AIDS; social movement theory; gender studies; and media studies. She is coeditor of *Queer Diasporas* (2000) and a special issue of *Cultural Studies* on Pierre Bourdieu (2003). She is the author of such works as *Globalizing AIDS* (2002), *Cinematic Identity: Anatomy of a Problem Film* (1997), *Fatal Advice: How Safe-Sex Education Went Wrong* (1996), and *Inventing AIDS* (1990), and *LA Plays Itself/Boys in the Sand: A Queer Film Classic* (2014).

Margaret Rhee is a feminist experimental poet, new media artist, and scholar. Her research focuses on technology and on intersections with feminist, queer, and ethnic studies. She has a special interest in digital participatory action research and pedagogy. She is the author of the chapbooks *Yellow* (2011) and *Radio Heart; or, How Robots Fall Out of Love* (2016) and the poetry collection *Love, Robot* (2017). She currently serves as managing editor of *Mixed Blood*, a literary journal on race and experimental poetry. She coedited the collections *Here Is a Pen: An Anthology of West Coast Kundiman Poets* (2009) and online anthology *Glitter Tongue: Queer and Trans Love Poems* (2012). She was the Institute of American Cultures Visiting Researcher in Asian American Studies at UCLA for 2014–15. From 2004 to 2006, she worked as an editor for publications *YOLK Magazine*, *Chopblock.com*, and *Backstage*. Currently she is a College Fellow at Harvard University in the Department of English and Assistant Professor at SUNY Buffalo in the Department of Media Study.

Juana María Rodríguez is Professor of Ethnic Studies and Performance Studies at the University of California, Berkeley. She is the author of two books, *Queer Latinidad: Identity Practices, Discursive Spaces* (2003) and *Sexual Futures, Queer Gestures, and Other Latina Longings* (2014), which won the Alan Bray Memorial Book Prize at the Modern Language Association and was a Lambda Literary Award finalist for LGBTQ Studies. In 2019 she coedited a special issue of TSQ: *Transgender Studies Quarterly* on "Trans Studies en las Americas." She is currently completing a new manuscript, *Puta Life: Seeing Latinas, Working Sex.*

Sarah Schulman is a novelist, playwright, nonfiction writer, screenwriter, and AIDS historian. Her twenty books include *Let the Record Show*, a history of ACT UP (forthcoming). She is the cofounder of MIX NYC: Queer Experimental Film and Video Festival, co-director of ACT UP Oral History Project, and the US Coordinator of the first LGBT Delegation to Palestine. Schulman has published ten novels, among them *The Cosmopolitans* (2016), *The Mere Future* (2010), and *People in Trouble* (1990); and six works of nonfiction, including *Conflict Is Not Abuse* (2016), *Gentrification of the Mind* (2012), and *Stagestruck* (1998). She has received various awards and honors, including a Guggenheim, a Fulbright, and the Kessler Prize for Sustained Contribution to LGBT Studies.

Nishant Shahani is Associate Professor of Women's, Gender, and Sexuality Studies at the Department of English at Washington State University. His teaching and research interests focus on LGBT studies, queer theory, AIDS historiographies, and transnational sexualities. His first monograph was *Queer Retrosexualities: The Politics of Reparative Return* (2013). He is currently working on his second monograph, tentatively titled *Pink Revolutions: Queer Triangles in Contemporary India*, on the connections between queer politics in India with globalization and the emergence of Hindu fundamentalism. He has published articles in venues such as GLQ, *Modern Fiction Studies, Genders, Postcolonial Studies, Journal of Popular Culture, South Asia Multidisciplinary Academic Journal*, and QED: A Journal of LGBTQ World Making.

C. Riley Snorton is Professor in the Department of English Language and Literature and the Center for Gender and Sexuality Studies at the University of Chicago. He is the author of *Nobody Is Supposed to Know: Black Sexuality on the Down Low* (2014) and *Black on Both Sides: A Racial History of Trans Identity* (2017), winner of the Lambda Literary Award for Transgender Nonfiction and an American Library Association Stonewall Honor Book in Nonfiction. The book has also been recognized by the Organization of American Historians, the Modern Language Association, and the Institute for Humanities Research. Snorton's next monograph, tentatively titled *Mud: Ecologies of Racial Meaning*, examines the constitutive presence of swamps in racial practices and formations in the Americas. He is currently coediting *Saturation: Race, Art, and the Circulation of Value* and *The Flesh of the Matter: A Critical Reader on Hortense Spillers* and has coedited several special issues of journals, including "Blackness" for *Transgender Studies Quarterly* (2017), "The Queerness of Hip Hop / The Hip Hop of Queerness" for *Palimpsest: A Journal on Women, Gender, and the Black*

International (2013), and "Media Reform" for the *International Journal of Communication* (2009).

Eric A. Stanley is Assistant Professor in the Department of Gender and Women's Studies at the University of California, Berkeley. In collaboration with Chris Vargas, they directed the films *Homotopia* (2006) and *Criminal Queers* (2019). Stanley is also a coeditor of *Trap Door: Trans Cultural Production and the Politics of Visibility* (2017, with Tourmaline and Johanna Burton), and *Captive Genders: Trans Embodiment and the Prison Industrial Complex* (2015, with Nat Smith).

Jessica Whitbread works in the realm of social practice and community art, often merging art and activism to engage a diversity of audiences in critical dialogue. Whitbread often uses her own body and experience as a queer woman living with HIV as the primary site of her work. Her ongoing projects include "No Pants No Problem," "Tea Time," "PosterVIRUS," and "Love Positive Women." She is the author of *Tea Time: Mapping Informal Networks of Women Living with HIV* (2014) and the coeditor of *The HIV Howler: Transmitting Art and Activism*. Whitbread was the youngest and first queer woman to be elected as the Global Chair for the International Community of Women Living with HIV/AIDS (ICW) (2012) and is the founder of the first International Chapter of Young Women, Adolescents and Girls living with HIV (2010).

Quito Ziegler is an artist and curator who has worked at the intersection of art and community organizing for two decades. They currently teach about the future and social movements at the School of Visual Arts, and have several film projects in the works. They are a founding member of the WRRQ Collective, an intergenerational queer/trans community that makes art and food together for visual resistance and collective healing. Ziegler has curated exhibitions at the International Center of Photography, where they are currently engaged in "Decolonize ICP" conversations. For nine years (on and off) they produced exhibitions and grant programs at the Open Society Foundations Documentary Photography Project.

INDEX